"In this excellent book on group therapy, De Haas provides a great service to the field. This textbook integrates new knowledge and accrued clinical wisdom, richly illustrated with clinical examples that group therapists at all stages of their career can utilize to deepen and maximize the effectiveness of their work. De Haas provides a clear path to improving access for patients to high-quality mental healthcare delivered in therapy groups of all forms and structures."

Molyn Leszcz, MD, FRCPC, CGP, AGPA-DF,
professor of psychiatry, University of Toronto, past president,
American Group Psychotherapy Association

Group Therapy and Group Dynamic Theory

Group Therapy and Group Dynamic Theory offers an innovative approach to group therapy with an integrated and highly practical method. It is written for all group therapists. The book offers a solid base for professionals practicing group psychotherapy and for professionals working with structured, educational, or training-oriented therapy groups.

The method discussed in this book is based on the core knowledge about groups: group dynamic theory. This theory is used to clarify the variety of group processes and is translated into practical techniques to highlight the benefits of these processes within group therapy. Each chapter contains concrete interventions, skill labs, and a practical manual where corresponding techniques are further demonstrated with lively examples and practical exercises. The book concludes with a troubleshooting guide to offer solutions to complex problems group therapists may encounter.

Group Therapy and Group Dynamic Theory is the translation of a best-selling book about group therapy in the Netherlands. It is in line with the Dutch and American Practice Guidelines for Group Psychotherapy and is used in the official group therapy training in the Netherlands.

Willem de Haas is a clinical psychologist and psychotherapist with his own practice. He is an expert in the field of groups and group dynamics and has many years of experience as a group therapist and team leader in mental health care. He teaches group therapy, group dynamics, and team leadership for psychologists, psychiatrists, and other professionals at post-master institutes of the University of Amsterdam and the University of Groningen and regularly gives in-company lectures, training courses, and supervision at various organizations in the health care sector. For extra tips, techniques, questions, or comments about the book, please visit www.dehaasgroepsdynamica.nl.

Group Therapy and Group Dynamic Theory

A Professional Method for All Group-Based Treatment

Willem de Haas

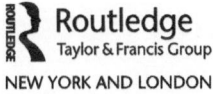

Routledge
Taylor & Francis Group

NEW YORK AND LONDON

Designed cover image: © Getty Images.

First published in English 2025
by Routledge
605 Third Avenue, New York, NY 10158

and by Routledge
4 Park Square, Milton Park, Abingdon, Oxon, OX14 4RN

Routledge is an imprint of the Taylor & Francis Group, an informa business

© 2025 Willem de Haas
Translated by Delia Burggraaf

First published in Dutch *Groepsbehandeling en Teambegeleiding in
de Zorg* by Boom Uitgevers, 2020.

Library of Congress Cataloging-in-Publication Data
Names: Haas, Willem de, 1947– author. | Burggraaf, Delia, translator.
Title: Group therapy and group dynamic theory : a professional
    method for all group-based treatment / Willem de Haas ;
    translated by Delia Burggraaf.
Other titles: Groepsbehandeling en Teambegeleiding in de Zorg. English
Description: New York, NY : Routledge, 2025. | "First published
    in Dutch as Groepsbehandeling en Teambegeleiding in de
    Zorg by Boom Uitgevers, 2020"—Title page verso. | Includes
    bibliographical references and index.
Identifiers: LCCN 2024034509 (print) | LCCN 2024034510
    (ebook) | ISBN 9781032437729 (hardback) | ISBN
    9781032437712 (paperback) | ISBN 9781003368786 (ebook)
Subjects: LCSH: Group psychotherapy.
Classification: LCC RC488 .H3313 2025 (print) | LCC RC488
    (ebook) | DDC 616.89/152—dc23/eng/20240816
LC record available at https://lccn.loc.gov/2024034509
LC ebook record available at https://lccn.loc.gov/2024034510

ISBN: 978-1-032-43772-9 (hbk)
ISBN: 978-1-032-43771-2 (pbk)
ISBN: 978-1-003-36878-6 (ebk)

DOI: 10.4324/9781003368786

Typeset in Times New Roman
by Apex CoVantage, LLC

Access the support material via the Routledge website:
routledge.com/9781032437729

'There is nothing as practical as a good theory'[1]
Kurt Lewin, founder of group dynamic theory

*To my dearest group: Pauline, Bas and Maaike,
and to my most endearing group: Thomas, Jonathan,
Melle and Felix*

1 Lewin K (1943).

Contents

Acknowledgements

All my life I have been interested in groups. They fascinate me, and since I have been professionally involved with groups, that fascination has only increased. It has become a scientific fascination. As a student I started with sociology, followed by psychology, resulting in a profession as group therapist. What exactly happens in groups, and how can that be helpful for group therapy: these questions keep me busy during my professional activities as group therapist, trainer, supervisor, researcher, and writer. I am grateful that I have been able to describe and share that fascination, and I am also grateful that it is read and used with interest. The original book in 2008, the second edition in 2020, and now an English version.

The direct reason to embark on this English writing adventure is the 'Dutch Design' group of the Dutch association of group psychotherapy colleagues, with whom I presented our approach and guidelines for group therapy at three conventions of the American Group Psychotherapy Association. Thank you Silvia Pol, Charles Huffstadt, Anne-Marie Claassen, Laura van Groenendael and last but not least Rob Koks for your professional enthusiasm and your conviviality during these conferences, especially the last one in New York. And very stimulating was the AGPA who invited us several times, with an enthusiastic reception to our presentations. Special thanks go to group therapist and author Molyn Leszcz, who was always enthusiastic and stimulating about our presentations. It's great that he was willing to write an endorsement.

More people have been a source of inspiration or help in the creation of this English version of my book.

I owe a great debt of gratitude to the translator Delia Burggraaf, with whom I went through all those sentences and words together and, sometimes after the necessary discussion, established them.

I would like to thank Routledge representatives Ellie Broadhurst and Amanda Savage for their assistance and help with the complex process of writing and publishing.

A lot of gratitude goes out to Charlie Pohl, fellow group therapist in Idaho, whom I met at the various AGPA conventions. He was willing to read the manuscript and provide USA inside commentary. I am immensely grateful to him for his continued support throughout the project, including his down-to-earth questions, practical advice, and his careful attention to language and word use.

Thanks also to Abie Tremblay, fellow group therapist in New Hampshire, for reading carefully the first three chapters and giving accurate advice.

Anton Hafkenscheid has meant a lot to me by patiently explaining the complex aspects of the IPC model and the research involved.

Thanks also go to the authors who kindly made their figures or examples available for inclusion in this book. Thanks Jan Remmerswaal, and thanks Marloes van Beersum of Boom Publishers; thanks also to Cor de Jong, Wim van den Brink, Anneke Jansma, and for using the example of their Adoptive Psychotherapy group; many thanks go to Malou Geenevasen and Anna Bartak.

I am very grateful to Alfred Burema for the kind and expert way in which he helped me to design all those complicated figures and tables.

I would like to thank Daniel Lechner, who also played an important role in this book, namely thinking about the proposal that eventually led to this publication.

Instructive and pleasant are the contacts with my fellow teachers of the many courses that we give together, and in which the use and thinking about my book is always part of it. Thank you Miriam Saschowa, Agatha Hollander, Margriete de Jong, Mayaris Zepeda Mendes, Helga Aalders, Marc Daemen, Titus van Os, Roelof Wolters, and Salvatore Vitale.

I am also grateful for the many years of fruitful contacts in the professional field of group therapy: the many group therapy clients, all those trainees in courses, the many supervision trainees, and all those incredibly wise and nice group therapy colleagues of the NVGP, who give and inspire me so much in cooperation and contact.

And I can't be grateful enough to Pauline for her patient and lasting support of this time- and attention-consuming job.

Preface

This book describes an innovative approach to group therapy with a striking concrete and powerful method. It is written for *all* group therapists. The book provides a solid foundation for professionals who practice group psychotherapy and is also very useful for professionals who work with structured, educational, or training-oriented therapy groups.

The purpose of this book is to show how to lead a therapy group in a professional way. That means in the first place based on guidelines, research, and expert knowledge. But it also means leading a therapy group with a clear, consistent, and integrated method. The method described is based on the core knowledge about groups: group dynamic theory. This field of science offers the best specialized knowledge currently available about groups, moreover, knowledge that also translates very well into practically applicable tools. The detailed practical techniques in this book will help every group therapist to recognize, utilize, and where necessary limit the natural group dynamic processes in service of the therapy group.

The book is the translation of a well-known textbook on group therapy in the Netherlands. It is in line with the Dutch and American Practice Guidelines for Group Psychotherapy. In the Netherlands it is used in the official group therapy training nationwide. This Dutch approach to group therapy has been well received during several presentations at recent AGPA conferences.

The 12 chapters are divided into three parts. Part 1 is about the importance of group dynamic processes for group therapy, and about the great advantage of a powerful organization and start of a therapy group. Part 2 is entirely devoted to the group therapist, leading and steering the therapy group. In Part 3, all important group dynamic processes, such as cohesion, norms, roles, etc., are discussed, each as the main subject of its own chapter. Each concept is clearly described with an explanation of how a group therapist can use it in group therapy. Every chapter concludes with a Practical Manual, which describes the associated techniques, with vivid examples and practical tools. The book concludes with a Troubleshooting guide that provides solutions to the most complex problems a group therapist may encounter. For extra tips, techniques, questions, or comments about the book, please visit www.dehaasgroepsdynamica.nl or reach out to the author at info@dehaasgroepsdynamica.nl.

Part 1

Before the start
of the group

Chapter 1

Group dynamic processes as a natural source of power

1.1 Introduction: the group as therapeutic instrument

Perhaps not every group therapist may realize this, but group therapy always works with two theoretical frames of reference (De Haas, 2020). First, the theoretical frame of reference of the group itself. This frame of reference is the universal part of any group therapy and has its own theoretical basis, namely group dynamic theory, *group dynamics* in short. When I speak of group dynamics, I mean all the relevant scientific knowledge about the small group[1] derived from group dynamics, social psychology, and sociology (Dion, 2000; Forsyth, 2017). This field of science offers the best specialized knowledge that currently exists about groups. It includes a comprehensive and integrated theory about the small group, which also translates very well into practical tools. Needless to say, all this knowledge is necessary because the group is, after all, the fundamental and professional tool with which every group therapist works. The group therapist uses what I call 'the group as therapeutic instrument' (De Haas, 2020). Therefore a group therapist must really understand groups, be a 'master of groups' in the first place. Solid education in the Group Dynamic frame of reference is a 'must' for any group therapist in order to feel competent and comfortable with his essential and often complex therapeutic instrument. In addition, the universal basis of the group dynamic frame of reference also ensures a common identity of group therapy in the varied field.

The second frame of reference every group therapist uses is the chosen therapeutic frame of reference, or therapeutic method if you will. These methods are often proven or validated methods from individual (psycho)therapy that are also applied within group therapy. They provide important theoretical concepts about pathology and healing of the individual client, including important 'change-agents.' In health care today we see a wide variety of methods being applied in group therapy, conducted by a wide variety of professionals. Some examples: a psychotherapist providing group therapy for people with Personality Disorder using the Interpersonal method, a social worker providing Emotion

DOI: 10.4324/9781003368786-2

Regulation Group Therapy using the DBT method, a psychologist providing an online group therapy for students with severe fear of failure using the CBT method, a psychiatric nurse providing Social Skills Group Therapy, a psychologist providing Educational Group Therapy for patients with Acquired Brain Injury, a psychiatrist providing group therapy for people with depression using the IPT-Group method, a psychologist providing an Educational Group Therapy for veterans with PTSS.

Two frames of reference are not that strange

Two frames of reference may seem strange, but this is also true for individual therapy. In individual therapy, the therapeutic method is applied using the therapeutic relationship, the working alliance between client and therapist, as the instrument. Here, too, the relationship must be handled correctly for the therapeutic method to be applied productively. We know from research on individual therapy that professional handling of that therapeutic relationship contributes significantly to the outcome of therapy (Hafkenscheid, 2014). Burlingame et al. (2018) and Yalom and Leszcz (2020) describe how the handling of group cohesion, the network of group relationships, within group therapy has a similar function and contributes to the outcome.

Thus, a competent group therapist is an expert in the field of groups, and an expert in the chosen method, and knows how to apply the method within the group instrument. This incorporates the skill to integrate the method and group dynamics in a fruitful way, ensuring the right amount of interaction for the therapeutic method.

This book focuses deliberately on the first frame of reference, group dynamic theory, and how a group therapist can organize and use the group as therapeutic instrument for his method. Although the methods are also very important, I do not go into detail about them. For clarity in the text and examples I use my categorization of different types of group therapy, taken over from the first Dutch edition (2008) of this book. See Table 1.1.

This broad vision on group therapy is nowadays the standard in the Netherlands, adopted in 2004 and formalized in Practice Guidelines in 2019 by the Dutch Association of Group Dynamics and Group Psychotherapy.[2] In this book I use the same broad vision: all forms of treatment groups, within health care, conducted by a health care professional using a serious (validated) therapy method is genuine 'group therapy'. And the professional who leads a professional therapy group is called group therapist.[3]

Table 1.1 Different types of group therapy in health care. With permission from Boom Uitgevers Amsterdam adapted from W. De Haas (2008) *Groepsbegeleiding en groepsbehandeling in de gezondheidszorg*. Soest: Nelissen. Translation by the author.

Four levels of Target groups with different types of group therapy

Client target group	Major group goal	Method and working method	Task and use of group dynamic process and Interaction	Different types of group therapy	Example
1. People with permanent condition People involved with the client (kin, social network, help network)	Support Compassion Expansion of coping capabilities Eduction	Individual support Fellow sufferers support Coping training FACT method	Individual treatment in the group sometimes with interaction between members	**Support Group Therapy Coping Group Therapy**	Support or coping group therapy for clients with: Acquired Brain Injury Schizophrenia Dementia
2. People with a recently acquired serious complaint	Symptom reduction Coping Insight and knowledge in a theme	Information Education Advice Targeted symptom treatment Theme discussion	Individual treatment in the group with appropriate interaction between members	**Eductional Group Therapy**	Educational group therapy for clients with ADHD Trauma Course Addiction Course 'Substance detox'
3. People with maladaptive but changeable behavior	New behavior	Skill training	Protocol-working method with appropriate interaction	**Skill Training Group Therapy**	Social Skills group therapy DBT Aggression Regulation Group Therapy

(Continued)

Table 1.1 (Continued)

Four levels of Target groups with different types of group therapy

Client target group	Major group goal	Method and working method	Task and use of group dynamic process and Interaction	Different types of group therapy	Example
4. People with maladaptive but changeable feelings and cognitions about themselves	Insight and change in personal feelings, cognitions, self-image, and self-esteem	Thinking Feeling Analyzing Role-play Experimenting with new behavior	Protocol interactional	**Protocol-Based Interactional Group Psychotherapy**	CBT Group psychotherapy for anxiety disorder Schema Focus Group psychotherapy for personality disorder
		Interpersonal Experiencing Feeling Thinking Analyzing Experimenting with new behavior	Using a lot of group dynamic process and interaction	**Intensive interactional Group Psychotherapy**	Interpersonal Group psychotherapy for personality disorder Psycho Dynamic Group psychotherapy for mood disorder

It is interesting to see that the international authoritative researchers on group therapy, Gary Burlingame and Bernard Strauss, use a similar broad view on group therapy in their thorough ten-year group therapy research review in *Bergin and Garfield's Handbook of Psychotherapy and Behavior Change*[4] (2021). They include therapy groups from not only mental health but also from addictive and somatic care, dedicated to specific client populations with specific psychiatric and somatic disorders. They also include different used methods and also made a categorization to bring more clarity to this wide field of group therapy. Their classification includes three main forms of therapeutic groups: leaderless groups, educational groups, and psychotherapy groups.

1.2 What does 'group dynamics' or 'group processes' mean?

Group dynamic processes arise in every group

In all of the knowledge about groups, group dynamic processes always play a leading role. Group dynamic processes are the most typical and essential feature of any group; they are always present and always have a significant influence. But what exactly are these group dynamic processes?

There are forces at play in each group that are not immediately apparent but are highly influential nonetheless. We call these group forces the *group process* or *group dynamics*.[5] They arise in every group as a result of the motives (individual dynamics) the participants bring into the group. All group members have their own desires, thoughts, fears, emotions, and expectations. Motives that, once they come together in the group, interact and create a collective dynamic field. Kurt Lewin (1951/1997), a pioneer in social psychology and small group research, introduced the term 'group dynamics' for this interplay of forces. By this, he meant the interplay between positive and negative forces in the group (Dion, 2000; Lewin, 1951/1997). In every group, this group dynamic interplay of forces develops into various group processes, all of which are discussed in this book.

Apart from the more or less hidden forces, group dynamics are *natural-spontaneous* forces. We cannot instantly grasp them. They arise from all the group members together, but, once the group is functioning, they take on a life of their own. For example: a very reserved group member notices that the incredibly enthusiastic group atmosphere excites him, too, whether he wants it to or not.

The evolutionary origins of group dynamics

Because group dynamic processes have evolutionary origins, we experience them as natural and self-evident. They are life processes. Groups and group dynamics cannot be separated from our human nature and evolutionary origins. Our current group behavior exhibits many similarities with that of our relatives in the primate family, the chimpanzees and bonobos (De Waal, 2005; Van Vught and Ahuja, 2010). Characteristically, primates utilize the group for preserving the species. Working together in groups increases the chances of finding food, provides protection from outside threats, and provides the necessary secure base for raising young. Early human history also shows that our species needed groups to survive (Brewer and Caporael, 2006). Finding food, defending against attackers, and trekking across the landscape are primarily cooperative activities and thus involve group processes. From this perspective, group processes such as cohesion, norms, and roles, for example, are well understood as structures with survival value. Our species became cooperative and interdependent out of necessity (Brewer and Caporael, 2006). Evolution has equipped humans, through mutation and selection, with a natural ability to form groups, make them safe, and preserve themselves in groups (Boyd and Silk, 2008; Goudsblom, 2000). Thus, utilizing groups and moving within them are evolutionarily acquired abilities embedded in our DNA (Kameda and Tindale, in Schaller, 2006).

Nowadays, we mostly do not literally need each other for practical things like finding food but rather for our psychological and social needs, such as cooperation, being accepted, and a sense of belonging. Years of adaptation and selection have produced human beings who are social, even though there always are cultural differences and individual exceptions. Our self-esteem largely depends on social acceptance, the degree to which we are accepted and recognized by others or the group (Leary et al., 1995). Our need for affective connection is an innate human trait, as fundamental as the drive for food, drink, and sex (Baumeister and Leary, 1995; Bowlby, 1969). Conversely, social rejection and ostracism are extremely stressful. Several experiments indicate that social exclusion causes the same biological responses of fear, pain, and distress as physical injury (Williams, 2007). Even though connectedness is an essential need, the ever-present risk of rejection and ostracism makes establishing new contacts a tense and ambiguous undertaking. Therefore, the avoidance of rejection and ostracism is as strong a 'drive' as the desire for acceptance and connection (Williams, 2007).

Man is not only a being with a need to belong. Besides wanting to 'belong,' human nature also has the need for individuality and uniqueness. Identity and 'self' are also psychological phenomena with evolutionary origins. Sedikides et al. (2006) make a plausible case for how, in evolution, a developing self has been essential for preserving the species thanks to capacities such as self-awareness, taking initiative, and self-reflection. Preserving the group and the species is due not only to our collective abilities to cooperate but also to the performance of useful individual functions and roles within that cooperation. This means that, evolutionarily, we have learned not only how to behave socially but also how to maintain our individuality within groups (Brewer and Caporael, 2006).

Despite our 'social nature,' groups do not always progress peacefully. According to primatologist Wrangham (2019), both altruism and cruelty are in our human genes, and we bring these traits to our groups where they can collectively reinforce themselves. Our history and daily life show plenty of examples of groups or group members who are noble, sacrificial, and accepting, or just the opposite: destructive, hateful, and mean. This duality can also be seen in experiments and research on group dynamics (Burlingame et al., 2018; Milgram, 1974; Zimbardo, 1969). Thus, we can assume that we will also encounter this human reality of positive and negative processes in our therapy groups.

Fear and avoidance of group processes

Even though we experience group dynamics as natural and self-evident, for a professional who has to lead a group, they can be tricky sometimes. Allowing and accommodating the typical spontaneity of group dynamics is especially challenging for many group therapists. One often hears group therapists lament that they have no influence on the course of events in the therapy group. 'The group is not doing what I want!' This feeling of powerlessness can lead to fear of the group, causing them to avoid this spontaneous process side. In such a case, group therapists tend to fall back on their formal leadership role and lead the group primarily from a dominant role. They control the group by pushing or pulling it in their direction, sometimes against the group's wishes. Sometimes the group starts to resist the directive attitude, and a fight ensues. Otherwise, the group becomes very passive, which is also not conducive to the group result at all. Avoidance and fear of spontaneous group processes are thus quite normal – certainly for novice group therapists (Billow, 2001; Shay, 2021). The fact that clients – especially in the beginning – always feel fear of the group reinforces that fear in the group therapist.

Another reason for apprehension regarding group processes is their complexity. It is often difficult to oversee exactly what is happening in a therapy group because there is always so much going on at once. One or two therapists, eight or more participants, a jumble of interactions, and sometimes complicated layered processes often make it difficult to grasp exactly what is happening. Even then, we see how some group therapists start to control the group out of uncertainty or revert to 'individual therapy' within the group. For example, the group therapist keeps asking questions to each group member individually, with very little interaction occurring among the group members. Sessions become awkward, the group therapist actually does all the work and is exhausted afterward.

The potentially negative impact of group processes is also a reason for fear and avoidance. I described previously that negative group processes are a human reality. Everyone experiences negative group processes in childhood or adulthood and knows how disruptive and intimidating they can be. Group processes can develop so negatively that group members become unable to engage in the group task. Consider an unsafe therapy group in which no one dares to say something or a group in which a destructive power struggle between two informal leaders or two subgroups dominates everything, or in which participants are bullied or excluded. In a therapy group like this, work is no longer productive, and the potential for harm is high. The great insecurity that results can also paralyze the group therapist and cause him to revert to excessive control.

Finally, a group therapist could also 'accidentally' leave group dynamics unutilized and avoid them because, for example, he is unaware of them or assumes that group dynamics are unimportant. This leads to difficulties sooner than later because group dynamics are *always* there and simply cannot be ignored.

Let me share an example:

A while after starting an educational therapy group on obsessive compulsive disorder, a novice group therapist noticed that the group members were not participating in the discussions very enthusiastically. He responds by trying harder, providing more explanations, and conveying the information even more clearly. But to no avail. The energy level of the group discussions remained low, and the number of group members actively participating decreased rather than increased. Dissatisfaction among group members became palpable. When attendance also declines, the group therapist decides to seek advice from an experienced colleague. The latter also does not know why the group is reacting so lukewarmly, but he advises the group therapist to take a break from the topics and discuss the group members' behavior with them. A very tense group therapist implements this plan at the next meeting. After a short silence, a conversation ensues in which more group members participate than was the case in the earlier sessions. They express different opinions about the group. In general, most participants find the informative topics useful, but they tend to drag on a bit too long. They would like to have time to exchange information with each other about how they cope with the effects their obsessions and what problems they encounter. The group therapist is pleased with the clear information and decides at the end of the meeting to use the various responses to adjust the method.

Thus, it is important for every group therapist to face group processes as a reality, to become familiar with them. To feel when to bend or stop negative processes or when to give fruitful processes room. Then he won't have to control or suppress them anymore. Paradoxically, the group therapist will find that he has more control over the group if he can let go of the group processes than if they try to keep them under control. The group therapist will notice that he can benefit from these group dynamic processes, precisely by first allowing them and giving them space.

Learning to utilize group dynamics

Most people know that group processes can have negative effects, but few know that they can also be very useful and valuable. Negative group processes simply stand out more because of their drama and strong emotional value (think of movies like *The Experiment* [Scheuring, 2010] or *One Flew Over the Cuckoo's Nest* [Forman, 1975]). But that does not make them more important than positive processes. In this book, I pay attention to both: how the group therapist can learn to recognize, bend, or limit negative group processes and, especially, how a group therapist can use these spontaneous processes to facilitate an effective therapy group.

Spontaneous group dynamics offer many useful applications to support the group therapy task. In Part 3 of this book, I demonstrate in detail how the group therapist can benefit from sub-processes like group cohesion, norms, and roles. Shortly, I give a general account of how group dynamics can work positively. That can happen in four ways.

First, group *dynamics* provide the drive, energy, and thus *autonomy* that allows the therapy group to move. Group dynamics is an important engine that provides movement, vitality, and development: all energies that we do not want to lose and from which we can benefit. Thanks to their interactive dynamics, group members make the therapy group an independent and living social entity that will develop a power of its own.

Second, spontaneous group processes foster learning within therapy groups. By their very nature, group processes are interactional processes, and when the group therapist gives them appropriate space, it stimulates interactive learning processes all by itself. Thanks to spontaneous group dynamics, group members bring in their own material and respond spontaneously to the input of others. As we know, members can be good therapeutic helpers, advisors, or influencers; they believe each other more easily than they believe the group therapist. In this context, it helps to think of the group as an 'information processing system' (Swogger, 1981). The more information is introduced, the more the system of group members is stimulated to process that information. In a group with sufficient interactive space, participants resonate and respond spontaneously and associatively to each other, creating a chain of interactions, which produces all kinds of useful information. Think of a member in a therapy group for people with contact problems who excitedly shares that she broke up with her friend yesterday. This evokes a lot of reactions (and reaction to reaction), such as compassion, questions about the reason, associations with one's own partner relationship, a discussion about being single, separation, and bonding anxiety, memories of old partner relationships, and so on. In spontaneous interactive processes, a lot of information is created that participants will think about and can learn from.

Third, group processes provide an important entry point for steering the group. Group processes are very influential and thus a tool of influence and leadership. To illustrate: in an educational group therapy, several group members cancel too often, giving the group therapist the impression that a bad habit (norm) is developing. The group therapist who understands the process topic of group norms can then turn a nonfunctional norm into a functional norm.

Finally, the group processes ensure that the learning processes in the therapy group take root and are well applicable in the outside world. Thanks to vibrant group dynamics, the therapy group becomes a microcosm (mini-world) similar to the real world (Yalom and Leszcz, 2020). Therefore, the learning processes have a natural quality so that the results easily stick and are readily transferable to the real world. For example, skills that group members learn in a social skills group therapy are easily translatable to the home situation.

There are more than enough reasons to cherish these group processes as a great asset for our therapy groups and not to oppose, neglect, or dismiss them. Fortunately, group dynamic theory offers a lot of knowledge on this subject, and the art of using group dynamics can be learned. It is the motto of this book: *become skillful in using group processes by subtly strengthening them and cleverly utilizing them for the therapeutic task of the group.*

Group processes in online group therapy

Online group therapy means missing the nonverbal essentials for group process development, such as eye contact, body-to-body interaction, physical presence, and proximity. Despite this difference, the group processes and techniques described in this book are recognizable and applicable to online group therapy. But there are differences: the group processes form more slowly and sometimes achieve less depth. Thanks to the experience with online group therapy in recent years, there is more knowledge about the way in which the group therapist can compensate for and handle the lack of nonverbal characteristics. Where relevant in the text, I will briefly explain this and illustrate how a group therapist can handle such an online situation. I base this on my own experience with supervision and training groups and on existing expertise. For specific and comprehensive knowledge about online group therapy, I would like to refer to experts such as Weinberg (Weinberg, 2024; Weinberg and Rolnick, 2020).

Group, individual, and group processes

Groups and group processes are collective phenomena, but of course the unique individual is and remains the focus and value in this special way of treatment. The group doesn't have a depression, but each individual person in a depression group has their own unique mood disorder. Group therapy is no more than the applied method, and sometimes the best method to make individuals better.

Thus, group therapy and group processes are important and useful for the individual members, but the same applies vice versa. Individuals are always important for the group, the developing group processes, and for the group therapy itself. Some individual members are very useful thanks to their knowledge about the therapeutic task. Other members foster the development of group processes with their personality traits. Consider individuals who bond well, thus facilitating cohesion development, or role development, which cannot possibly occur without a diversity of personalities within the group. And consider individuals who dare to make contact and work together, stimulating interaction.

1.3   How does group therapy work?

Participants in a therapy group learn from interactions with each other

Interactions occur among group members due to the development of group dynamics. The different desires, visions, and thoughts expressed by group members evoke equally different reactions from other group members. Such a 'back-and-forth' reaction between group members is called an interaction (Bales, 1950). We see interactions occur between group members, between group members and the group therapist, and between group members and the entire group. Thus, a group consists of numerous strands and networks of inter-actions. The goal of a therapy group is for these interactions to work thera-peutically for each individual group member. A characteristic feature of group therapy is that group members learn from each other rather than from the group therapist. The more the group members can genuinely encounter each other in such a group, the better because then the opportunity for learning experiences increases.

> **Group members more easily accept something from each other than from the group therapist**
>
> Not only could group members learn a lot from each other, but they will also accept something from each other more easily than from the group therapist. It is a fact based on experience that I regularly hear from profes-sionals I meet in my group dynamics or group therapy training.
>
> I still clearly remember a situation from one of my psychotherapy groups. One of the group members had a strong tendency to get defensive when receiving feedback. His standard response was, 'Yeah, you can say that, but it feels different to me!' When I tried to make that pattern clear to him, he naturally responded just as defensively as usual: 'You say I'm get-ting defensive, but that's not true at all. Maybe it seems that way, but . . .' The striking thing was that fifteen minutes later, he did open up to a fel-low group member, who had said almost the same to him that I had said a moment before: 'You keep saying, 'Yes, but . . . ' to everything that is being said to.' The group member responded with: 'You mean I'm defen-sive? Am I . . .?'
>
> I have discussed this phenomenon with the group members of many different groups. I generally got the following responses: 'We understand each other better than you understand us because we are in the same boat. You don't know our problems.' 'You are in a different position than we

are?' 'When one of us responds supportively, it feels real; you respond from your therapist role.' And they are correct, of course. They are peers; we are professionals. However, that does not mean we cannot understand them well. We are all human.

Research on the efficacy of group therapy

What do we know about the efficacy of these interactional learning experiences? How effective is group therapy?

That group therapy works for various complaints or diagnoses has been demonstrated conclusively (Burlingame and Strauss, 2021; Burlingame and Jensen, 2017). *How* group therapy works exactly and how those learning experiences lead to results are subject to ongoing research. The effective factors of the therapeutic method used are mostly well known, but I find the efficacy of the general factors of the group instrument itself and, in particular, of the group processes especially important. What is the effect of clear group norms, and how important is role differentiation? What is the influence of cohesion on the efficacy of group therapy?

What do we already know? As for cohesion, that process has been proven to play a vital role in the outcome of group therapy. Burlingame et al. (2018) found that cohesion is not only a prerequisite for successful group therapy, but it is also a therapeutic factor. Therapy groups in which the therapist pays extra attention to cohesion have significantly better outcomes than therapy groups lacking this extra attention. Chapman and Kivlighan (2019) demonstrated that sufficient group development had a positive cohesion-outcome effect.

Plenty of qualitative research has been done. Older research, but certainly still important, is the qualitative research on 'therapeutic factors' in group therapy. According to Yalom and Leszcz (Yalom and Leszcz, 2020, 10) a therapeutic factor is an '*intricate interplay of human experiences*' that fosters the complex process of therapeutic change. Several group therapy researchers who started in the early years of group therapy have systematically described how group therapy works (Bloch and Crouch, 1985; Corsini and Rosenberg, 1955; Yalom, 1975; Yalom and Leszcz, 2020). Based on previous research, interviews with clients about their most valuable therapeutic experiences, and their own clinical expertise, these authors each constructed a list of therapeutic factors.

In this book I use a modified version of the list of therapeutic factors by Yalom and Leszcz (2020). In Table 1.2, I describe ten therapeutic factors. This list incorporates a broad variety of affective, cognitive, and behavioral aspects of therapeutic learning in group therapy. They occur in all therapy groups, although the most effective factors may vary from group to group. Each factor describes a group member's learning experience during a therapeutic interaction.

Table 1.2 Ten therapeutic factors. Modified version of the therapeutic factors, with permission inspired by Yalom and Leszcz (2020).

Therapeutic factor in group therapy	Group member experience
Acceptance (cohesion)	If a group member experiences acceptance by group members and/or the group for who he is, that he belongs, feels supported
Universality	When a group member experiences profound recognition of the same problems, experiences, feelings in one or more group members; he notices he is not the only one with that problem
Altruism	A group member gets a positive feeling about himself after hearing that his advice, reaction, or experience has really helped another person
Hope	When a group member believes the positive, uplifting, successful experiences from other group members
Guidance	When a group member receives information, advice, guidance that helps or leads to solutions
Learning from exemplary behavior (modeling)	When a group member adopts another group member's behavior as a solution for themselves and is happy about it Or When a group member strongly identifies with another group member
Learning through insight	When a group member perceives valuable, useful, new insights within his own experience and thoughts
Learning through feedback	When a group member hears from someone else how they come across specifically. Using this new information about themselves, the group member can try out new behaviors
Self-disclosure	When a group member shares an experience, feeling, fantasy, or secret and feels more understood as a result thereof
Catharsis	When a group member experiences great relief after being emotionally unleashed for a moment

Not only is this concept of multiple therapeutic factors important for research, but it also provides insight into how group therapy learning occurs in practice.

How does such a therapeutic factor work in practice?

How do we recognize an interaction involving a therapeutic learning moment? Group members learn from each other by exchanging information on the themes, exercises, and discussions in their therapy group. The mutual interactions create new information from which they can benefit. By information I not only mean the cognitive but also feelings, emotions, and behavior; anything that comes along in a therapy group can serve as new input. If a group member is willing to open up, he can absorb new information and start processing it. When the new information properly sinks in, we see it in the emotional expression due to 'the penny dropping,' the relief or surprise, or the feeling of being led astray. Group members then say something like: 'Wow, I didn't know that was possible. I'm going to try that, too.' 'Are you serious? I'm amazed!' or 'Jeez, that's a relief. I thought it was much worse.' This is what we call a *therapeutic moment.* We can recognize a therapeutic moment in a group member by the *emotional expression* that always accompanies such a moment. It is always an *unsettling moment of reflection and emotion at the same time.* Learning from each other in a therapy group is both a cognitive and an emotional process. If a group member returns to a therapeutic experience a short time later, that's a good sign. It shows that the therapeutic experience was strong enough to stick and anchor within. Whether the new learning eventually sticks depends again on the next step, namely how the individual group member processes and integrates the new information. This often requires the repetition of similar learning moments.

Suppose we observe the therapy group or interview participants afterward. We can then assign each observed or reported therapeutic experience to one of the therapeutic factors. For example, one group member's experience clearly matches 'Learning through insight,' and another group member's experience clearly matches 'Acceptance.' Next are two examples of a learning experience.

Learning through universality and learning from model behavior
Juan attends an intensive interactional psychotherapy group because he is always very tense when he is among people. He can't imagine that there are people who feel as miserable as he does during, i.e., a birthday party. Everyone sees how relieved Juan is when Ireen tells him she feels exactly the same way. He feels less alone now; it gives him hope. In doing so, he is genuinely surprised by Ireen's way of coping with her fear and tension. In fact, he sees that Ireen handles it differently than he does. It makes him reflect on his own fear and how he deals with it.

Learning through feedback
Dylan knows he has diabetes but is tremendously resistant toward the educational therapy group in which he is participating. When the group therapists explain something, he opposes it with lengthy explanations. He also expresses his resistance nonverbally with a negative, uninterested attitude. Annoyance grows among the other participants during the course of the sessions.

By the fourth session, Casper is fed up: 'Dylan, what are you doing here, man? Your negative attitude is killing me! I don't like being sick either or injecting myself and watching what I eat, but I know I have to accept it. I don't think you even dare to face your illness!'

Dylan is completely taken aback and does not utter a word for the rest of the session. At the next meeting, he says he has been thinking and has discovered that Casper is right: he cannot accept that he has diabetes.

Therapeutic factors in different groups

If we look at the list of therapeutic factors, we see a wide variation in the type of efficacy. Depending on the working method, certain therapeutic factors will stand out in one form of group therapy, while other factors will emerge in another form. For example, in intensive interactional group psychotherapy, factors such as 'Learning by insight' and 'Learning by feedback' play an important role. In a social skill therapy group, it is mainly about learning from behavior, which means that we will encounter the factors 'Learning from exemplary behavior' or 'Guidance' more often. But despite the factors that stand out, the other therapeutic factors are always effective as well. Therapeutic factors such as 'Acceptance' and 'Universality' are so fundamental that they support learning in any group.

The fact that there are always more effective factors simultaneously adds to the group's strength. We can compare the action of this range of factors to that of a *broad-spectrum antibiotic* (several antibiotics in one pill): if one factor does not work on a group member, chances are that another factor will. And there is synergy, factors can reinforce each other. For example, a member of a therapy group for social anxiety learns even more powerfully if, in addition to explanations from the group therapist ('Guidance'), he sees that other group members can relate to his problems ('Universality'). A therapy group thus has a great helping potential.

Notes

1 Groups up to about 15 people.
2 In the Netherlands group therapy was recognized in 2014 as a specialty by the NVP (Dutch Association of Psychotherapy; Factsheet Groepstherapie, 2019). In the US group therapy is recognized as a specialty by the APA (Whittington et al., 2021).
3 Foulkes (1977) spoke of 'conductor' to indicate how the group therapist makes use of the input of the group members, just like in an orchestra. It is often referred to as a group leader. My preference is to use the professional title Group Therapist for the professional leader of a professional therapy group.
4 Burlingame and Strauss (2021). Chapter 17 Efficacy of Small Group Treatments: Foundation for Evidence-Based Practice. In: *Bergin and Garfield's Handbook of Psychotherapy and Behavior Change* (2021).
5 In this book, the terms 'process,' 'group processes,' 'group dynamics,' and 'group dynamic process' have the same meaning.

Chapter 2

Mapping interaction

2.1 Introduction

In the previous chapter, I explained how participants in a group naturally respond to each other. This is called interaction: behavior in one person evokes behavior in another and vice versa (Bales, 1950).

Interaction

Bales (1950), a social psychologist at Harvard University at the time, was the first to systematically study interactions within small groups. He defined interaction as an action by one person to which at least one reaction follows from another person (verbal or nonverbal).

In group therapy interaction is extra important. After all, group therapy is *learning from each other*; effective learning takes place during the interactions between the members. Think of feedback between members after an exercise, reactions of members to a presented problem of one of them, or discussing a meaningful theme. Of course every group therapist has to steer and influence those interactions, but that's not as easy as it seems. Interaction in, for example, a group of eight members and one or two therapists is complex simply because of the multitude of possibilities. Interaction is not limited to a simple one to one between two people but usually expands into a series of interactions. And when others get involved, a whole network of interactions emerges. Moreover, these encounters between group members involve not only words but also nonverbal interaction, interaction through behavior. That's why every group therapist needs an instrument or model to understand how interaction works and to keep a handle on it. This chapter is about such a model. And thanks to its practical usefulness the model is one of the important red threads throughout the book.

The most well-known and reliable tool for this is the model nowadays known as the Interpersonal Circumplex or Circle: in short, IPC (Kiesler, 1983). This model was developed in the 1950s by clinical psychologist Timothy Leary and

DOI: 10.4324/9781003368786-3

fellow researchers (Leary, 1957). These researchers drew from the Interpersonal Psychiatry of the influential psychiatrist Harry Stack Sullivan. Both Sullivan and Leary view humans as fundamentally social and relational beings (Leary, 1957; Sullivan, 1940, in Berk, 2005, 93). An individual's behavior can only be understood when the relational context is included. This view of humankind is entirely consistent with group dynamics and social psychology, the core scientific tenets of this book. Leary (1957) based his theory on evolutionary principles, concluding that our relational abilities are of survival significance to the individual: 'We view the interpersonal behavior of an individual as the machinery by means of which he wards off anxiety and maintains a multilevel balance of self-enhancement' (Leary, 1957, 15).

The IPC model has been researched and modernized over the years, resulting in different versions with their own terminology, purpose, and, in some cases, questionnaires, which have been derived from it (Kiesler, 1983; Horowitz et al., 1988; Remmerswaal, 2003; Van Dijk et al., 2019; Hafkenscheid and Timmerman, 2023). In the modern versions, the original model of Leary is still recognizable. At the end of this chapter I present some of the questionnaires.

2.2   The Interpersonal Circle: the theory and the model

Two fundamental relational desires

According to the IPC theory, human interaction always involves two basic *dimensional relational* desires.

One desire concerns the *degree* of *influence* or *control* we want to have in the interaction with another person, and the other desire concerns the *degree* of *affiliation* or *attachment* we desire in interaction with the other.

- Influence-Control: a person wants to influence the other person and sense that the other person conforms, follows, and takes them seriously or, the opposite, a person wants to be helped, given advice, or be allowed to be dependent and to follow.
- Affiliation-Attachment: a person wants contact and proximity, to be close and accepted by the other, to belong. Or they want the possibility to be on their own, free, left alone, or keep their distance.

When people meet, they mutually convey these relational desires to each other in their interaction. People not only do this with words, but always with behavior. Interaction is verbal as well as nonverbal behavior as we said at the start of this chapter. In this respect, nonverbal behavior is extra important because in a relationship it strongly affects the other person. Nonverbal interaction – the interaction through behavior, attitude, and tone – is a powerful means of making our relational desires clear to the other person.

Some examples from everyday life: two friends meet in a café. One of them is very enthusiastic about a movie he saw and wants to convince (*influence*) his friend to see the movie too. He will express this in many ways, for example, by convincing in words why this movie is so good, reinforcing his words with behavior, like enthusiastic gestures and voice. He will be glad when he succeeds in his influencing behavior, seeing that his friend gets enthusiastic and says he will see the movie the next day. Another example: a teacher in a class wants to correct a boy who is repeatedly bullying a vulnerable classmate. He behaves directive and limiting (*influence*) to the boy and is glad when the boy startles and says he will stop his aggressive behavior. Or consider a team meeting where everybody is very joyful, hugging each other (*affiliation*) because the team received a medal of honor. And we see it in our therapy groups: a group member who feels and behaves very insecurely (*influence*), and thus evokes a lot of advice and tips, a group member who shows a very distancing attitude (*affiliation*) by sitting out of the circle, not participating in the group discussion, looking irritated. The others keep their distance from this member. Or a group member always showing a lot of empathic behavior (*affiliation*) to members with pain or sorrow.

Because people vary in their personal desire for affiliation or influence, both fundamental desires are represented in a dimensional line. This creates the so-called influence line, which indicates how much desire for influence a person shows in his behavior.

The *extremes* of that line are Above behavior ('I want to have a lot of influence over you') and Under behavior ('I want to receive a lot of guidance from you').

The second line is the affiliation line, with the *extremes* being Distant/Counter behavior ('Stay away from me') and Near behavior ('I like it when you are close with me'). We can place each person somewhere on those lines according to their *relative* need for influence and affiliation. Table 2.1 illustrates those two-dimensional lines.

Influence line

Above. . . . . .Under

A person can be placed somewhere on this line depending on the degree of influence expressed by their behavior/attitude

Affiliation line

Distant/Counter. . . . . .Near/Close

A person can be placed somewhere on this line depending on the degree of closeness expressed by their behavior/attitude

---

Table 2.1 The dimensional influence line and dimensional affiliation line.

In interaction, the desires for influence and affiliation always play a role simultaneously and affect each other. Leary shaped this by connecting the two lines to form a cross. He placed the line of influence behavior vertically and the line of affiliation behavior horizontally. Thus, we get the basic model of the Interpersonal Circle, with the two crossed lines and the four basic interaction behaviors (see Figure 2.1).

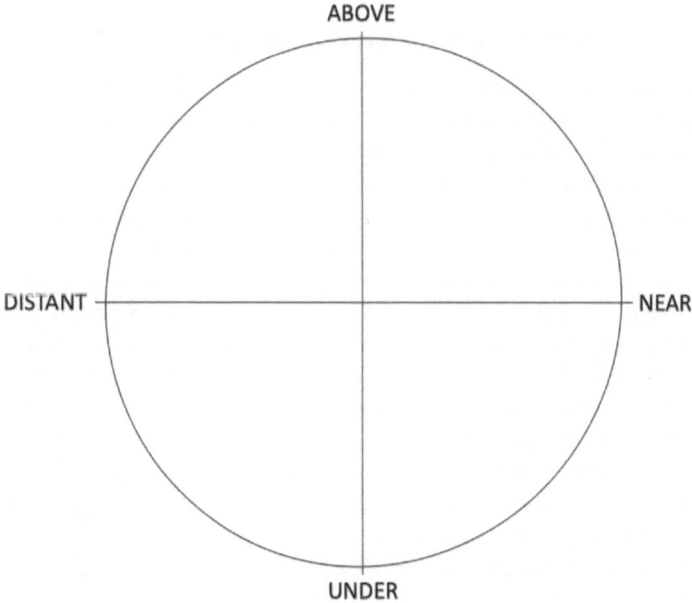

Figure 2.1 IPC basic model: four basic interactional behaviors. Figure by the author.

These four basic interactional behaviors or attitudes can be described in general terms as follows:
1. A person with Above (dominant) behavior: I want to take a leading position toward you and expect you to follow me.
2. A person with Under (following) behavior: I want to be dependent on you and want you to guide me.
3. A person with Near (contact-seeking) behavior: I want to get closer to you and hope you want that too.
4. A person with Distant (counter) behavior: I want to keep my distance from you and expect you to keep distance too.

In group therapy, we tend to favor horizontal relationships because proximity, safety, cohesion, and interpersonal openness are so important. But every group therapist knows from experience that vertical relationships always come into play alongside horizontal ones. Some clients stand out because of their pleasant natural leadership or, in the extreme case, because of their dominant position.

Other clients show cooperative supportive behavior, or in the extreme case can be docile, yearning to be helped and guided. The beauty of the IPC model is that it explains that fact so clearly. Influence is a basic human need, as is affiliation. In Chapter 4 (Leadership) and Chapter 10 (Roles) I demonstrate how those vertical relationships and positions are quite normal and also provide another useful foothold for the group therapist to steer the group.

The interactional laws of the Interpersonal Circle

The expression of a relational desire by one person inevitably means that, at the same time, a particular behavior is desired and evoked in the other. There is always a *relationship definition* incorporated in interactional behavior. For example, if someone expresses a desire for closeness, that person automatically desires closeness from the other person as well. That other person can meet that relational appeal or not, based on their own relational desires.

If we look at the lines in Figure 2.1 and the behavioral descriptions, we can more easily explain what behavior is expected and evoked in the other person. We see that Above behavior evokes Under behavior and vice versa. This *complementary* reaction makes sense: a leader needs a follower and vice versa. On the affiliation line we see a *symmetric* pattern: a hostile attitude evokes a hostile or defensive attitude in the other person. Distant/Counter behavior evokes Distant/Counter behavior. Similarly, Near behavior evokes Near behavior. We are familiar with this experience when we encounter a friendly person who has a disarming effect on us, making it easier for us to open up to that person. These are the four interactional laws involved in the IPC model. Next, we provide an example of each of these laws.

Above behavior evokes Under behavior
The group is seated and ready to begin the psychotherapy group. But the door is still open. Group therapist Maria kindly commands group member Cyndi to close the door. 'You're the closest, Cyndi!' Cyndi stands up and says in a friendly tone as she closes the door, 'Okay, Maria, if you say so.'

Under behavior evokes Above behavior
Sharon complains a lot in the therapy group. The group members take notice of Sharon's plight and try to help by giving her advice and support. When the complaining does not lessen, the group members' advice becomes increasingly resolute and coercive.

Near behavior evokes Near behavior
Kate rewards Jordan who reports in the therapy group about his assertive 'action' to his boss who sometimes belittles him. Jordan thanks Kate and says he is very glad about her support.

Distant (Counter) behavior evokes Distant (Counter) behavior
Maya announces in an angry tone that she is fed up with the uninterested
way Ahmed behaves in the therapy group, and that he should 'look in the
mirror.' Ahmed angrily responds that he is fed up with her bickering and
that she should look at her own behavior.

The standard IPC model

In the standard IPC model, each of the four quadrants is split to create eight behavioral sectors (Figure 2.2). The eight interactional behavioral variants each have
their own combination of influence and affiliation behaviors, with one of those two
behavioral characteristics predominating in each case. Each sector represents a
possible interactional behavioral variant based on the combination of its position-
ing on the horizontal and vertical axes. An appropriate behavioral indicator from
our daily lives was identified for each of these eight behavioral variants.

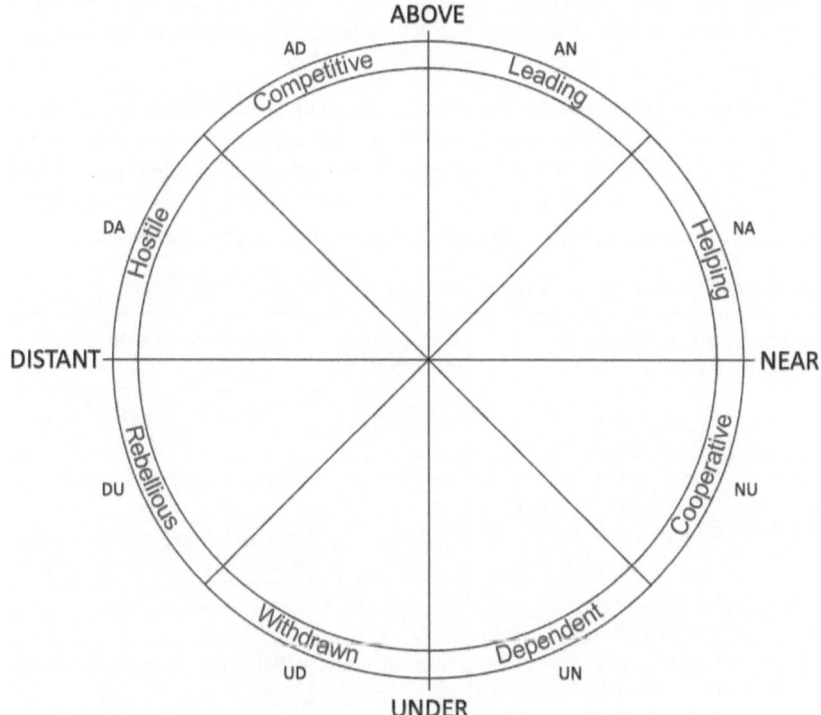

Figure 2.2 The standard Interpersonal Circle model

With permission adapted from: Remmerswaal J (2003) *Handboek groepsdynamica*. Soest:
Nelissen. Translation by the author.

The Interpersonal Circle is a neutral and validated instrument.

Each behavioral variation could be an adequate response by a person to a particular interactional situation at some point. For example, Withdrawn could be an adequate response in a very threatening situation, and Competitive may be necessary if your interests are being undermined.

Experience shows that people experience a negative or positive regard for certain behavioral variants. This is related to the behavioral designations chosen and the valuation placed on certain behaviors in society or in professions. For example, in a professional domain such as the military, offensive behavior is more often valued positively, whereas such behavior is generally undesirable within the health care sector. There, for example, people value helping behavior.

An important fact is that research showed that the so-called Circumplex structure of eight behavioral interaction variants is a validated representation of human interactional behavior (Van Dijk et al., 2019; Hafkenscheid and Timmerman, 2023).

In Table 2.2, I present each IPC behavioral variant with the behavioral designation from everyday life and some typical behavioral examples. For example, for the behavioral variant 'Near-Above,' HELPING is the behavioral designation. A person who fits that behavioral variant will stand out because he or she 'reacts empathic' to the other person and 'helps' them by giving support or practical advice.

Table 2.2 The eight behavioral variants of the Interpersonal Circle.

Sector	IPC behavioral variant	Behavioral designation	Behavioral examples
AN	Above-Near Above predominates	Leading	Lead, take initiative, direct
NA	Near-Above Near predominates	Helping	Help, support, protect
NU	Near-Under Near predominates	Cooperative	Agree, admire, accommodate, be modest
UN	Under-Near Under predominates	Dependent	Wait, lean on, adapt, ask
UD	Under-Distant Under predominates	Withdrawn	Withdraw, hide, keep silent
DU	Distant-Under Distant predominates	Rebellious	Resist, passive-aggressive, Distrustful
DA	Distant-Above Distant predominates	Hostile	Showing anger, aggression, Attack
AD	Above-Distant Above predominates	Competitive	Being high-minded, competing, humiliate

We can extend this table by adding the interaction aspect – the effect on the other person. After all, our behavior toward the other always implies a relationship definition: in our behavior toward the other, we display how we see ourselves, but also what behavior we expect from the other. The interactional laws of the model (Above evokes Under and so on) are decisive here. I illustrate what those interactions look like in Table 2.3. For each behavioral variant, you can see which relationship definition (*for clarity, in a somewhat extreme form here*) is communicated to the other person and which corresponding behaviors are initially evoked in the other person. For example, the behavioral definition of DEPENDENT shows how someone who acts in a 'wait-and-see' manner automatically evokes LEADING behavior in another person.

Table 2.3 The behavioral variants showing the evoked behavior in the other person.

Behavioral designation	Associated behavior	Associated relationship definition	Evoked behavior in the other person
Leading	Lead, take the initiative, self-confidence	'I am strong, and you are weak; just do as I say'	Follow, wait, receive, obedience, dependence
Helping	Help, support, protect, solidarity	'I can help you, and you need help; we fit together'	Receive, absorb, cooperate
Cooperative	Agree, admire, accommodate, modesty	'I can't do everything myself, and you are very good; please tell me what to do'	Reward, support, help
Dependent	Wait, lean on, adapt, ask, be uncertain	'I can't do anything, and you can do everything; you have to help me'	Lead, direct, advise
Withdrawn	Withdraw, hide, keep silent, distrustful	'I feel worthless, and you can't be trusted; forget about me'	Disregard, reject, ignore
Rebellious	Resist, passive-aggressive, rebelliousness	'I don't want to, and you are forcing me; I won't do what you want'	Suppress, aggression, condemn

(Continued)

Table 2.3 (Continued)

Behavioral designation	Associated behavior	Associated relationship definition	Evoked behavior in the other person
Hostile	Aggression, offensive, distance	'I am angry, and you are wrong; we do not tolerate each other'	Rebelliousness, defend, attack
Competitive	Being high-minded, humiliate	'I don't want to, and you are forcing me; I won't do what you want'	Suppress, aggression, condemn

Modified version, with permission adapted from: Remmerswaal J (2003) Handboek groepsdynamica. Soest: Nelissen. Translation by the author.

These interactional laws always show variation in the reality of encounters between people, and sometimes they do not materialize. It depends on the relationship definition of the receiving party whether the evoked behavior is adopted. Fortunately, individuals are autonomous, and it does happen that someone behaves differently than the initiator of the interaction wishes and expects. But with very strong behavior, it is not easy to disregard the expected response. We all know the highly domineering other we will follow regardless, even though we don't want to or that excessively friendly person who entices us to share things we really want to keep to ourselves. This brings us to the relative strength of the behavior in the Interpersonal Circle.

Qualities and pitfalls in the Interpersonal Circle

Leary completed the model with the possibility of representing the relative strength of an individual's interactional behavior. To do this, he divided the circle into four concentric rings. He reserved the two outer rings of the IPC for the strong behavioral variants by sector and the inner two rings for the mild forms. In Figure 2.3, I show the IPC in this form, describing the behavior in varying strengths. You can view the inner two rings as the qualities of behavior in a sector and the outer two rings (in grey) as the pitfalls ('too much of a good thing') of that behavior.

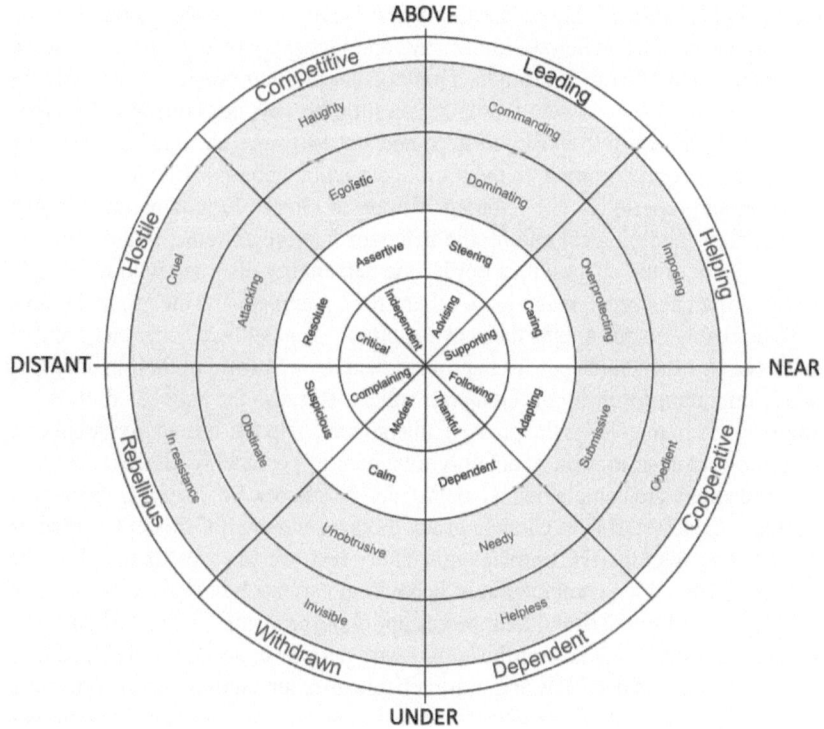

ABOVE

Competitive · Leading

Haughty · Commanding

Egoistic · Dominating

Hostile · Helping

Cruel · Imposing

Assertive · Steering

Attacking · Overprotecting

Resolute · Advising · Caring

Critical · Independent · Supporting

DISTANT — Suspicious · Complaining · Following · Adapting — NEAR

Obstinate · Modest · Thankful · Submissive

In resistance · Calm · Dependent · Obedient

Rebellious · Cooperative

Unobtrusive · Needy

Invisible · Helpless

Withdrawn · Dependent

UNDER

Figure 2.3 The Interpersonal Circle with qualities and pitfalls.

2.3   The Interpersonal Circle as practical instrument

Now that we know how interaction works, we arrive at the question of how we can apply the Interpersonal Circle theory and model during group therapy.

There are four ways of using the interaction table for practical work in group therapy: the Interpersonal Circle as diagnostic instrument, as therapeutic instrument, as technical instrument and as didactic instrument. We discuss each of these functions next.

1.   The Interpersonal Circle as diagnostic instrument: mapping the interaction style or habitual attitude of a person and registering repetitive interaction patterns

The IPC offers us two important diagnostic options: first, mapping someone's *habitual attitude/behavior* and, second, registering and understanding *repetitive interaction* patterns in the therapy group.

With a person's *habitual attitude* we mean the typical interaction style and characteristic social behavior someone initially presents to another person. Every human being has their own habitual social attitude. Our social behavior is an important aspect of our personality, our character (Carson, 1969). Our habitual attitude is our 'social business card,' the first behavior we make contact with and show to one another. When we know someone longer we recognize that person by that characteristic habitual attitude. Think of the familiar people in our daily life: our hairdresser Johanna, who typically is a little bit shy; our colleague Memphis, who mostly is heartfelt and interested; and not to forget our neighbor Suzanne, who is always quite grumpy. In the normal case, that habitual attitude shows some variation and repertoire. The habitual attitude of clients, by comparison, is striking due to its pathological nature; the behavior is more extreme, fixated, and less varied. Think of the client with a borderline personality disorder, who is fixated in strong 'attract and repel' behavior to other group members and the group therapist.

Remarkably no one knows their own habitual social attitude completely, and clients have an extra blind spot for that matter. But being aware of their habitual attitude is important for every group therapy client. Because the habitual attitude is so striking and often includes the problem clients seek help for, it is an important entry point for treatment, especially not only treatment of personality disorders but often also when there are complaints like depression or anxiety. So, mapping the habitual attitude is a good start for a client in group therapy, and the IPC model is perfect for this purpose. With the IPC and the explanatory text, we can score the habitual attitude, assessing which combination of behavioral variants best represents the client, and help them to understand themselves and their problems better. And of course we can use a questionnaire for this aim. Leary and his colleagues developed a test battery no longer in use. New and more reliable questionnaires about the IPC model have been produced. A commonly used questionnaire in the USA is the: Inventory of Interpersonal Problems, or IIP (Horowitz et al., 1988, 2000, www.mindgarden.com).

The model or questionnaire can be used as well as self-scoring, or other-scoring instrument. Such a questionnaire produces a profile characteristic of the person's habitual social attitude. See Figure 2.4 for two examples, in this case, based on the Dutch questionnaire ICL-R (De Jong et al., 2000).

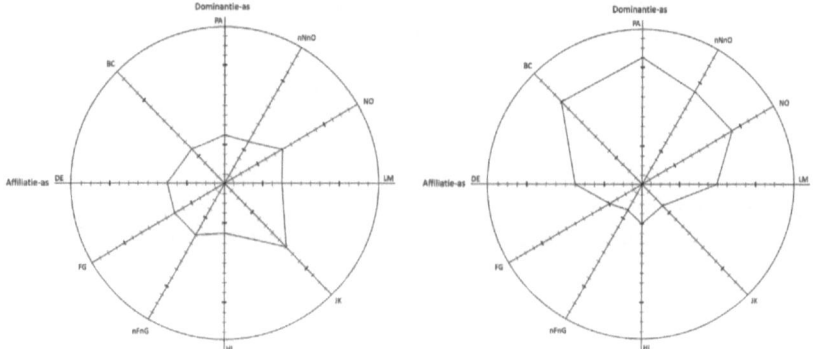

Figure 2.4 Two examples of different personal IPC profiles. With permission adapted from de Jong C A J., Van den Brink W, and Jansma A (2000) *ICL-R: Handleiding bij de vernieuwde Nederlandse versie van de Interpersonal Checklist (ICL).* Sint Oedenrode: Novadic.

What immediately stands out in such a profile is the direction of habitual social behavior; is someone primarily a leading type or a follower, or does someone possess a bit of everything? We also gain insight into the variety of someone's social-behavioral repertoire. This way, the group therapist gets information and insight into the habitual attitude and an impression of the individual's social flexibility within the therapy group.

The second diagnostic function of the IPC model is that it helps to explain and understand the notable and repeating interaction patterns that are happening between group members. From the model, we know that certain behavioral variants evoke each other. For example, if Paul's personality often presents a strong victim attitude (DEPENDENT), then it wouldn't come as a surprise that Suzy, who has a genuinely helping character, always has to rescue him (HELPING). As such, it is a useful diagnostic tool for notable interaction patterns. In Chapter 7, 'Interaction lines and relationship patterns,' I show how a group therapist, after a group therapy session, can plot the members in the IPC model, which gives insight in the interactional turmoil in the therapy group.

2. The Interpersonal Circle as therapeutic instrument for group therapy clients

As I said previously, this instrument can also be used therapeutically in group therapy. It involves the group therapist scoring with the IPC model, or exploring with a questionnaire, in which sector a member recognizes themselves in terms of their habitual attitude. As an alternative the group therapist can ask the members to score themselves. Then it is valuable to have the group members exchange their scoring and tell each other whether they would place their fellow group members in the same sectors. The group therapist can then invite the group to explore why each member presents precisely that habitual attitude and not a different one. This will give the group therapist and the group member a good idea of the latter's missing social behavioral repertoire and interactional flexibility. The group member could then set personal goals to experiment with the unfamiliar behavioral variants within the group therapy. At the end of their group therapy the client can repeat the IPC scoring to evaluate the growth in their behavior repertoire.

3. The Interpersonal Circle as a technical instrument for the group therapist

As we know, interaction is a basic activity in group therapy. With the Interpersonal Circle, the group therapist has an instrument with which she can influence the interactions in the group. Also, the group therapist is continuously part of the interactional field and reacts to the behavior of the group and its members through her interactional attitude. She can exploit that fact by using that attitude 'strategically.' By this, we mean that, with the help of the IPC model, the group therapist can adopt a specific attitude in order to achieve and keep the desired collaborative relationship with a group or group member. For example, suppose the group is always rather passive and waiting; the group therapist is then tempted to be active and leading. That attitude is not helpful if the group therapist desires an active and engaged group. To promote that, it is best for the group therapist to 'strategically' behave in a reserved and passive DEPENDENT manner, provoking the group to take the initiative and re-establish a productive collaborative relationship.

Optimizing the collaborative relationship is one of the three basic leadership techniques that I explain in more detail in Chapter 4 under '*Relationship technique.*'

4. The Interpersonal Circle as didactic instrument in a group therapy training: 'scoring your own habitual interaction style'

Because interaction is such an important tool in group therapy, every group therapist should have insight in their own habitual attitude and interaction style. That's why in the Netherlands the IPC model is often used for this didactic goal in group therapy training. The students are asked to examine – or use a questionnaire to discover – which behavioral variants the person best recognizes themselves when imagining herself in a safe, social environment: for example, a very pleasant work team in which the person can be themselves. One then discovers their own personal habitual attitude. The profile shows the qualities of the students' habitual interaction style, makes clear what behaviors are less familiar, and helps make goals to broaden and strengthen their repertoire.

And of course any experienced group therapist is never too late to investigate her own interaction style, especially when difficult interactional situations or countertransference feelings play up. In this respect it is useful to mention the Impact Message Inventory Circumplex (IMI-C; Manual: www.mindgarden. com; Kiesler and Schmidt, 1993). This IPC-based questionnaire is intended to trace objective countertransference, the feelings and behavioral tendencies that a client or a group evokes in the group therapist (Hafkenscheid, 2014).

Chapter 3

Organizing a therapy group

3.1 The foundation of any therapy group: group task and group process

Introduction: the dichotomy of task and process

In Chapter 1, I explained that group processes are at play in every group. Whether it's a health care team, a neighborhood club, a drama society, or a therapy group, group processes are always involved, ensuring the spontaneous relational and emotional interplay between the people working together. But the process side is only half the story. A group also always has a task. The task is the most important part; it is the reason a group exists. A group is created to achieve an agreed goal from which the group task arises.

'Task and process' is a typical example of a dichotomy, a duality. Task and process are different but always coexist in any group. It is very useful to be able to distinguish them if we want to understand behavior within a group. We discover the task by looking at *what* group members do, and we can detect the process if we look at *how* (the way) the group members do it. For instance, we know from experience that group therapy, with exactly the same themes and assignments, always progresses differently in one group than in another. The task, the *what*, is the same, but the process, *how* the task is carried out, differs from group to group.

Task and process each have their own source

The distinction between task and process becomes more insightful when we realize that both have an entirely separate source. The task aspect stems from what has been agreed upon regarding the goal and task of the group, that is, from the organization. The process has an entirely different source, namely, the people: the persons with their characters, their feelings, and their mutual relations. The task is conceived and agreed upon, thus more or less predictable, but the process is spontaneous and unpredictable. The task is the 'makeable' part of the group, one can organize a group task; the process is the spontaneous 'not-makeable' part; you never can organize process.

DOI: 10.4324/9781003368786-4

Task and Process

The distinction between task and process is referred to in various terms throughout the history of social sciences. Social psychologist Bales (1950) was the first to state the distinction. His research concluded differences between 'task-related' and 'person-related' interactions and roles. Communication scientist Watzlawick (1973) referred to the differences between 'content and relation,' and Remmerswaal (2015) refers to the 'task level and social-emotional level.' Hersey (2007) distinguished 'task and relationship' in his research on leadership. In group dynamics (Carron, 1988; Dion, 2000), the distinction between task and process has since been seen as a universal phenomenon in human interaction and group formation.

Both aspects of human interaction are always simultaneously present in the group members behaviors, like two sides of a coin (Remmerswaal, 2015). So, referring to a task-based or process-based group is confusing and incorrect. Of course, some therapy groups make use of the processes a lot, but that is then part of that group's working method and task. Even in such a group, you can always see the duality of task and process during the sessions. A non-task-based group does not exist. In Table 3.1, I summarize the distinction between task and process.

Table 3.1 The distinction between task and process.

Task	Process
WHAT	**HOW**
Arises from the organization	Arises from the people
Facts	Feelings
Conceived	Spontaneous
Business-like	Personal and relational
Makeable	Not-makeable

Task structure and process structure

Both the task and process side of a group exhibit a structure of elements. On the task side, we see elements related to the group's organization; on the process side, we see elements related to the human aspect of the group. Table 3.2 shows the elements of both structures.

Table 3.2 Task structure and process structure.

Task	Process
Task Structure	**Process Structure**
TARGET GROUP A selected group of people with a corresponding help request	**GROUP COHESION** A group's attachment network and its positive perception by the group members
GROUP GOALS and INDIVIDUAL GOALS What group members want to have achieved by the end of the group therapy	**INTERACTION and RELATIONSHIP PATTERNS** Interaction among group members lead to certain relationship patterns
THERAPEUTIC METHOD and WORKING METHOD Therapeutic method and the concrete procedure by which goals are pursued	**DEVELOPMENT STAGES** The group's course of development
THE GROUP MEMBERS' TASK The task actions that all group members are expected to perform	**NORMS and SOCIAL INFLUENCE** The emergence of group norms and a group culture
IMPLEMENTATION Organizing the group implementation, such as composition, duration, frequency, and the setting	**ROLES** The manifestation of roles among different group members
EVALUATION/RESULT How the outcome is evaluated or measured	**TERMINATION PROCESSES** The process of parting and participants detaching
AN APPROPRIATE NAME A clear and logical name	

The seven elements of the task structure show a logical order. The starting point is always the *target group*, the selected group of people with a corresponding help request. The next step is the *group goal*: the group to be set up must have a goal that is the answer to the help request. Within that group goal, the participants create *individual goals*. These goals are pursued using a specific *method and procedure*, which means that group members are given a necessary *task*. All this can be *implemented* in a specific way. To determine effectiveness, the group result is *evaluated*. Finally, an appropriate *name* gives the group recognition and identity.

The task structure is always conceived and agreed upon, and the group therapist shapes it based on expert knowledge about the target group. In Section 3.2, we discuss the task elements in detail because they form the basis for organizing a group.

In the right-hand column of Table 3.2, you can see the structure of process elements. The process stems from the people's personal motives: feelings, desires, fears, opinions, and views. Motives that, once they come together in the group, interact and, over time, crystallize into typical group processes, which we call the process structure. In any group that meets more frequently, a sense of *cohesion develops*, and cooperation among group members develops through *interaction* and *relationship patterns*; we see incremental *development*, and *roles* and *norms* crystallize through *social influence*. And when the group or a participant stops, it is accompanied by a natural process of *parting* and *detachment*. Thanks to extensive theoretical and experimental research over the past 80 years (Forsyth, 2017; Nijstad, 2009), the science of social psychology and group dynamics has discovered those processes and demonstrated that they are universal; that is, they occur spontaneously in every group, independent of the task. These processes and their usefulness for group therapy are the core around which this book revolves. In Part 3, I discuss all of them in depth.

An unclear task

In a therapy group for people with addiction problems, three people who have not yet 'finished' stop within a short period of time. The group therapist spends a lot of time worrying about what the problem could be. When number four leaves, the therapist expresses his concern to the group members about the group falling apart. They share his concern. During the conversation, they indicate that it is not clear what the group is about. The goal and task appear to be unclear. The group therapist then again explains the purpose of the group and is surprised by the nescience and lack of clarity among the group members. The next session proceeds very differently. The motivation to get started and persevere is much more palpable among all the remaining group members.

Perceiving the distinction between task and process

Task and process have different sources but are always coexistent. This means that a group member's behavior always has a task component and a process component. How do we see these two aspects? By what do we recognize the distinction? Because a task and process each have their own source, we perceive them with different receivers – the task (WHAT, the businesslike and conceived aspect of the group) with our mind, our ratio, and the process side (HOW, the human aspect of the group) with our feelings, senses.

Here's an example. You participate in a team meeting that has to make a difficult decision. If you perceive with your mind and concentrate on *what* factual is happening, you see that the team is engaged in the task, exchanging arguments, discussing different options, and so on. If you watch and listen with your feelings and intuition, you can sense *how* the group is engaged in the task. Levi is going out of her way in the meeting to ask others' opinions, and the rest of the group members sit back without taking initiative. You realize this imbalance in the group annoys you.

Being consciously aware of this distinction is an advantage for a group therapist. Because task and process are so obvious, group members are often unaware of this distinction. If the group is doing well, this conscious knowledge is
unnecessary. However, it is necessary when the group becomes stagnant or out
of sync. When misunderstandings and ambiguities arise in the group, the confusion between the task and the process almost always comes into play. Then the
group therapist, aware of this distinction, has a powerful tool to use. Because of
the distinction between task and process, he can often quickly understand and
sense what is happening and use his observations to help the group. Not only are
task and process and the distinction between them fundamental to understanding
what is going on in the group, but it also provides the basis for influencing the
group (see Chapters 4 and 5).

A notable distinction between task and process
In a veteran recovery center, an educational group therapy on PTSS and
trauma is an important component. The group therapy is well structured and
always receives excellent reviews from participants afterward. A few weeks
ago, the two experienced group therapists started a new group. However, they
noticed their usual enthusiasm quickly faded with the current group. During
the debriefing of the third session, the two group therapists noticed that there
was a strange atmosphere in this group. Everyone is neatly on time and duti-
fully participates, but they never ask questions, and when the therapists invite
them to participate in mutual discussions, they rarely do so. The atmosphere
is inhibited; group members avoid eye contact and sit with crossed arms. It
seems as if the group is afraid or holding something back. The group therapists
resolve to first discuss this process side with the group at the next session.

3.2   Organizing a therapy group, step 1: designing the task organization on paper

The seven-step plan for concretizing a group task organization

A group never simply exists. It owes its existence to the function it fulfills for
the participants and for the organization it belongs to. If the group manages to
achieve its goals, then the participants are glad, and the group gains in its existence. Thus, a therapy group known to be efficient and result-promising will be
attractive to potential participants and referrers. Therefore, it is very important that we organize a group that functions as productive as possible (AGPA,
Practice Guidelines for Group Psychotherapy,[1] 2007; De Haas and Van Hest,
in NVGP *Praktijkrichtlinen Groepsbehandeling voor de (Geestelijke) Gezondheidszorg*,[2] 2019).

How do we do that? The premise of group dynamics, the dichotomy between
task and process, offers us a solution. We know that the task side stems from

group organization; it is the makeable part of the group. It is therefore wise to organize that task as best as we can. It helps to see its organization as a 'two-stage rocket' with two distinguishable moments. The first moment is the preliminary phase in which the therapy group is well thought out and designed, *the group task on paper*. Later, when the therapy group actually begins, followed by the second moment, the convincing *start of the therapy group*. In this section, I demonstrate how to best conceptualize and design the group on paper. At the end of this chapter, I discuss the convincing start, the second moment of group organization.

In the previous paragraph, I demonstrated that the row of task elements depicts a logical order in the organization of the task side of a group. We can make use of this when designing the group. We can build the seven elements step by step. In doing so, the target group, our *clients*, is always the starting point. Each subsequent step can be derived from that starting point and the concreteness of the previous step. And here, the more concrete and consequent the logical coherence, the better. Claassen and Janzing (2014) use the term 'coherent treatment' for this purpose, a concept that fits well with the aim of this chapter. A therapy group works best when it is organized in such a way that the entire task organization forms a logically coherent whole for all users: the client, the group therapist, and the relevant organization. Such a successful organizational setup is also called a 'design.'

The design

In organizational science, we use the term 'design,' meaning that the task organization is a beautiful, coherent, and functional design (Bellerby, 2017).

As we will see in Chapter 6, 'Cohesion in group therapy,' such a coherent organization is not only good for organizing a concrete group task but also conducive to process development. It directly fosters the emergence of both group cohesion and the holding environment for the group therapy itself.

In the following, I explain how a group therapist can use the seven task elements of Table 3.2 to organize a new group step by step.

Step 1:   Concretizing the target group
Organizing a therapy group is a client-oriented and demand-driven undertaking, and the corresponding help request of the client target group is always the starting point. It is important to be as clear as possible when describing the target group because everything that follows in the step-by-step group organization thereafter is based on this initial beginning. Anything that goes wrong here is

difficult to correct in the subsequent concretization steps. In my practice, I have found that drawing an imaginary circle around the people who qualify is helpful. The question is then, Do these people all have the same help request or problem? If so, I can continue. A concrete description of the target group provides immediate practical benefits. In practice, it makes selecting participants easy by making it clear who does and does not fall within the circle. The boundary is then also immediately clear. Because a target group that is described too broadly carries the risk that the group formed is too diverse in nature and becomes unproductive. By not recognizing each other's problems sufficiently, cohesion cannot develop, and it then becomes difficult to formulate a common group goal.

In health care, such a description is always based on two criteria: the participants' precise help request, problem, or chief complaint and the professional's diagnostic criteria, often a *DSM* disorder. For example, suppose a psychologist wants to set up a therapy group in her own practice for people who seek relief from their depression symptoms. In that case, she will have to think carefully beforehand when defining the target group. She must clearly define the *DSM* criteria for depression symptoms she wants to treat. But also what exactly the participants expect from a group and their help request. A successful outcome is only possible if the offered group therapy matches those two criteria.

Concretizing the boundary of a target group
A psychogeriatrics department is experimenting with an education therapy group for loved ones of a family member with dementia. The target group includes both partners and children of a person with dementia. After having conducted the course three times, the group therapists conclude that the combination of partners and children as a target group does not work that well. The peer contact in the course shows that the partners benefit most from the experience of other partners, and the same is true for the children. Therefore, the group therapists decide to make the target group a little more homogeneous. There is enough interest to easily form two separate education groups, one for partners and one for children. Next, they will investigate whether this works better in practice.

Homogeneous or heterogeneous

This touches on the question of a homogeneous or heterogeneous composition of a therapy group. As the corresponding help request of the target group is always the starting point for group organization, every therapy group is, in principle, a homogeneous group in terms of the help request, complaint, or problem. Without this common basis, a fruitful group organization will not succeed. In addition, it always involves heterogeneous characteristics. Better said, both characteristics are important for the working method. If we look at the list of therapeutic factors (Chapter 1) we see that participants learn from the similarities with each other ('recognition'), as well as from the differences between them ('feedback,' 'learning from exemplary behavior'). However, it is true that in some therapy groups, learning from differences in working methods stands out, while learning from similarity and recognition is somewhat more important in another group. It's all about a balance with differences in emphasis. A homogeneous therapy group dealing with PTSS, for example, benefits from different persons, each with their distinct personalities, backgrounds, cultures, and solution strategies, while a heterogeneous intensive interactional group psychotherapy needs homogeneous characteristics, such as equal ego-strength. Homogeneous or heterogeneous is not unimportant as an organizational criterion, but the distinction is relative. As long as we remember to always organize the basis of the therapy group – the help request of the target group – homogeneously.

Step 2:   Concretizing the group goals with your essential intention; organizing individual goals

The corresponding help request of the *target group* automatically leads to the *group goals*. The reason for setting up a therapy group already refers to a desired outcome. This is the focus point of the group organization, where you want to go together with the group. What goals would you want to have achieved by the end? The concrete formulation of that desired end result is extremely important because it lays the foundation for the participants' practical work. Three things can help us do that. The first is, the value of group goals: the more the formulation of the goal defines the participant's help request, wishes, or expectations, the more valuable the group becomes. I call this main goal 'the essential intention' (Hart, 2017). This essential intention is easy to formulate for a target group with a single complaint. The help request is often enough to formulate a concrete group goal, usually symptom reduction or improved functioning. Clients in a therapy group for anxiety disorders will be happy with a significant decrease in their anxiety symptoms. For target groups with complex problems, this is more complicated. Consider a group for adolescents with intellectual disabilities combined with schizophrenia. A group therapist will not succeed in reducing symptoms or curing them. In that case, formulating an appropriate group goal requires more creative thinking, and the idea of essential intention will be helpful.

A group therapist will discover his essential intention by reflecting on the target group and on his own role as a help professional. What are my clients suffering from the most? What achievable outcome would allow these participants to suffer less and lead a better life? What do research and treatment practice say about these complaints? What realistic outcome would make me happy as a help professional? The essential intention thus touches on the motivation of the members as well as the motivation of the group therapist. Hence, organizing a group is also a value-oriented undertaking; what is this group really about, and what is the real value or relevance of this whole-group undertaking? Being aware of that essential value of your group makes it easier to set concrete and essential goals, and you will then know definitively that those are relevant goals for the members.

The second aspect in concretizing the group goals is considering feasibility so that the goal realistically matches what the target group can achieve. Some problems or disorders can be cured, but in many cases, that is often not possible. Based on their expertise, a group therapist must then consider what is and is not possible and align group goals accordingly. Essential intentions can help identify alternatives when curing is not possible. Consider a group for people with acquired brain injury where curing is not possible, but providing better coping skills is feasible.

Finally, when concretizing the group goals, it is important to formulate them SMART[3] and in end terms. Or, rather, 'at the end of this group therapy, you will feel more positive more often' than 'the goal of this group therapy is to reduce feelings of depression.' Concrete goals make evaluating or measuring the treatment outcome at the end of the group therapy easier.

Individual goals

In any therapy group, there are always individual goals in addition to a group goal. More importantly, individual goals are what every therapy group is about. It is not the group that has an anxiety disorder but the individuals who each suffer from anxiety symptoms in their own way and want to be helped in a personalized way. That is why individual goals are so essential. In a well-organized therapy group, the individual goals will match up well with the group goal, and the synergy of the two makes it a strong therapy group. On the one hand, participants feel the support of the commonality of their symptoms; on the other hand, individual differences are afforded recognition and space. This allows the participant to formulate his personal emphases related to the group goal, which will enhance motivation.

To safeguard this individual focus, not only are the individual goals important, but it also helps if the group therapist keeps an eye on whether each group member is sufficiently addressed. In any treatment, the clients can avoid attention, and a typical avoidance method in group therapy is that participants go 'diving,' keeping themselves in the background in the group without noticing. Because this individual attention is so important, Ormont nearly made it a group rule when he stated: 'The contract calls for each member to take a part of the total talking time; that is, in a group of eight, each member speaks approximately one-eighth of all time over a period of weeks or months' (Ormont, 1968, 153).

Individual goals

The main goal of a psychotherapy group for students with depressive symptoms is to gain better control of their moods. Therein, participants can place different personal emphases to form relevant personal goals. For example, Jocelyn's personal goal is to 'keep in touch with friends even when I am in danger of becoming depressed.' She knows she tends to withdraw when her mood drops, making it worse. Rochelle's personal goal is to 'stay active' because she knows that is the best way to keep her mood balanced. And Ben has chosen 'to be allowed to feel my anger and stand up for myself' as a personal goal. He has learned that giving in to his shyness and sub-assertiveness makes him feel somber.

To consciously form personal goals, a separate moment is often needed with a focused conversation or targeted questionnaire in which the participant can indicate their personal goals. In (mental) health care, personal goals are usually set in a treatment plan even before group therapy starts. This can be done as a working hypothesis, but a better time for this is shortly after the start when the participant has experienced the therapy group sufficiently long to know what it has to offer. Personal goals can always be adjusted later, for instance, because they develop and change throughout the group therapy.

An evolving personal goal
Gordon needed time to get used to the working method in his intensive interactional psychotherapy group. He initially expected his symptoms to disappear quickly, but as he began to feel more secure in the group, his expectations changed. He noticed that his anxiety and feelings of depression became important sources of information for how he felt on the inside. Getting to know himself better gradually became his main goal, and his symptoms became less important.

Step 3:   Concretizing the therapeutic method and working method
A therapeutic method is always required to work toward group goals. The method is often based on a therapeutic frame of reference, established for a target group based on scientific research, and often dictated by guidelines. For example, for patients with borderline disorders, an often used therapeutic method in the USA is Dialectical Behavior Therapy (Linehan, 1993), which is also applied in group therapy. The working method is derived from this, with matching therapy procedures and interventions. In Chapter 1, I explained that the efficacy of group therapy is attributable to the proper handling of group processes (the group as therapeutic instrument) in combination with such a methodical therapeutic framework.

If such a therapeutic framework is lacking, knowledge about the target group helps the group therapist to devise a tailored working method. For example, a group for young adults with ADHD benefits from a method and procedure with concrete protocols in a consistent order because this target group learns best in a low-stimulation and transparent environment.

The therapeutic method and working method also includes the degree of structure in the approach. The more protocols, techniques, ground rules, and dos and don'ts, the more structure and vice versa. The degree of structure must match what the target group needs and suit the group goal so that the entire task organization becomes a logically coherent whole. When describing the working method, the group therapist also takes into account his own task, how he works, which techniques he uses, and what his role is (see also Chapter 4, 'Leading a therapy group,' and Chapter 10, 'Role behavior in a therapy group').

A clear working method

A social worker and addiction counselor are the co-group therapists of the so-called cleaning-up-the-mess therapy group, a part of a clinical addiction program. After all, many clients have made a mess of things during their addiction: jobless, dropped out of school, debts, no benefit entitlement, no permanent residence, and so on. When setting up the therapy group, careful thought is given to the target group and the type of help the group members need. The group's goal is twofold: start cleaning up their societal life and learn ways to keep that life on track. The group works with a clear and appropriate working methodology, the 'assignment method.' Before group participation, each resident details the state of their affairs with the social worker and then agrees on concrete targets. In each weekly session, each participant chooses a *concrete* and *achievable* step in the remediation process. The following week, he reports on how the assignment went. The methodology further emphasizes success, working with the principles of rewarding desirable behavior, and ignoring undesirable behavior. Members praise each other extensively when the assignment has succeeded and help each other make an assignment achievable. When a member fails to meet the assignment the group therapist informs briefly to understand why: was the assignment concrete enough, feasible enough, and relevant enough for the client. The group therapist then keeps the communication short and neutral to prevent rewarding the fail behavior too much.

Step 4: Concretizing the group members' task

The task is the crux of what it is all about: the performative work, what the group members must do together to achieve the intended result. This task is a logical consequence of the therapeutic and working method or is even already contained therein. In the example mentioned previously, the group uses the assignment methodology. The participants' resulting task, among other things, includes discussing a concrete assignment aloud, helping each other make the assignment concrete and achievable, praising a fellow group member when he has completed his assignment successfully, and not reacting to the complaining behavior of a fellow group member. Thus, the task is the concrete interactional cooperative behavior established in the method and what the group therapist and the participants expect from each other.

The task often involves multiple actions. For example, during social skills training, participants are expected to read information beforehand, be prepared to role-play together, give each other feedback, and practice new behaviors at home. It is important to include all of these actions in the task description; this also makes it clear which task is inappropriate and which is not expected. In social skills group therapy, one does not expect participants to delve extensively into their past and tell their life history. The more clearly the task is made explicit to participants, the clearer the required work in the group will be. Over time, the procedures become ingrained within experienced group members, facilitating task performance.

An important aspect of the task description is the desired form and degree of interaction among group members. Because interactive learning is so self-evident in group therapy, therapists tend to forget to mention this part of the task. Thus, the group therapist must always indicate within the task description exactly what interaction is expected of the participants. Because the desired form of interaction determines how much the group members make use of the group dynamics. If the desired form of interaction is free and unstructured, it allows for ample spontaneous group dynamics, and group members use them frequently in task performance. In contrast, if the desired form of interaction is highly structured, group members will make little use of group dynamics. In an educational therapy group, interaction mainly occurs between the group therapist and the group, and less interaction usually occurs between the group members themselves. By comparison, a psychotherapy group is mainly based on the exchange of feelings and opinions, so there will be a lot of mutual interaction. Some groups work 'individually within the group.' In this case, interaction occurs mainly between the group therapist and alternating individual participants, with other members as spectators or role-players. Psycho-drama group therapy is an example of this.

It is most effective when the type and degree of interaction match the target group and the method. It will be a shame if too little interaction occurs because the participants are not challenged sufficiently. If too much interaction occurs, they may be overloaded, causing too much anxiety.

Some groups work on a task with protocol forms of interaction set within the working method. For example, the interaction task of group members in a CBT group consists of systematically exploring and writing down their cognitions, feelings, behaviors, and consequences. Role-playing or doing exercises together suits a social skills therapy group. In many groups, the group task consists of a combination of different forms of interaction.

The group therapy task can be complex. Especially for a first-time group member, it is often still unclear what is expected of him or her. The task is sometimes complicated and may involve various forms of interaction. Group therapists often misjudge this lack of clarity among group members. For this reason, it can do no harm, especially in a beginning group, to regularly explain and discuss the logic of the task and the various forms of interaction.

Re-explaining the task

A 'working points' group therapy in a day clinical program for clients with personality disorders is not progressing well. In this group, each participant talks about their working point involving domestic contacts; for example, 'I don't do everything on my own, but ask a friend to help me.' The intention is for participants to discuss their assignments on their own initiative and to respond to each other.

But that doesn't happen. All the participants wait until the group therapist designates the next person who may talk about their working point. At the end of the session, the group therapist asks the group their opinion about the group therapy. 'It's okay,' Jamila says. And Milan adds that he finds it boring and doesn't understand the point of it all. 'Shall I re-explain the intention and goals of the therapy?' the group therapist asks. 'Sure,' Milan says. When the group therapist has re-explained that the intention is for everyone to discuss their working point, for the others to give feedback on it, and that not everyone necessarily has to take their turn every time, the group members react. 'Oh, is that the idea!' Jamila exclaims. 'So, we may respond to each other?' Robert asks. 'I thought we were supposed to wait our turn,' Milan responds.

The next session is still not running quite as smoothly but not nearly as awkwardly as before. At the end, when the group therapist revisits the task and intention, the group members indicate that it is clear to them now and that they appreciate that.

In a target group with many vulnerable characteristics, it may even be necessary to re-explain the task many times. For example, in an inpatient therapy group for clients with acute psychiatric problems like severe depression or psychotic disorder, repeating the members' tasks every session is helping and necessary, even though it is the same information each time.

Step 5: Concretizing the implementation of a therapy group
Concretizing the implementation means that a group therapist determines what the therapy group organization will look like in detail. He must define the following five variables:
1. Group size
2. A therapy group with fixed or changing composition (closed or open group)

3. The duration of the therapy group – continuous or limited
4. The frequency and length of the sessions (intensity)
5. The spatial setting.

1. Group size

Research indicates that group size affects the quality of group therapy. In a small group, the task is accomplished more easily, and cohesion develops more quickly (Evans and Dion, 2012; Mullen and Copper, 1994). Unfortunately, there is no scientific measure for the optimal therapy group size. We currently have to make do with our experience. For example, we know that our capacity for productive interaction in relationships is limited. In addition, a large group feels less safe to participants. The appropriate group size is also determined by the group's function. In my experience, in groups where task-oriented collaboration and interaction are required, that is, an educational group, effective task performance becomes difficult when there are more than 18 participants. Groups in which highly personal exchange is required, such as in an Interpersonal or Psychodynamic psychotherapy group, preferably do not have more than nine participants (Fay et al., 2000). Experience shows that a group that is too small is also less effective. For example, if a group has only four participants, they often focus more on the group therapist than on each other. The group then has too little 'body.'

2. A group with a set or changing composition

A therapy group with a set composition of participants does not admit new members during the duration, whereas a therapy group with a changing composition admits new members each time someone leaves. A set composition suits many types of therapy groups within health care like an educational or skill training group therapy. A group with a set composition almost always has a limited duration, while a group with a changing composition is always ongoing. Within the field of group therapy, we refer to it as an open group (changing composition) or closed group (set composition).

The 'out together, home together' effect of a therapy group with a set composition reinforces the task and group goal. All group members work parallel on the same task and goal in the same amount of time. This also has a beneficial effect on process development. The set composition, undisturbed by the entrance of newcomers, promotes the process of group cohesion and development, enhancing the group's efficacy.

A therapy group with a changing composition best suits clients who need a longer trajectory. The advantage of this form is that group members can determine their own participation time. Because the end of group participation is not preset, concretizing group (and certainly individual) goals is especially important in the open form to prevent group members from becoming 'stuck.'

A semi-open form exists between these two forms. A semi-open group is closed to new participants for an agreed period (e.g., three months) to ensure sufficient opportunity for group development. At the end of each closed period, people can stop and leave the group. This is followed by a short open period (say, two weeks) during which the group accepts new participants. This intermediate form was devised primarily to eliminate the disadvantages of the two other forms. The semi-open form reduces the agitation of new-comers by ensuring closed duration periods. In addition, the semi-open form prevents long waits for potential participants. A variant of the semi-open therapy group is one with an overlapping composition. Each time after a set period (e.g., six months), half of the group leaves to make room for half a group of newcomers. This method allows the group to always consist of half seniors and half juniors, a combination with the added benefit of making it easier to maintain the therapeutic culture, and the benefit to learn to say goodbye.

3. The duration of the group

The point is determining whether a short or more prolonged treatment best suits the target group, task, and method. For example, five sessions for a therapy group for people with complex grief problems is insufficient; they need prolonged treatment. The duration of the group is linked to the decision of whether to use a limited or unlimited format. In a limited group, the number of sessions is set, and the end date is predetermined. In an unlimited group, a participant can basically continue indefinitely. A limited group almost always has a set composition of participants. We can derive the preference for a limited or unlimited form of group therapy from the characteristics of the working method. For example, for a group with a training goal and working method, a limited number of sessions is the best choice.

4. The frequency and length of a session (intensity)

The length of a session and the time between sessions together determine the intensity of a group. Some target groups require an intense and short group approach. A group of people with addiction problems is better treated in a concentrated frequency because we know that avoidance becomes too prevalent in stand-alone sessions. Hence, addiction therapy often takes place in closed, regularly scheduled groups. In inpatient addiction therapy and inpatient psychotherapy, we apply 'high-pressure group therapy,' in which a person essentially undergoes therapy 24 hours a day. Attendance at the treatment unit is entirely devoted to clinical group therapy. An example of a group where a less intensive approach is appropriate would be a group of elderly psychiatric patients with depression symptoms. The group sessions should not last more than 45 minutes for these participants because their concentration could decrease significantly after that. Allowing a longer time between sessions will also be better for this target group. From experience we know that, for a lot of therapy groups, a 90-minute session once a week is appropriate.

5. The spatial setting

Jongerius (1993) describes the desired furnishings and settings for group therapy. For a psychotherapy group, for example, he recommends a setting in a spacious room without distracting furnishings and with not too many windows. Chairs that are not overly comfortable are placed inside the room at arm's length from each other in an open circle. The circle emphasizes the group-like character of the therapy and the associated holding environment; the distance between the armrests marks the space afforded to each individual to whom the group therapy is ultimately aimed. The therapist does not always sit at the head of the circle or the table, but often just between the group members, and when there are two of them, they face each other. As we previously noted about length and frequency, the group therapist can vary with the spatial setting to achieve the group goals. The spatial setting can also be a circle of chairs around a table or mats in a gym. It is up to him to deduce from the target group, group goal, and group task which setting is appropriate for which group. See the following example.

With online group therapy, extra attention to the setting is necessary, because the therapist has less influence on it, and because the self-evident safe physical circle is missing. Weinberg (2024) advises providing additional explanations and targeted technical assistance with questions, advising on how people find a safe space, how best to sit behind the camera, that they name names, and so on.

A dual spatial setting

A therapy group for men with burnout symptoms and persistent neurotic problems follows a combination group therapy. For the first three-quarters of an hour, the group does various confrontational exercises in the gym under the guidance of a psychomotor therapist, which are also recorded on video. In the second 45 minutes, the group, led by a group therapist, elaborates on the avoidance behaviors seen in the video, focusing on new solutions for each individual. During that group conversation, the men sit in an open circle of U-shaped chairs, facing the video screen at the front.

Step 6:   Concretizing the evaluation
A therapy group is always a results-oriented undertaking. Therefore, choosing an appropriate evaluation or outcome-measuring instrument is an integral part of organizing a therapy group. Successfully formulating clear goals in concrete SMART end terms will make it easier to compile an evaluation questionnaire. Given what we have said in this section about the group and individual goals, we need two evaluation instruments: one to measure group effectiveness and one to measure personal goals. For example, in the Netherlands mandatory ROM (Routine Outcome Monitoring) data are used to measure treatment outcomes (Hafkenscheid, in NVGP, 2019; Koementas-de Vos et al., 2018) in the mental health system. I revisit the subject of evaluation in Chapter 11, 'Termination,' but I do not elaborate on the subject of measuring instruments as it is beyond the scope of this book.

Step 7:   Coming up with an appropriate name
The final element of group organization is deciding on an appropriate name, which is more important than we think. It would be helpful to come up with a concrete, logical, and distinctive name. It gives the group identity and recognition, which is pleasant for participants and referrers. This is important as group therapy needs a constant flow of new clients. The name could refer to typical characteristics such as the target group ('Tired Heroes' Group), the problem ('the Group for Depression Issues'), the method ('the DBT Group,' 'the Psycho-Dynamic Group'), or the result (the 'No More Fear' Group).

The group design

In health care, we frequently see design combinations when we organize therapy groups. For example, we often encounter a short-term closed-limited combination in therapy groups that use education or training as their working method. But the purpose of this step is mainly to show that you can play with all these design parameters and combine and vary them to create a tailored offer for the target group. Knowing the target group well often provides enough material to determine that uniquely appropriate form.

Table 3.3 provides an overview of the step-by-step organization of a therapy group. The left column lists the seven task elements, and the second and third columns indicate, in each case in greater detail, the concretization. You can shape your new group with the help of this table by looking at all the important task elements from top to bottom and concretizing each task element from left to right.

Table 3.3 The group design; organizing a therapy group in seven steps, and two concretization levels (the group on paper).

Group Design

Task Elements	Concretization Level 1 General		Concretization Level 2 Operational	
	Client demand			
1. Target group	What is the corresponding help request from the participants?		Emphasis on a heterogeneous or homogeneous group?	
2. Group goals	The essential intention (the core purpose)	In end terms and words based on the client's experience	Tool for individual goals in end terms	Valuable behavior
				Achievable
	Other goals			Concrete (SMART)
	Professional supply offered by the group therapist			
3. Method	What therapeutic frame of reference suits the target group?		An appropriate working method	
			Concrete procedures of the method	
			An appropriate amount of structure	
4. Group Task	What actions are expected of all group members?		Presenting your problems	
			Responding to each other	
			Exploring/analyzing the problems	
	What type of interaction among group members is the most suitable?		Interaction between the group therapist and each group member (individually in the group)	
			Interaction between the group therapist and the whole group (classroom)	
			Interaction based on a protocol	
			Free interaction	
	What group rules are agreed upon?		Confidentiality	
			Attendance	
			Working undisturbed	
			The group as workplace	
			Other group rules	

(Continued)

Table 3.3 (Continued)

Group Design

Task Elements	Concretization Level 1 General	Concretization Level 2 Operational
5. Implementation	An appropriate group size	
	Open/closed group	
	An appropriate group duration	Limited or unlimited
		Duration of the group
		Length of the session
	An appropriate intensity	The time between sessions (frequency)
		Number of sessions
	Setting	Type of room (therapy room, gymnasium, living room, etc.)
		Decoration in the room
		Chairs in an open circle
		At the table
6. Evaluation/result	Group goals	An appropriate measuring instrument
	Individual goals	An appropriate evaluation method
7. Appropriate name		A name that makes clear what participants can expect and/or hope for and that has a recruiting effect on referrers

Step-by-step organization of a therapy group (based on Table 3.3)

Target group (people with similar help requests)

Adult clients with an adoption background, who get stuck because they suffer from shame and a negative sense of self, don't dare to show themselves, have difficulty accessing their emotions, and have difficulty connecting with others. They hope that group therapy can help them feel more positive about themselves, take up more space for themselves, and dare to bond more with others.

Diagnostically, there are often mood and/or anxiety complaints and often personality problems (attachment problems) from the B or C cluster.

Group goals: after the group therapy, the clients have/are:

- A stronger self-identity and self-esteem
- More self-compassion
- More in touch with one's own emotions and needs, including needs that may have been lacking in the (early) past.
- More satisfying relationships with others
- More satisfaction with the way they shape their lives.

Individual goals

Each group member formulates some individual goals at the beginning of the therapy group that are concrete enough to be easily evaluated at the end.

Therapeutic Method

Affect Phobia Therapy (Mc Cullough Vaillant, 1997). The Affect Phobia Therapy method aims to help clients experience their healthy feelings and needs as fully as possible. To do this, they need to recognize and dare to let go of their avoidance behavior and feelings of fear. At appropriate moments, the therapists provide psychoeducation about adoption and trauma-specific psychological development and its consequences on current functioning.

Working method

Intensive open interactional group therapy method. The group members spontaneously bring in their problems, respond to each other's input, and investigate with each other and the therapists the background of the destructive patterns they show.

Group task

- Bringing in your own topics, questions, and problems and being open to and responding to the input of others
- Honestly communicate what is going on inside you, what you feel, and what others bring about in yourself
- Curious and nonjudgmental attitude (toward the other and toward oneself)
- Confronting each other with the defensive patterns in a respectful way
- Investigate the patterns together with each other and the therapists
- Trying out new behavior in the group and in one's own environment
- Group rules: Attendance, confidentiality, 'group as workplace' (i.e., no interactions outside the group)

Implementation

Nine months of weekly 1.5-hour group psychotherapy in a closed group of six participants. Chairs in the circle (with empty chairs in case of any absent group members).

Name

Roots Before Branches[4]

3.3   Preparing the therapy group: selecting and preparing clients

For the therapy group on paper to become an actual group, the group therapist must still fulfill three necessary organizational conditions:
1. Selecting clients and group composition
2. Prepare the clients
3. Make agreements and establish the group rules

1.   Selecting clients and group composition

For proper selection, the group therapist should answer the following questions in consultation with the potential client:
- Is the therapy group the right answer to the client's request for help or diagnosed problems? Does the potential client fall within the criteria of the target group?
- What is the best composition of the therapy group?
- Is the potential client unsuitable for group therapy?
- Can the group therapist and potential client enter into an agreement?

Group therapy is demand-driven care: *which group fits the client instead of does the client fit the group.* In consultation with the potential participant, the group therapist determines in a targeted interview whether the therapy group matches their help request. Two sources of information are important here: on the one hand, the client's problem, help request, and expectation and, on the other, the diagnostic expertise of the group therapist. The group therapist uncovers the first aspect with an inviting attitude toward the potential member and targeted questions. What is the problem, what do they want to achieve, and what is the desired end result? Afterward, the group therapist assesses the second aspect by testing the collected information against his diagnostic knowledge.

Regarding the composition, the chosen target group with its corresponding help request has already set the group's composition advance. Therefore, when selecting, you first and foremost assess whether the client meets the minimum entry requirements of the group. Does the potential group member has corresponding issues? Does the potential member fall within the chosen age limits (e.g., in the case of an adolescent group)? Does he have the relevant diagnosis (e.g., in a diagnosis-based therapy group)?

When composing a therapy group, the choice between homogeneous or heterogeneous comes into play. In a homogeneous group, the corresponding characteristics of the participants are additional important therapeutic factors, whereas, in a heterogeneous group, these are the differences between the participants. See also what is written about this subject in Section 3.2.

So far, we have talked about inclusion criteria. What do we know about exclusion criteria? Although research results on this matter leave much to be desired, we may conclude that some people are unsuited for group therapy (De Haas and Van Hest, in NVGP, 2019). A very clear exclusion criterion is the potential member's attachment style. Mikulincer (2007) demonstrates in a study on the relationship between cohesion and attachment that avoidant-attached clients are so afraid of proximity to others that they are highly likely to drop out of group therapy. They are better off not being included, not only because they will not benefit but also because their fear could significantly inhibit the process in the whole therapy group.

When it comes to intensive interactional group psychotherapy, it is better to exclude these clients: clients with severe comorbid somatic (brain injury) or psychiatric problems like hypochondria, paranoia, psychopathy, psychosis, and participation under the influence of substances (De Haas and Van Hest, in NVGP, 2019; Yalom and Leszcz, 2020). Group therapy is less appropriate for a client with very complex and multiple problems because the group can offer too little recognition and effectiveness. Individual therapy is then preferable (Berk, 2005).

How can we describe the selection procedure? The selection task may seem to be a one-sided activity on the part of the group therapist, but this is certainly not the case. It always involves 'Shared Decision Making' (Elwyn et al., 2012). Of course, the group therapist is and remains responsible for the design, composition, and implementation of the group, but during the selection interviews and the group therapy itself, commitment from the client is imperative. That is why it is so important to inform the potential participant during the selection interviews about what is expected of him in the therapy group in terms of his own contribution, self-efficacy, and commitment to the group rules and to ask him if he is willing to commit. The selection thus involves both parties.

It is best to consider the selection interview an orientation meeting between a client and a provider. After mutually informing and gauging each other, both parties form their opinions about the usefulness of participation and the associated cooperation. If the parties decide to cooperate, they have entered into an agreement with each other. In case of slight doubt about the expected result, the group therapist and the client can agree on a limited trial period with a predetermined evaluation moment.

Sometimes a referrer conducts (part of) these interviews. In this case, it would be preferable that they be well informed about the availability and working methods of the various therapy groups. The group therapist should conduct the selection interviews, especially the contract interview (Kauff, 2015), as these interviews form the basis for establishing a working relationship between the client and group therapist (De Haas and Van Hest in NVGP, 2019). An additional advantage is that the group therapist can best assess whether the new client will fit in well with the other members. Because a selection procedure serves multiple purposes, it usually involves more interviews. Many group therapists assume at least three sessions (Sanders, 2010).

2.   Preparing the clients

The selection interviews also work as preparation interviews, but that is not enough. When client and group therapist have made an agreement on participation, a special preparatory meeting is necessary. All the relevant information about the group therapy, like the goals, the method, and what tasks are expected of the new member are explained. Special attention is given to the fear of groups and therapy groups, which often is a preoccupation of the new member.

Fear of participating in the group
It is normal for the prospective group member to experience anxiety about participating in a therapy group (Shay, 2021). The first concern that occupies every new group member beforehand (as well as during the beginning phase of a group) is whether the group and group members will accept him. As I illustrated in Chapter 1, the fear of not belonging or being excluded is so fundamental

that people always want to avoid it. Logically, this fear surfaces when starting in a group with strangers. The group therapist must explain to the prospective member that therapy groups can be very safe and that acceptance and cohesion always have the highest priority in group therapy. 'Will there be enough space and attention for me?' and 'Will I be able to learn something from other group members?' are also common concerns expressed by prospective group members. It is helpful to sympathize with this normal tension. Unrealistic concerns can be dispelled by giving the prospective member matter-of-fact information and clarifying misconceptions about group therapy (Jongerius, 1993). This anxiety often stems from preconceptions about group therapy, such as

- 'Real professional care is given individually; group treatment is second-rate.'
- 'Group therapy is diluted therapy; you only get a part of the attention you need from the expert/group therapist.'
- 'Group members can't help each other; only professionals can.'

These prejudices and misconceptions, not only among clients but often also among referrers, give a false impression about what group therapy has to offer. Therefore, it requires realistic education and explanation to both parties. Group therapy is regularly the first choice in health care practice, and the group approach is in general as effective as individual therapy (Burlingame and Strauss, 2021). Group therapy works differently from individual therapy; it is learning from each other rather than from the group therapist. In practice, group members prove to be excellent at helping each other. They do this not so much by being each other's therapist but instead by being themselves and being honest about their problems, solutions, and feedback to each other. The honest encounter of fellow sufferers and experience experts in the group generates a rich variety of instructive and therapeutic factors, as we learned from Chapter 1.

Information and dropout prevention

The preparation meeting provides an opportunity to gain insight into the prospective participant and the difficulties that one could possibly expect. Suppose there is a lot of anxiety and a high risk of dropping out. In that case, the group therapist can identify in advance a way for the participant to indicate that things are not going well so that the group therapist can offer help on time.

Fear of the group

Omar is a shy 16-year-old boy. He attends a social skills therapy group at the mental health youth center. The group therapist understands that Omar is very reluctant to participate in role-playing because his shyness gets in the way. Omar would like to participate in the skills training under conditions. 'Can I also participate without role-playing?' he asks. 'You can't, Omar,' says the group therapist. 'It is the most important part of the training; you learn the most from that activity. That is why it is a prerequisite that everyone must participate.' The group therapist pauses as he sees Omar pondering. 'That's what I thought,' says Omar. 'Too bad.'

'What can we do to make your participation in the role-play less challenging?' the group therapist asks. Omar frowns thoughtfully and says, 'I don't know.' The group therapist replies, 'You can tell the group beforehand how stressful it is for you, or you can agree with me on a signal for when you wish to stop the role-play.' 'Okay,' Omar says. 'I guess that does make it easier to participate. But I'd like to think about that and come back to you. Is that okay?' 'Of course,' the group therapist says.

3. Making agreements and setting group rules

Agreeing on group rules in advance with each member about the preconditions for the therapy group's progress will prove beneficial. In most groups, this involves the following aspects:

Continuity – The group member must realize that the therapy group cannot function if he is absent too often and must commit to maximum attendance. This includes any vacation arrangements.

Privacy – The group member must adhere to the privacy rule. This means he is prohibited from disclosing anything that could make another group member identifiable. This rule is not necessary for all groups. For example, not all members at a mental health day activity center will consider privacy necessary, but clients at a rehab clinic most assuredly will.

Respect each other as individuals – The group therapist must ensure safety by explaining that every group member will respect each group member's opinions and feelings. That differences of opinion are logical and that any conflicts will always be resolved through discussion. Any physical action toward each other is prohibited.

The group as workplace – In many therapy groups, it is important to agree that the group sessions are the only place for meeting up and not anywhere (both off- and online) outside the group. It is important to explain to participants that this agreement is not so much about a ban but mainly about a safe social contract within the therapy group. It counteracts the negative effect of gossiping about group members in subgroups outside the group. Even though it happens that therapy groups use an app-group in addition to the therapy group, that too cannot be done without safety agreements such as that everyone participate and that real problems not be discussed there but only in the therapy group itself.

'The group as workplace' is also a useful group rule when the therapy group needs adjustment because it is not progressing well. When explaining this group rule, it helps to tell the members that if they feel unhappy about how things are going in the therapy group, you, as a group therapist, expect them to share this with the group so that it can be discussed. This way, members know straight away that talking about the group-self is normal and even necessary in some situations.

Crisis – For some therapy groups, it is important to indicate what members can do in case of a crisis. For example, who can be reached on which phone number and when?

Working undisturbed – 'Cell phones off' is, for example, an important agreement to guarantee undisturbed work. In many therapy groups, 'no eating' and 'no drinking' also fall under this group rule.

What tasks are expected of the group member? – The new group member's expected contribution is discussed during the selection interviews. If these tasks are very specific and an important part of the group therapy, including them in the group rules will be wise.

Duration, frequency, and termination – The number of sessions and frequency, the length of a session, the average duration of the group therapy, and how members can end their treatment (see, for details Chapter 11, 'Termination').

House rules – When the therapy group is part of a clinical or day clinical setting, house rules may be part of the group rules or exist separately from them.

Practical – Group rules should also provide practical information, such as when the group starts, the location, start and end times of the group sessions, the number of sessions and frequency, how to cancel in case of illness, and, if necessary, payment details.

Finally, an important note on this topic. The preparation interviews are about essential problems and hopeful solutions and are therefore not considered superficial conversations. Intensive contact naturally develops between the group therapist and the potential group member. That encounter instantly becomes a test case for cooperation and – if the potential member continues into the therapy group – forms the basis for a good cooperative relationship.

Being able to work undisturbed in an online psychotherapy group
In an online psychotherapy group, two participants find it difficult to work undisturbed. One of them is sitting at her laptop in the kitchen; the other is sitting at his PC in the bedroom. Emma, who's in the kitchen, is regularly disturbed by family members who walk into the view because they need something from the kitchen; Mason, in his bedroom, has a cat on his lap that is snoring loudly. Those involved are unaware of any harm, but it is increasingly disturbing to other participants. Group therapist Romero notices agitation and suspects that it relates to these disturbances. He turns his attention to one of the troubled group members: 'Is something wrong,

Charles? You seem irritated.' Charles: 'Yes, sorry, Emma, I can feel that it irritates me that people keep entering your space all the time, I mean, it's your space, your kitchen, I think, but it seems to be distracting you, and it distracts me too.' Emma: 'Okay, yes, you are right, Charles. It doesn't bother me, but I understand it can be a nuisance to others.' Marisol: 'I also feel it is unacceptable, but because of our privacy, Emma.' Emma: 'Okay, if it's that objectionable, I will look for another space later. That won't be easy; maybe our bedroom . . . but then I also want to say something to Mason. Mason, your cat is on your lap, snoring all the time. That bothers me a lot.' Mason: 'Really, Emma? It's very cozy, and besides, this is a 'relaxed' online group; we don't have to take this so seriously, do we?' After that remark, Mason gets told off by the whole group, saying that it's bad form to drag the group down like this and that others actually want to take the group seriously. In response, Mason relents and promises not to let 'Tiger' spend any more time in his bedroom during the group sessions.

3.4 Organizing a therapy group, step 2: starting the group with the 'pitch'

Once the group therapist has organized the therapy group properly on paper and selected the clients, we can officially get started. Being together as a whole group for the first time in real life is a tense and important moment. It is best to think of the start as part of the organization of the group. Group organization is in fact a 'two-stage rocket.' The concrete therapy group on paper is stage 1, but the organization can only be completed with stage 2, which is a clear and concise summary of the group's essential intention at the start, the end result you want to go to together with the group. I call that the 'pitch.'[5] A pitch follows the same steps as the 'therapy group on paper' but is concrete, encouraging, and guiding at this 'moment supreme' at the start. Such a 'pitch' fits extra well with the start of an online therapy group in which concreteness as well as 'presence' and transparency of the group therapist are so helpful (Weinberg, 2024).

Since the start is such an enormously important and influential moment, there is no harm in explaining to members once again what the common problem and help request is (the target group), what the group therapist hopes to achieve with the group therapy (the essential intention and group goals), what method and techniques will be used by the group therapist, what is expected of the client (the task), and what the group rules are. Especially at that moment, this 'pitch' has some important benefits:

1. Clarity about what is expected of them is what new group members typically need at the tense start. Not turning the task expectation into a puzzle decreases anxiety in the therapy group, and participants' activity gains momentum.

2. Especially at the start, with all the ambivalent feelings associated with it, it is appropriate to provide information about what the therapy group can accomplish. It gives hope for improvement, which can boost members' motivation.
3. Third, this concrete explanation at that specific moment is the perfect opportunity to reaffirm the contract regarding the task and group rules with all clients together (Kauff, 2015).
4. Finally, this starting ritual also has an immediate unifying effect, which is good for initiating group cohesion and therapeutic norms.

Not only is such a pitch necessary at the start of a new therapy group, but it is also very useful at many other times in the group's life, for example, when a new member enters an ongoing therapy group or at a time when the group is about to restart, such as after a long break, or just in between when the group has lost its way. As a group therapist, you can never give direction and explain the intention compellingly too often.

Here is an example of a pitch to a beginning therapy group.

Pitch at the start of a therapy group for seniors who have recently lost a partner

'Welcome, everyone. I met all of you individually in the preliminary process, and now we are together as a group for the first time. Exciting because you don't know each other yet. So, we will begin by introducing ourselves. Who wants to start by saying their name, why they are participating in this group, and what they hope to achieve?'

~after the introduction ~

'It was nice to hear everybody's introductions. Before we really get started, I'd like to take a moment to review the purpose of this therapy group with you, what we hope to accomplish, what is expected of you, and the applicable group rules.

1. You have come to this group because you all suffered a loss, the loss of your partner. This is a profound experience for each of you, resulting in grief, mourning, and loneliness. Some of you have become depressed because of it. *(Embracing the target group)*
2. I sincerely hope that at the end of the group therapy, the grief and mourning will no longer be prominent, that you will be able to deal with it better, and that you will have renewed energy to undertake things in your daily lives. *(The essential intention and group goals)*
3. To realize those goals, we will meet ten times for two hours on Monday mornings, every two weeks. Next to group discussions, we will use a practical method to help you cope better with grief and mourning, and we will help you re-engage in activities. *(The method)*

4. In doing so, we need your active participation. All ten meetings have a topic. You have read about the topics in the leaflet we distributed. Before each session, we ask you to read about certain topics on the internet and watch certain videos that we will discuss during the session. In most sessions we will start with an exercise and, after that, take time for discussion, sharing experiences and offering each other advice and tips. As you all know, the intention is for you to talk about yourself and also to listen and respond to others' contributions. *(The task)*

5. Group therapy does not work without some group rules. Those group rules are primarily designed to create a safe and trusting environment for active participation. Confidentiality is an important ground rule. We agree together that we will never disclose any information about the other members outside the group. Another important group rule is attendance. Because we need each other for group therapy, we agree to attend every session. Finally, we have the 'the group as workplace' rule. This means we agree to only meet up in the group and not anywhere outside of it. And if there is something you feel dissatisfied or unhappy about, the intention is to discuss it here. *(The group rules)*

6. Can you go along with this, and can we agree on this with each other?' *(The contract)*

Notes

1 When repeated, abbreviated as AGPA, 2007.
2 When repeated, abbreviated as NVGP, 2019.
3 Specific, Measurable, Acceptable, Realistic, Time-bound (Wikipedia).
4 Information from fellow group therapists Malou Geenevasen and Anna Bartak.
5 Derived from 'Elevator pitch': Explaining your essential intension within the few minutes of an elevator drive (source: Wikipedia).

Part 2

Influencing the group

Chapter 4

Leading a therapy group

4.1 Introduction

Every group therapist must realize that she is not only a group *therapist* but always a group *leader*. If you work with groups, you must first and foremost understand the art of leading a group. Fortunately, group dynamic theory offers much knowledge on leadership. This chapter mainly deals with the general aspects of group leadership. In the next chapter, 'Steering a therapy group,' we apply that knowledge in practice in an ongoing group therapy session.

The following topics are addressed:
- Leadership and leading groups
- How a group therapist gains influence
- Three basic leadership techniques of the group therapist
- Co-therapy leadership
- The personality of a group therapist

4.2 Leadership and leading groups

Not only does the therapy group has a task, but so does the group therapist herself. The most important task is, of course, that of carrying out the group therapy, with all the attention paid to the execution of the tasks and the use of the group processes. But there are two other important tasks. In the previous chapter we saw how important the task of organizing the therapy group is. And in the course of this book, we will see how important the educating task of the group therapist is, explaining to the group members how group therapy works and what is expected of them. The group therapist performs these tasks thanks to her leadership of the therapy group.

Chemers (2000) defines leadership as 'a process of social influence in which one person is able to enlist the aid and support of others in the accomplishment of a common task.' The essence of leadership is that a group is following the leader, thanks to the interaction (social influence) between leader and group. Group members themselves and the group leader can influence each other in two

DOI: 10.4324/9781003368786-6

ways: by convincing the other (informational social influence), or by approval or rejection of the other's behavior (normative social influence). Because 'social influence' is closely connected to the concept of group norms, I develop this subject in Chapter 9, 'Norms and social influence.'

'Leading and following' is a relational phenomenon that arises spontaneously in the group process. In every group we see, after some time, leaders and followers as emerging roles. We then speak of informal leadership. We are all familiar with informal leadership within our daily lives: in every group − whether it is a group traveling together or a team taking part in a pub quiz − an informal leader emerges after a while who tries to direct, with others (initially) following that person.

Besides informal leadership, there is also formal leadership. Within the typically hierarchically organized health care, we encounter formal leadership roles with titles such as director, socio-therapist, treatment coordinator, team leader, group therapist, manager, mindfulness coach, and so on. Such a formal leadership role comes with a defined authority to influence the group and members, such as giving assignments, coordinating collaboration, and removing members from the group. The group is in principle *obliged* to follow a formal leader. In organizational science, we call this formally defined authority the formal mandate. However, we have an informal mandate arising from the process, which I call the relational mandate (Cauffman, 2003). This involves the influence that the group and members *concede* to the leader, not because it is formally required but because they *want* to follow that person as their leader.

In practice, there is almost always a combination of formal and relational mandate. The benefit of a formal mandate is that it provides clarity about who is officially responsible as a leader. However, a formal leader only has real influence when a combination with the relational mandate exists. This is not something a group therapist simply gets − she must earn it. That brings us to the question of how the group therapist gains her influence − her authority − and which factors contribute to it.

4.3   How a group therapist gains influence

Why can some leaders gain influence with little effort while others struggle to succeed? Several factors are at play. This section discusses the six main factors:
1. The formal leadership role
2. Competence in relationships and group processes
3. Professional expertise
4. Organizational skillfulness
5. The group therapist as model
6. Personal factors

As the leader of a therapy group, you are not required to master all these, but having more than one will be beneficial.

1. The formal leadership role

Every therapy group functions within the context of an organization (forensic psychiatry department, psychogeriatric center, mental health, addiction, youth care, somatic care, etc.). The group therapist is part of that organization, and her group leadership stems from that official position and mandate to influence. This position is always organized as a formal role. Having that clarity about who is responsible as a leader is comforting for all parties: the client and the organization know whom to talk to in case of needs or problems. The group therapist is the group's 'boss.' She organizes the therapy group and is responsible for the outcome, both to the group members and to the organization that created the group. This formal position gives a group therapist authority, for instance when designing the task organization, selecting new members, and running the therapy group. And if the therapy group's progress is in danger of being jeopardized, the group therapist can fall back on her formal leadership role and direct from a position of control and authority. From her formal position, the group therapist monitors the parameters for the safety and functionality of the group. For example, suppose group therapy is not the right solution for a group member's problems. In that case, it is always her responsibility to help that group member leave this group therapy and provide them with a suitable alternative. Or if some group members no longer feel safe, then it is her job to restore safety within the group.

It sometimes happens that a group therapist, that is, out of insecurity, hesitates to use her formal mandate. That truly is a shame. Insecure leadership creates ambiguity around task performance and can awaken undesirable processes. Dominant group members will walk all over a weak leader, creating confusion and provoking negative feelings such as rivalry. Therefore, I advise always: if you hold a formal leadership role, assume it with full conviction and leverage it.

2. Competence in relationships and group processes

In the previous section, I described the relational mandate, meaning the influence bestowed upon the group therapist by the members. How does that work? What makes people in your group want to commit to you, follow you and work with you? One straightforward important factor is kindness. We have all experienced this in everyday life: if a customer service employee does not help you in a friendly way or does not take your problem seriously, you will shop at a different store next time. Cialdini (2014) found that kindness, respect, and acceptance are crucial for customers to remain loyal to a company. Kindness, respect, and acceptance are even more crucial in therapy groups. It directly promotes attachment between all members and so the development of cohesion and safety, all indispensable prerequisites for effective group therapy. If clients feel that they are taken seriously, accepted, and understood, they will quickly develop a positive feeling about the group and the group therapist and will subsequently be eager to participate.

A group therapist also derives relational influence from being 'skillful and competent' in relationships. A group therapist who has knowledge of group dynamics and can methodically utilize group dynamics, and handle relationships and group processes well is one step ahead of a less competent person and will thus gain influence.

3. Professional expertise

Being proficient in the subject matter is the next key influence factor for a leader. According to social identity theory (Turner et al., 1994), each group has a specific identity. Members who are familiar with these typical traits or know much about them automatically gain authority and leadership (Karakowsky and Siegel, 1999, in Nijstad, 2009, 189–190). In a group of friends who regularly watch soccer together, the person who has played soccer at a high level automatically has more authority. It works the same way in health care. The group therapist, as a professional, is usually an expert on the target group. An expert on mood disorders is more easily followed as a group therapist of a therapy group for depression than someone without that knowledge.

4. Organizational skillfulness

The therapy group setting is always more complex than the individual therapy setting. The job of a group therapist in health care involves many organizational responsibilities. Consider a group in which outcomes are evaluated. Organizing a group and monitoring the purposefulness 'along the way' is just as important. Good organizational skills always make a group therapist stronger and more influential.

5. The group therapist as model

'Learning by modeling' is one of the therapeutic factors I described in Chapter 1. This therapeutic factor occurs when a group member copies something from another group member. At that moment, that group member is seen as *example*, as *model*. The group therapist regularly serves as an example to the group in exactly the same way and that is a significant influence factor. For example, if the group therapist often responds openly and honestly to group members, there is a good chance that that behavior will be adopted.

The group therapist is in a position where people look up to her. People hold her behavior in high regard and observe her closely. They identify with her, observe her behavior, and imitate her mannerisms. As a result, group members may start using the same words, mirroring poses, or dressing the same as the therapist. Such learning processes cannot be organized as a task; they occur spontaneously (usually not even consciously) as part of the group process.

It is important that the group therapist realizes that the group members constantly observe and view everything she does – her professional behavior and the personal attitude that resonates therein – as an example. For instance, a group therapist with a personal habit of arriving late for everything and regularly does so to group sessions should not be surprised when group members no longer come on time either.

6. Personal factors

Personality also involves factors that afford a professional influence when leading a group. Research shows that intelligence is a precondition for someone who wants to lead a group (Nijstad, 2009). Being able to think quickly and clearly and combine and act cleverly helps the group therapist with the complexity of organizational tasks involved in working with groups.

Another personal factor that promotes influence as a leader is the ability to 'serve.' A group therapist must be capable of fully committing and, in doing so, sacrificing her personal interests. In prehistoric times, group leaders who exhibited servant leadership were more effective than leaders who primarily utilized ego and power (Van Vught and Wildschut, 2012). A group therapist who needs a lot of affirmation from the group will quickly be perceived by members as narcissistic and thus less likely to be followed. In Section 4.6, 'The personality of a group therapist,' I discuss the personal aspects of group leadership in more detail.

4.4 Three basic leadership techniques of the group therapist

Some of the factors mentioned previously (intelligence, a not-too-narcissistic personality) are given to you as a person, other factors can be learned through practicing specific group dynamics techniques. This section explains what techniques a group therapist can master to gain influence.

In Chapter 1, I wrote that 'learning within a group' happens during member interactions. During those interactions, new information arises that can have therapeutic effects. For example, in a group on self-esteem, a member becomes brave enough to adjust his negative self-worth after really listening to the corrective feedback from the other members and taking it seriously. If the group therapist wants to influence the group, then the interactions between the members are the main leveraging points. She naturally wants to help to make those interactions as fruitful as possible. Because the group therapist is part of the interactional field, she can intervene in group members' interactions and guide them in the desired direction. How does a group therapist do that?

To influence interactions, the group therapist uses three techniques: organizational technique, verbal technique, and relationship (or attitude) technique. Organizational technique concerns properly organizing a therapy group in advance, and monitoring that organization during the course of the therapy group. Once the group has started, the group therapist applies verbal technique and relationship technique. Verbal technique means that a group therapist uses language and words to effectively process and direct all that task and process information that group therapy entails. Relationship or attitude technique aims to support the collaborative relationship. Relationship technique is the nonverbal aspect of the interaction with which the group therapist directs and influences. Organizational, verbal, and relationship (attitude) techniques are three essential influencers, which together form the basic tools of any group therapist. Next, I discuss each of the three techniques individually.

1. Organization technique

A lot of prerequisite work is done before a group actually becomes up and running. In Chapter 3, I pointed out that before we implement a group, we first consider it in thought and then work it out on paper, followed by active preparation and, ultimately, implementation. The better the group organization (the 'design') matches the target group's help requests, the better the group will function. The important aspects we must establish beforehand are the task aspects of the group: target group, goals and working method, member task, member selection, and group composition.

The result is partly predetermined

During an ongoing therapy group, people sometimes forget that the result of a therapy group is largely determined before the group has even started. A group therapist in a poorly run group could, for example, critically ask herself what she is doing incorrectly at that moment, although the shortcoming may not be attributable to her actions now but may have been caused beforehand by, for instance, poor member selection.

We call this essential prerequisite work *organization technique*. The emphasis of the group therapist's organizational activity is on the preliminary phase when she starts designing the group. That said, the group therapist also needs to perform organizational work during an ongoing group. Examples include selecting a new group member for an ongoing group and evaluating and adjusting the group rules, and it is necessary to monitor the task organization during the course of a group therapy and regularly re-explain the task through a 'pitch' (see Chapter 3). This may be necessary, for example, when a new group member joins or when it appears that members do not understand how things work in the group. It may also be necessary to adjust the task organization because the target group has different needs than initially agreed upon. Hence, organization technique forms a continuous essential part of the group therapist's mindset and actions.

Organization technique also directly supports the group therapist's leadership. If she has organized the group clearly and convincingly, there is a good chance that the working method and member task will become normative and embedded in the therapeutic culture. In case the of deviant behavior, the group members will very quickly correct each other, and it will not be necessary for the group therapist to take remedial action. The natural task organization then takes over that part of the group therapist's leadership work.

And when there is a need for the group therapist to correct deviant behavior, a clear task organization is a very strong case to *convince* group members to change their minds and their doing.

Correction by the group thanks to the embedded task organization in the therapeutic culture

In a psychotherapy group for veterans with anxiety and mood complaints, Eric is a new member. In his third session he announces that he is quitting the therapy because he has no more symptoms. The other group members are surprised and ask questions to understand why Eric wants to quit so soon. Sala: 'I don't understand your intention, Eric, do you really think you're there yet? Are there no more questions or problems to sort out?' Eric: 'Definitely, but I think you should stop when your symptoms are over, that's how Gerard (the group therapist) explained it to me . . . but I still have all kinds of questions about myself and, of course, about that confusing military profession of ours . . . only I'm not depressed anymore.' Gordon: 'Aah, dude, that belongs here too, we all struggle with those questions, and they are not separate from our complaints.' Eric: 'That's confusing, can I still stay here Gerard (looks quizzically at the group therapist)?' Gerard: 'I think so Eric, . . . but first of all, how nice that you feel less depressed . . . and indeed this psychotherapy group is not only meant to reduce the complaints but also to see what is underneath those complaints, such as those questions of yours, so be welcome with that.'

The relationship between task structure and process space when organizing a therapy group

As I wrote at the beginning of this book, every group therapist works with two frames of reference: the frame of reference of the group as therapeutic instrument (the theory of group dynamics) and the chosen therapeutic frame of reference: CBT, Psychoeducational, a social skill method, Interpersonal, Psychodynamic, and others. A therapy group works best when these two frames of reference are optimally combined. And that starts with the organization of the therapy group. In Chapter 3, I demonstrated how the method used determines how much task structure and free process space in the working method of that group therapy is appropriate. One group has a working method that involves using the group process a lot, while in another group, the method hardly requires any group process. An interactional psychotherapy group for people with social anxiety will function best with a small task structure, ensuring the maximum opportunity for insightful encounters and confrontation. In contrast, in an educational therapy group for adolescents with ADHD, too much spontaneous group dynamics and interaction is unnecessary and possibly even disruptive to the task.

The images in Figure 4.1 symbolize the organization of two types of therapy groups, each with a different ratio of task structure and space for interaction and group process. The left image represents a group with a small task structure and a lot of space for free group dynamic interaction. The right image shows a group with a large task structure, many protocols, and agreed-upon themes and a small space for spontaneous processes.

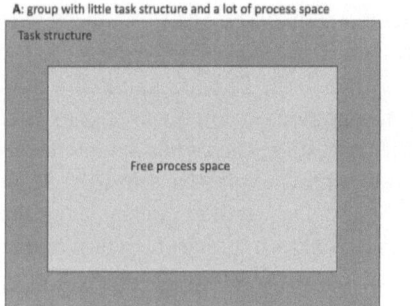
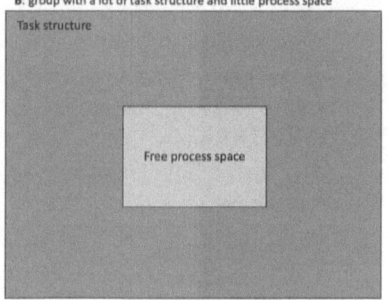

A: group with little task structure and a lot of process space

Task structure

Free process space

B: group with a lot of task structure and little process space

Task structure

Free process space

Figure 4.1 Two groups with a different balance of task structure and free process space. Figure by the author.

The detailed organization of that appropriate ratio occurs in many different ways and is still evolving within group therapy. As yet, there is little evidence as to which combination works best. But some forms are beginning to crystallize.

- Group therapy with a working method incorporating lots of open interactive space that uses the language of the method consistently (i.e., Interpersonal group psychotherapy; Psychodynamic, group psychotherapy).

- Group therapy with a working method incorporating an open interactive space after exercises (occurs, e.g., in CBT group therapy) to broaden and deepen what has been learned.
- Split group therapy: first, half a session protocol-based, followed by half a session free group therapy (regularly occurs with Schema-Focused group therapy).
- A combination of two types of group therapy: first a protocol group therapy and, later on in the same week, an open interactive group therapy or vice versa.

A group with the right degree of structure in its working method

Early in my career as a group therapist in mental health care I was asked to set up an outpatient group for psychiatric patients after their clinical admission. This was novel at the time. The existing outpatient therapy groups focused exclusively on people with mild personality problems; outpatient therapy groups for people with more severe psychiatric problems simply did not exist. This experiment worked out surprisingly well, mainly due to the structure of the working method. This aftercare group became a big success using a simple, clear, and solution-oriented working method and a suitable attitude from my co-therapist and me. The working method entailed that no group member walked out the door without a very concrete, appropriate, and achievable self-conceived assignment and that extra attention was devoted the following week to the successful assignments. Our fitting approach consisted of an active, supportive, and transparent attitude mixed with as much relativity and humor as possible (De Haas, 1987).

2. Verbal technique

Language is one of the influence tools group therapists use the most. Words are basic human properties to express oneself and to connect with other human beings, to communicate.

The power of words, the art of language

Words can have a major impact. Choosing the correct word is often an art form. A correctly chosen word or phrase can make us feel 'understood,' while a different word could evoke fear or cause pain. Words can wield power. For example, they can direct, reflect commands, be an invitation, or limit someone. Words and language are indispensable in the arena of diverse encounters within a therapy group.

Furthermore, language is the instrument for transmitting, receiving, and processing information and indispensable for any group therapy. When performing the group task and the processes arising from it, a lot of information is exchanged between the group therapist and members, and among the group members themselves, which stimulates the natural mechanism of 'the group as information processing system' (see Chapter 1). These information exchanges are essential because they contain the potential new therapeutic information that members in a therapy group profit from. Through their specific meaning and impact, words have an essential function within a group in clarifying the exchanges that take place in the many group interactions.

An insightful group conversation in a psychotherapy group

Daisy tries to explain why she feels so depressed, but because of her insecurity, she talks very softly and in general terms. She possibly does not even understand why she is this depressed. Joshua sympathizes with Daisy and tries to understand what is troubling her. Joshua: 'I don't understand you, Daisy. Are you feeling lonely because you have no friends?' Daisy: 'Sorry, Joshua, I don't really understand it either. All I just know is that I have been feeling incredibly awful lately, and maybe it's because of this group.' Joshua: 'Because of this group? Now I don't understand it at all anymore. I actually believe that you are less lonely here.' Daisy: 'That's true, Joshua, . . . but since I have been feeling better in the group, I feel worse at home. I now realize I have no one in my personal life who really understands me, which makes me very sad' (starts to cry). Group therapist: 'Daisy, it's very brave of you to tell us this. Now we understand why you are feeling so down. And well done, Joshua, for helping Daisy in such a good way.'

This is all the more true for the group therapist who wants to influence interactions professionally. As the leader of a therapy group, she always keeps the therapeutic task of the group in mind. She helps direct verbal interaction between group members accordingly by establishing contact, stimulating, clarifying, or unraveling. Sometimes, she is a listener; at other times, a messenger; and at times a translator or educator. In this respect, words, and the verbal techniques derived from them, are fundamental directive instruments for the group therapist. Further on in this section, I present an overview of specific *verbal techniques* for targeted use by a group therapist.

Sometimes, she will use her verbal interventions to direct task information, for example, by discussing ground rules with the group, explaining an exercise, educating important therapeutic concepts, giving advice, or evaluating a group member's treatment outcome. In other cases, she will deem it necessary to use her verbal interventions to direct attention to the process information. For example, by exploring emotions, highlighting feelings of recognition between group members, or showing understanding for the experiences being shared. To be effective, a verbal intervention hinges on clear language and proper phrasing. An intervention has the most power when it meets a few characteristics, which I list shortly and illustrate with an example.

Table 4.1 Characteristics of an effective verbal intervention.

Language and phrasing	Example
Short	'You said that very clearly, Raymond!'
Concrete	'So, if I understand you correctly, Ali, you greatly appreciate this therapy group because you really feel that you become stronger and more assertive?'
Normal English words	'I understand that not all the words in the information leaflet are clear; feedback means giving us your opinion. And in our group therapy, feedback means that, after a role-play, you tell the players what behavior you noticed and how you experienced it.'
Matching exactly what a group member says	'You don't seem just a little angry, Paul. You are really furious.'
Call group members by name	'Ron, you are experiencing many similarities to Betty. Is that right?'
Group therapist uses herself as a reference point for an intervention	'Do I see well, Carl, that you are uncomfortable being here?'

Verbal interventions can be classified in three ways: according to the direction, form, and content of the interventions.

Distinction 1: The direction of interventions
The form of the interventions may be targeted at a single group member, at the group as a whole, or at an interaction. In therapy groups where the goal is always linked to individual improvement, the group therapist applies many individual interventions. However, group interventions are needed at certain times. This is the case, for example, when the group therapist needs to approach the group as a collective, such as in situations where the whole group is anxious and avoidant or, on the contrary, doing a very good job or when group norms (a typical group-as-a-whole issue) are involved. Often the group therapist can choose which form to use. This distinction is not always as important.

An individually directed intervention is listened to by the whole group. And vice versa, each group member can also experience a group intervention individually. The linguistic phrasing of a group or individual intervention is the same, except that the group therapist refers to the collective in one case and the individual in the other. For example, 'I notice that you are all very hesitant today. Can you tell me why?' or 'I notice, Ron, that you are very hesitant today. Can you tell me why?'

Each group therapist alternates individual, interactional, and group interventions regularly and in a playful manner. Interactional interventions come into play when the group therapist wants to draw attention to or encourage an important interaction. Examples of interactional interventions are *connecting* and *broadening*. An interactional intervention involves a specific technique that we explain in detail in Chapter 7, 'Interaction lines and relationship patterns.'

Distinction 2: Intervention forms
A group therapist can also choose to alternate between the stating and questioning forms of an intervention. The questioning verbal form, especially if accompanied by a questioning attitude, is inviting, disarming, and intriguing. For example, 'Do I feel it right that you have an idea why you feel so sad at the moment?' is more inviting than declarative phrasing: 'I'm sure you have some ideas where the sadness comes from.'

The questioning form is appropriate in situations where group members are invited to expand, deepen, or understand the conversation. A stating verbalization style proves functional when clarity or directness is especially important. For example, if the group therapist needs to constrain an undesirable situation, she will do so in a stating manner: 'Okay, I want to return to your important remark from just now, Mara: why is talking about yourself so difficult?'

Distinction 3: Content of the interventions
Verbal interventions may emphasize precisely the cognitive or highlight the affective. In a group discussion, the group therapist can choose to verbalize the intellectual, the cognitive aspect of the conversation, or just the affective aspect, depending on the situation. It is also possible to include both aspects, of course. For example, 'I don't know if I understand you correctly, John . . . um . . . do you keep doubting yourself, and did I hear you say that it also makes you depressed?'

Table 4.2 is an overview of verbal techniques that can be applied in therapy groups. Besides the name of the verbal technique (first column), I also listed the related behavior (second column). In the third column, I illustrate each verbal technique with an intervention example.

Table 4.2 Verbal techniques in group therapy. Table by author.

Overview of verbal techniques

Verbal technique	Verbal behavior	Example
Giving space (inviting) with silence	Leaning back, remaining silent, and looking around in a friendly manner	
Mirroring	Giving back exactly the content and/or feeling of what someone says or shows	'Do I understand that this topic doesn't interest you that much, Cecile?'
Connecting	Mirroring A's (hidden) message to B	'Anne? Are you telling Richard that – despite your disagreement – you still like him?'
Questioning	Using a question to extract information	'What do you mean by that, Donald?' 'Then how did that come about?' 'Suppose you could feel your anger – how would that be like in this group?'
Broadening	Ask about or note that other group members recognize similarities	'I remember last time more people in the group mentioned something similar.'
De-isolate	Ask whether someone recognizes a 'solo experience' or characteristic of a (solo) group member	'Does anyone else recognize that feeling of total loneliness that Jasmin is telling us about?'
Advise	Giving advice in a prescriptive or questioning manner	'In that case, I advise you not to think about it too long but just do it' 'How would you feel about asking Al yourself, Christa?'
Exploring (deepening, searching to sort out analyzing)	Ask or invite members to think about feelings, links, ideas, fantasies, and meanings based on what someone says	'What are your thoughts about the source of that nasty feeling that Peter has?'
Reward	Praising or allowing a group member to praise himself or others	'It seems to me you are quite proud of that achievement, Marian.'

(Continued)

Table 4.2 (Continued)

Overview of verbal techniques

Verbal technique	Verbal behavior	Example
Ignore	Not giving the group or a group member any attention by focusing on something or someone else	'And how did you experience that, Mandy?' (ignoring the other)
Structure	Create order with words/language	'It seems like a good idea to mention the group rules again.' 'Shall we discuss your point first, Omar, and then yours, Casper?'
Limit/inhibit	Set a limit with words/language	'We don't eat or drink here, Donald!'
Convince	Use arguments to try to change the thoughts or opinion of the group or group members	'I don't quite agree with you and would like to explain why.'
Challenge	Help test an assertion made by a group member against their own experience or that of others in the group	'Ask the others how they view you, Janet.'
Confront	Confront with or test against avoidant or contradictory statements, experiences, and behavior	'Are you also aware that all of you not just once but regularly show up late?'
Explain	Provide ample information on relevant topics	'That is exactly what is meant with group task in this case, namely, . . .'
Making connections	Present a possible clarifying link between visions, thoughts or feelings	'Those two things are very similar, don't you think?'
Attribute meaning	Establish a substantive link, give an interpretation, or attribute meaning to behaviors or experiences	'That's your perfectionism acting up again, Chris! And it's all related to those feelings of inferiority that you suppress with it.'

3. *Relationship or attitude technique (nonverbal)*

Leadership is also something you do with your attitude. Although words are important, they do not suffice on their own as leadership tool. The words of the group therapist only affect the members when there is a good working relationship (alliance) between them. Cooperation and trust are preconditions for influencing. Only such a secure relation will enable a group member to accept challenging (new) verbal information. The group therapist creates such a cooperative relationship using what I call the *relationship technique* or *attitude technique*.

Nonverbal interaction

When we interact, we don't just interact verbally. The way we convey something when interacting also exerts a big influence. That nonverbal part of our interaction is conveyed by our tone (the sound of our voice) and our posture, that is, what our body expresses. Everyone has at one time or another experienced just how much a message can be influenced by tone and posture. Someone might say something in a haughty tone, making us feel small and defensive. But the same message said by someone else in a friendly tone and with an inviting attitude will make us open up instead.

Setting the right tone with a tactful attitude is an art practiced by negotiators and diplomats. Evidently, attitude is a powerful tool when wanting someone to do something. Mastering this art gives the group therapist a powerful influencing tool. It directly affects the interaction and relationships within the group.

The essence of the relationship technique is that the group therapist plays with her interaction position in order to create and keep an optimal cooperative relationship and thus keep its influence. She ensures that the 'line' does not break, that the relationship with the group and the group members is maintained, and that the risk of a relationship rupture is minimal. She does this primarily through behavior, attitude, and tone, that is, through nonverbal interaction. This stems from what I presented in Chapter 2 about interaction in the Interpersonal Circle. I explained that it is mainly the nonverbal part of the interaction that determines the relationship between group members and the group therapist. For example, a more helping attitude is necessary when the level of anxiety in the therapy group is high, while a confrontational attitude creates the best relationship to influence the avoidance of group members. The varying group situations constantly require adjustment of that attitude. The group therapist provides *situational* leadership with her attitude (Hersey, 2007), and the relationship technique is the tool she uses for that process.

The relationship technique consists of two components. First, it consists of *sensing the attitudes of the group members*. And second, it consists of being able to easily vary her own attitude in a flexible manner. When using the relationship technique, the group leader fully applies the laws of the Interpersonal Circle model. Table 4.3 contains a quick recap.

Table 4.3 Interaction laws of the Interpersonal Circle.

Interpersonal Circle and the interactional laws

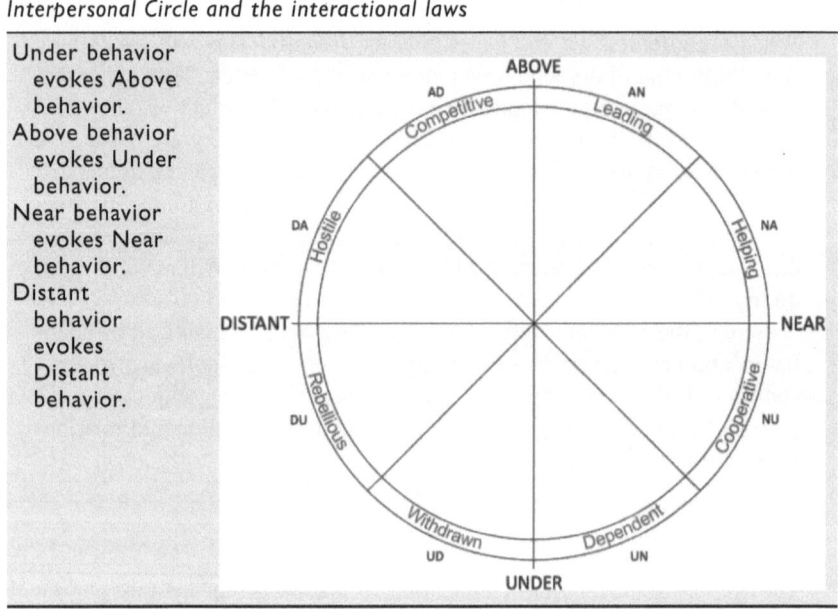

Under behavior evokes Above behavior.
Above behavior evokes Under behavior.
Near behavior evokes Near behavior.
Distant behavior evokes Distant behavior.

In the beginning, for example, group members expect a lot from the group therapist as their formal leader. Above behavior (LEADING) will then promote cooperation the most. The same is true in a crisis situation. Even then, members expect clear and decisive leadership (LEADING) from the group therapist to control the situation and curb anxiety and insecurity within the group. In many situations, Near behavior (HELPING or COOPERATIVE) by the group therapist will align best with group members: after all, a therapy group is meant to help those with problems.

But one can imagine several situations where a very different attitude may be required to achieve cooperation and influence. A strongly avoidant group may need directive confrontation (LEADING/COMPETITIVE) to maintain cooperation. And the group therapist can easily let a very independent group run its course. In such a case, a very accommodating attitude (COOPERATIVE) on the part of the group therapist will be most appropriate.

Situational leadership

Leadership used to equal directive behavior. Behavioral scientist and entrepreneur Hersey (2007) figured out that a situation sometimes requires different behavior from the leader than the traditional hierarchical approach. For example, a coaching style works more effectively with an autonomous team of professionals than a directive one. In organizational science, this is called situational leadership.

Also the group therapist must have a broader repertoire than just a directive attitude. As the IPC shows, there are more ways in which the group therapist can be influential. In a given situation, each behavioral variant can be the best-suited leadership attitude, from very directive to very expectant, from confrontational to very supportive.

Creating and maintaining the right collaborative relationship is continually at play, so relationship technique is always 'switched on.' This leadership technique is therefore one of the most powerful tools available to a group therapist. It is particularly useful in situations where the group or a group member has become fixated in a behavioral position. A fixated position causes a group or group member to get 'locked up,' which always harms the cooperative relationship. This is when the group therapist *strategically* applies the laws of IPC to restore the cooperative relationship. Once she has figured out a group member's undesirable behavioral position, she can discourage this behavior by deliberately avoiding *confirmatory* responses to that group member. Instead, the group therapist may engage in behaviors that evoke other, more desirable behaviors. The group or group member will then feel enticed or forced to let go of the position and change their behavior. We call this conscious predetermination of the position of influence *strategic* leadership. For example, in a group with a predominantly combative (HOSTILE) culture, we may strategically choose to approach the group with a friendly Near attitude (COOPERATIVE). This disarming attitude makes fighting more difficult and forces the group to cooperate. And if a group member reacts in a very passive and dependent (Under) manner, the group therapist can strategically approach that group member from an Under position (DEPENDANT), forcing that person into more Above behavior and thus less dependent behavior. Here are some examples of strategic leadership.

Under behavior evokes Above behavior
A passive culture has manifested in a therapy group for people with Somatic Symptom Disorder. Most group members are very dependent on the therapist and do not speak during the meetings. The group therapist cannot resist the group's strong plea and subsequently has to work really hard. But that only increases the passivity. After consulting with a colleague, she decides to take more of a back seat during the next session. When asked for explanations, she acts somewhat dependent on the group. 'I can't tell you off the top of my head,' she says in a hesitant tone. As time passes, a bit of unrest develops within the group, and group members start to get more actively involved in the process.

Near behavior evokes Near behavior
An anxious adolescent showers a group therapist with criticism (Distant). Instead of applying an evoked defense and counterattack response, the group therapist deliberately chooses to contact the group member in an understanding and cooperative manner (Near), thus reducing rather than increasing the tension. In a humble, friendly tone: 'Richard, I feel that you absolutely disagree with my approach, and that's ok, but I still don't quite understand why? Can you explain to me what it is that bothers you so much?'

Under behavior evokes Above behavior
Chantal has a dependent and helpless attitude and does nothing but complain. If the group therapist does not want to confirm this behavior, she can approach her from an Under position (DEPENDENT) to try to get her out of the victim position. The group therapist can say, for example: 'That's terrible, Chantal. I want to help you (a bit in a helpless tone), but I don't know what advice to give you anymore (sighing). How are you supposed to move forward? If only I knew (sighing again) . . . ' Chantal: 'Well, today is going better than yesterday, mind you.'

Above behavior evokes Under behavior
In a group therapy, group member Wynton tends to take over the group therapist's role. The group therapist initially allows this, but he intervenes when Wynton goes too far. Group therapist (straightens up in his chair):

'Wait a minute, Wynton, you're taking over my role now, and I don't want that, . . . okay?' Wynton: 'Well, fine, . . . as you wish, but . . .' Group therapist: 'Good, then I'll move on. I want to look further at your story Pamela and the negative convictions you mentioned.'

4.5   Co-therapy leadership

Introduction

Leadership of therapy groups is also done by two therapists together. In the USA, this so-called co-therapy is rare, but in the Netherlands, for example, it is almost standard. Too little research is known to determine which variant produces better results (Huffstadt and Remijsen, in NVGP, 2019). Despite the fact that co-therapy is common in the Netherlands, there are clear proponents and opponents based on practice-based experiences and arguments. A fervent opponent is Jongerius (1993). He has a point when he says that a therapy group is complicated enough as it is. Jongerius believes that group members do not benefit from a duplication of all interactions, with the added risk that the two group therapists each steer the group in a different direction because they do not share the same vision.

Also from an organizational point of view, double leadership in a therapy group is not very obvious. Two captains on one ship, that calls for disagreement. The two biggest risks of co-therapy lie in the two therapists' different views on the group task and in the personal rivalry that easily arises. If differences in vision and personal rivalry (which often go together) predominate, the group will certainly suffer. Plus, it's more expensive.

In addition to disadvantages, co-therapy also has obvious advantages. Take, for example, the continuity of the therapy group. If the group therapist is absent, the group will come to a standstill with a single group therapist, while with double leadership they can continue as usual. An important argument in favor of co-therapy is the complexity of a therapy group. With eight individual participants with their own goals, their mutual interactions, and spontaneous processes, an extra pair of eyes and ears comes in handy to observe what is happening. The debriefing is also given more depth with two group therapists. Huffstadt and Remijsen (in NVGP, 2019) mention as an advantage the stimulation of the professional development of both group therapists thanks to the reflection on joint leadership.

The most important party, the group members, are often positive about double group therapeutic leadership (Krijnen, 2004). Thanks to two professionals, they benefit from the increasing learning opportunities and often point out the importance of two different interaction styles and transference objects. In Table 4.4 I list the arguments for and against.

Table 4.4 Pros and cons of co-therapeutic leadership.

Pros	Cons
• Continuity. • Two see more than one • Two offer more learning opportunities than one, both for the clients and for the professionals themselves • Not one but two interaction styles for the group members • More transference objects • Deepening possible through the possibility of joint analysis of a meeting	• Chance of disagreement about the task • Chance of personal rivalry • Complexity of the field of interaction increases • More expensive

Co-therapeutic leadership in practice

How can two group therapists build and maintain a good collaborative relationship? Both professional and personal aspects have an influence on this. On a professional level, it is important that the group therapists are familiar with each other's working methods and vision of the group task. Of course, it is important that those visions are not too far apart. The shared vision determines where the group should go. On a professional level, the two group therapists should feel like one leader. If the two group therapists have different views on the direction and approach of the group, sooner or later this will lead to professional friction and rivalry. Think of two group therapists, one with the belief that you should only do group interventions while the colleague is trained in carrying out interactional and individual interventions. By comparison, on a personal level, differences are less onerous and often even welcome. Differences in style or attitude can complement each other to offer a broad repertoire of interventions.

However, dual leadership requires the personal ability to tolerate the other as a leader. Not all group therapists are able to do that. A group therapist who has a dominant interaction style will not easily exhibit the cooperative behavior (COOPERATING) that co-leadership requires alternately. You have to give your 'mate' space to determine the direction on a regular basis. Group therapists with a strong need for affirmation or admiration will also have a hard time with this. They prefer not to share the credits of group therapy leadership. With such co-therapy leaders, rivalry easily arises on a personal basis.

The collaboration is much easier with group therapists who bring a 'together' attitude. Such group therapists enjoy doing a group with a colleague and often prefer co-leadership to working alone. In order to maintain the relationship, it is important that both group therapists are willing to invest in that relationship.

For example, a scheduled regular reflection is a 'must.' That means taking the time to discuss each group meeting and immediately express and investigate any disagreement or resentment. Being able to tolerate and resolve a conflict with each other contributes greatly to a sustainable cooperative relationship. When group therapists work together for a long time, a long-lasting, reliable cooperative relationship can develop that can be very satisfying (Levine, 1979). If the following conditions are met, the risk of dysfunction of the co-leadership will be minimal:

- Both group therapists share the same vision on the group task and working method.
- Both group therapists are not too self-righteous, tolerate another person next to them, or find working with a colleague pleasant.
- After each group meeting, a short joint debriefing takes place in which the collaborative relationship can also be discussed.
- Differences of vision, disagreement, or annoyance are discussed by the group therapists immediately after the group and not in the group session.

Both group therapists are willing to agree on some technical rules for cooperation in intervening. The most important rules follow:

- Sit opposite each other and have regular eye contact.
- Don't intervene too quickly after each other (always let one or two reactions from group members pass before you respond to the same group member).
- Don't focus on the same group member for too long (if one group therapist is busy with a group member, the other looks around, 'monitoring').
- Let your colleague do her thing for a while when she is busy listening and connecting to a group member or the group: the 'tennis doubles tactic' (Remijsen and Huffstadt, in NVGP, 2019).
- When a group member shows or expresses strong negative or positive feelings toward one of the group therapists, the other group therapist takes an active stance to help clarify what is happening in the interaction between this member and the co-group therapist.

4.6   The personality of the group therapist

Much is required of a group therapist. Not only professionally but also personally. A group therapist must be able to oversee a complex group, vary between an active and a wait-and-see attitude, empathize with feelings, and deal with criticism. A group therapist uses herself as an instrument. And not only must that instrument be solid, but it must also be as pure and objective as possible.

Should a group therapy professional then be a superhuman? Thankfully, the answer is no. However, as a group professional, it is important that she be well trained in this profession and has gained insight into herself and her own qualities and pitfalls (Booij, in NVGP, 2019).

This section highlights some personal characteristics that would be useful for a professional person leading therapy groups.

Affinity with groups

If someone wants to work with groups, it helps to have a generally positive attitude toward groups. We learn this positive attitude toward groups by having enough positive experiences with them in our lives and by acquiring objective knowledge about what groups can and cannot do. Those who regularly work with groups in health care often develop this positive attitude through experience. First, because of the good results that group therapy produces on a wide range of problems and complaints (Burlingame and Strauss, 2021). Second, because many group therapists value their profession as they love the typical liveliness of the processes and the interactional microcosm (mini-world) unique to this method of treatment (NVGP, 2019).

Interpersonal skill and self-confidence

It helps if a group therapist can personally relate well to people. This diplomatic quality ranks at the top of the list of useful personal characteristics for a group therapist. After all, relationships and interactions are at the heart of any group therapy.

Therapy groups and their processes are fickle and unpredictable. As a person, a group therapy professional must be self-confident enough to tolerate some uncertainty, ambiguity, and anxiety and have enough flexibility to welcome and handle the typical spontaneous natural twists.

A group therapist is part of the interactional field. She must feel confident in meeting and interacting with group members. She must also be able to accept the fact that group members can see her personal side and deal with that during the interaction.

A group therapist must be able to tolerate and handle group members' feelings. These may be intense negative feelings, such as anger or distrust, or intimate feelings of vulnerability, such as sadness, anxiety, infatuation, or shyness. A group therapist must personally be sufficiently stable and strong. Enough personal self-confidence helps the professional group therapist, not to be too needy for affirmation, to be able to serve, and to be able to tolerate and handle critical comments directed at her. And in turn, she must dare to limit undesirable behavior by correcting the group or member in question.

Self-understanding

A group therapist must be interested in self-reflection and self-insight. She must be able and willing to reflect on and perceive her personal attitude and process characteristics. For example, the interaction position or role that she usually occupies within a group. In Chapter 2, I pointed out that each person has a characteristic attitude with which they initially approach someone. This also applies to each group therapist. It is thus important for a group therapist to know what position she naturally occupies in the Interpersonal Circle. But also how she responds, for example, to a dominant, dependent, or aggressive personality. For this reason, professionals who want to become group therapists should participate in a therapy training group as part of their education (Booij, in NVGP, 2019).

Transparency

A group therapist must be able to dose her personal openness and visibility (transparency). It is pleasing for a group to see that the group therapist emanates a personal style in her behavior. Professional behavior in which a personal style is reflected in addition to humaneness comes across as sincere and therefore trustworthy. Group members then relate more easily and follow the group therapist more readily. That said, a group therapist must often be able to restrain herself personally because too much visibility can hinder her professional task. After all, the point is to allow the group to function as independently as possible, and that intention does not succeed if the group therapist is too personally prominent. Group members then have the tendency to regard her opinion or feelings as too important and become dependent on them.

However, groups and group situations occur where the group therapist being very visible is actually desirable. For example, a group with a high level of anxiety needs a very prominent, supportive group therapist. A group therapist who is highly invisible and reserved in such a group increases the level of anxiety.

In summary, there are two ground rules when it comes to the group therapist's transparency. First, it is important that she is able to vary the degree of her openness as needed by the (target) group. Second, it is important that the group therapist realizes that her openness must always revolve around functionality for the group. She will regularly have to weigh up whether or not revealing her own opinion or feelings is useful. She will often have to reserve her true personal openness for interaction with colleagues or her private life (for more on transparency, see Chapter 12 on depth processes).

Chapter 5

Steering a therapy group

5.1 Introduction

In the previous chapter, I outlined the general knowledge and techniques available for a group therapist to lead a therapy group. This chapter is about how the group therapist can then influence an ongoing therapy group in practice. I explain that adaptive, flexible, and situational leadership is required in practice, and in addition, how crucial the *following* attitude is. That flexible leadership is what I call *steering* the therapy group.

The following topics are addressed:
- Task and process as leverage points for influencing
- The proper relationship between task and process: *the workgroup*
- Steering a therapy group

5.2 Two leverage points for influencing an ongoing therapy group: task and process

Before the therapy group starts, the group therapist only has to deal with the organization of the group task. Once the group is running, the process becomes a part of it, and he must monitor and influence the group task and process simultaneously. Task and process then intermingle and must be steered in combination. Nevertheless, being mindful of the distinction between the task and process during an ongoing therapy group is beneficial. In doing so, the group therapist gains influencing power. He does not have to influence the group as one complex thing but has two distinct leverage points which he can use. Because the task and process are so different in nature, the group therapist influences each of them in a different way. Shortly I explain these two ways of influencing.

The group task as leverage point: the concrete design

In Chapter 3, I explained that the task is the 'makeable' part of a therapy group. The clearer the group therapist defines its organization, the better. If he succeeds in doing that, it is essential also to maintain that clarity once the group is up and

DOI: 10.4324/9781003368786-7

running. After all, the group task is what it is all about; it contains the reason the therapy group is organized for. With a clear group task, the group therapist has an important leverage point to get the group moving in the right direction.

As the group task involves the actual business side of the therapy group, that encouragement will often be done in a factual, businesslike manner. Hence, the group goals often need to be re-explained (especially in the early days), working methods must be clarified again, and the members must be given instructions about their exact tasks. Sometimes during the course of a group, the task must be adjusted. These are all actions in which factual information must be exchanged.

But what about the group members? Don't they participate when it comes to directing the task? Most definitely. During an ongoing therapy group, the group therapist shares the responsibility of the task with the group as much as possible. Group members should be intensely involved in the task during group meetings. In the previous chapter and Chapter 10, I demonstrate that, in a therapy group that's been running for a while, this co-responsibility of the members arises naturally. The formal group therapist will always acquire fellowship with informal leaders due to their various useful roles within the collaboration.

That said, the group therapist remains the primary when the task is at hand. There are two reasons for this. First of all, as the expert of the therapy group, he remains at an advantage over the group members, even though they may grow in their expertise thanks to their experience. However, members are not expected to have *professional* expertise. Second, the group therapist always remains formally responsible, regardless of the amount of responsibility he shares with group members for task performance. This has consequences for his approach. When promoting the task, he will approach the group predominantly from the expert role and with a directive attitude, often using information-processing verbal techniques such as *explaining*, *questioning*, *convincing*, and *advising*. In short, when the group therapist promotes the task, he usually does so in a more or less directive manner (LEADING).

The group process as a leverage point: the art of following

Influencing the therapy group through the group process is quite different from the directive way the group therapist influences the group through the task. Group processes are the not-makeable part of the group and, therefore, unpredictable, distinctive, or even erratic. They can contribute a significant positive force but also counteract the task. Given that group processes are always present, it is not a luxury but a necessity that every group therapist be able to handle them in order to limit the negative effect and harness the positive effects. It is not possible to influence the process in a leading way as with the task. You cannot organize (make) or lead group dynamics in advance because they arise spontaneously by definition.

Then how can a group therapist influence the process side? He can influence group processes in a *following* manner by steering them as soon as they become perceptible. In task-oriented interventions, the group therapist often takes the lead as the 'initiator,' but in process-oriented interventions, he must primarily respond in a *following* manner. There are three ways in which a group therapist can direct the group process in a following manner.

The first thing he can do is *foster* spontaneous processes. This is where the paradox I mentioned in Chapter 1 comes into play: a group therapist has more steering influence − or control, if you will − when he lets go of controlling processes than when he tries to control them. Fostering initially entails allowing processes, affording them space, and then making contact with them. This sometimes means the group therapist literally has to sit back, listen curiously, turn on his 'feelings radar,' and respond when he starts to notice the process affecting him personally. After all, you observe processes with your feelings.

Being able to let go and follow is crucial when it comes to steering the process, even if the process is not immediately clear or going in the intended direction, is one of the skills every group therapist needs. If the process really becomes palpable, he can explore it by asking about it and trying to understand it. In doing so, he does not have to know what is going on right away. Then, questions like 'What is happening between you?' or 'It seems like you are not in the mood today, or am I mistaken?' are good openers to further explore and navigate the process.

The art of following, letting go, and giving space to processes is not only intended for the group therapists doing intensive interactive group psychotherapy, wherein the working method already incorporates using a lot of process. Also protocol-working group therapists must take into account regular process moments where a following attitude is required, for example, in the discussion after an exercise or just in between.

Following attitude of the group therapist in a protocol-working therapy group for adolescents with an eating disorder

After an exposure exercise, a lively discussion arises about the inconsistent eating habits of the clients in the family of origin. Because the theme feels relevant, the group therapist decides in a split second to postpone the next exercise until later and to give space for the spontaneously arising experiences and emotions. Strong feelings of incomprehension, anger, and sadness are shared. During the exchange, something special happens. Suddenly, a young woman says to another woman: 'I think we know each other from the past, from school, Chris, aren't you originally from Billings?' Chris: 'Uhh? Yes, I'm from Billings, but . . .' Group therapist: 'Let's reflect on this at the end of the session, and now let's go back to those weird eating habits at home and your anger about them.'

The second way is the exact opposite. If the group processes become too intense, the group therapist must *inhibit* them. That becomes necessary, for example, in a group overruled by anxiety, when there is a lot of arguing, or when things get a little too cozy. The processes then become so dominant that the task is obscured. The group therapist can control the intensity of group dynamics by fostering or inhibiting them. He ensures that there is neither too much nor too little intensity and that the intensity of the group dynamics fits the group goal and the group task.

The third way the group therapist can direct the group process is to make the group dynamics functional by *connecting them to the task*. He can do this by using verbal techniques (especially *connecting*) to direct the processes to the task and connect them to it. Sometimes just naming the process is enough to create a functional connection to the task. By restating important processes, such as feelings, interactions, and experiences, the group therapist emphatically reinserts process information into the group. This important emotional information is then openly available for the members, often encouraging the group to use it functionally. Take, for example, a member of a phobia group who, at an interim evaluation, says he still feels very tense during the sessions. When the group therapist verbalizes that group member's feeling, thereby reflecting it back to the group, there is a good chance that group members will respond. For example, a group member might say: 'How awful. I felt the same way in the beginning, but now I actually feel very safe in this group.' It is also conceivable for a group member to connect this with the task by asking, for example: 'How do you feel about the group? I mean, do you also benefit from this group; is it useful for you?'

Sometimes a situation arises where the group therapist can return the process to the group and also *actively* connect the process to the task. An example follows.

Steering the process (fostering it between the members and connecting it with the task)

In group therapy for people with generalized anxiety disorder, some group members become increasingly insecure because of a new group member who remains silent and quite gruff. When a group member expresses his insecurity once during an exercise evaluation, the group therapist devotes all his attention to this spontaneous interaction (*fostering the process*). He rewards the group member who expressed his feelings and asks the gruff group member to respond. The latter is not surprised and indicates that he is often told that he comes across as gruff and sulky. He then explains that he is afraid of letting people in and that his gruff attitude is his way of keeping people at a distance. The group therapist then rewards this group member for his openness and asks the group to respond (*fostering the process*). Many group members express relief as a result of this clarity and voice their admiration for the two group members' openness toward each other. The group therapist then connects these spontaneous processes to the group task. He extensively questions the two group members about their learning points during this interaction and connects them to their personal goals. Then he asks the other group members what they take away from this incident as a learning point (*connecting the process with the task*).

5.3   The right balance between task structure and free process space: the *workgroup*

(Therapy) groups without process do not exist. No matter how structured the therapeutic method of a therapy group is, there are always group dynamic processes a group therapist has to deal with. To give room to these dynamic processes every therapy group working method needs a certain degree of what I call 'free process space.' This free process space is necessary to give room for the spontaneous process development (cohesion, norms, roles, etc.) and room for the spontaneous interaction, which is an aspect of any working method. How much a group therapist makes use of these group processes, how much free process space the working method occupies, differs per therapy group. In the previous chapter, I described how the organization of each therapy group has its own balance between task structure and free process space as a starting point. That typical mix of task structure and free process space in the working method is an important stabilizing principle for every therapy group, but it is not fixed. It is dynamic and can, therefore, always be adjusted. During an ongoing group, a group therapist has the opportunity to change and reorganize the balance between the task structure and the free process space. For example, he may conclude that a group has too much task structure, causing group members to be inhibited in their spontaneous responses to task performance unnecessarily. During my supervisions, I often see group therapists dealing with the dilemma that the group wants to talk more freely while the protocol dictates the next exercise. He then has the choice of either stopping the spontaneous interaction and moving on to the next exercise or letting go of the task structure in order to allow this moment in the session to flow more freely and spontaneously. Conversely, a group therapist may notice that the therapy group is feeling anxious and vulnerable, with some clients behaving more regressively, with conspicuous passivity and relapse into complaints. In that case more task structure could be good to create more clarity and safety. Varying with structure is an integral part of the organizing technique of the steering group therapist of an ongoing group. I call this technique *structure dosing* to indicate that this is a playful precision tool. A group in which the intensity of the group process is functional will exhibit stability and work well on the task. We call that stage the *workgroup* (Bion, 1961). The group functions as a workgroup when a proper balance between task and process has been established within. The group members work together fruitfully because the degree of group dynamics is balanced: not too much or too little for the task. For example, a therapist of a therapy group for severe traumatized refugees may discover that its proposed open interactional method evokes too much anxiety and notice that the group members dare to contribute something and respond to each other more with the help of more structure.

Based on the target group, we expect a group therapist to know what balance of task-to-group dynamics is suitable for the workgroup. The variable balance between task structure and free process space for spontaneous group dynamics is best represented by Figure 5.1, reproduced from Figure 4.1 in Chapter 4. Here, we review that figure once more.

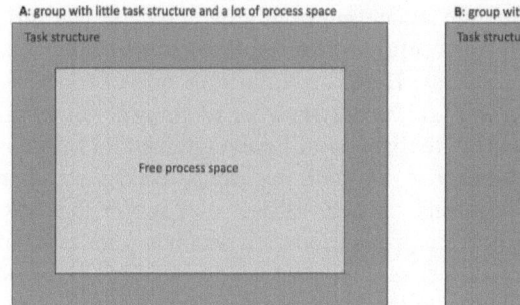 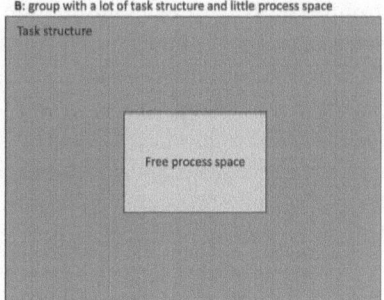

Figure 5.1 Two workgroups with a different balance between task structure and process space (the 'swimming pool'). Figure by the author.

This figure from Chapter 4 is also used as a metaphor, which I call the 'swimming pool.' It can be used for another meaning, namely, the position and steering of the group therapist in relation to the task structure and process space. The pool's edge is the firm task structure provided, and the water inside the pool is where the process occurs – sometimes calmly but sometimes intensely, with big waves or lots of splashing. The group therapist initially observes all this from the pool's edge, with his feet immersed in the water, allowing him to feel the emotional temperature of the process. If necessary, he will jump into the water to help someone who is being pushed under by someone else or to hold and slow down another swimming member. Then he returns to the pool's edge to continue to observe and feel what is happening.

5.4   Steering a therapy group

5.4.1   *The group task comes first; the group process serves the task*

When the group is up and running, the group therapist must influence the task and process combined and make the combination functional. To do this, the group therapist uses the two principles referred to in this chapter. First, he succeeds in influencing the group through both the task and process. Second, he knows how to find the right balance between the two. With the right balance, the group therapist can ensure that the group functions as a workgroup.

Typically, the way it works is that the group therapist directs the balance by fostering the desired side. He may pay attention to the group process when it is functional, for example, when very useful or, on the contrary, hindering processes are at play, or vice versa, emphasizing the task when necessary, when it is functional, when it is at risk of being overshadowed, when the task should be prioritized, or when the actual process is only partially predictable. A therapy group always remains a living organism. The group therapist must have the skill to be able to respond to what is happening within the therapy group with both reason and feeling. Sometimes the group task needs a little more attention; at other times, it is useful to focus on the process. It depends on what the group situation requires. Here, the following rule of thumb is helpful to the therapist: *the group task comes first; the group process serves the task.* The group task is always the focal point for everything that happens within the group. It always comes first; after all, the group task is the reason for the group's existence. The group process follows and serves the task. However, this does not mean that the group process is secondary in terms of importance; the group process is just as important as the task. The *thinking* order is what's important. The group therapist always has the task and the goal in mind in everything he does. The group task acts as a framework that directs the processes.

This does not mean that, in practice, he always pays attention to the task first and then the group dynamics. It may be fine for a group therapist to spend some time dealing only with group dynamics during a group meeting. But this must then always be done in light of the function of the task. Consider a team meeting that a valued colleague attends for the first time after a long period of illness. At such a moment, the team always feels the need to reconnect with, welcome and encourage their reintegrated colleague and restore cohesion. Then, not only is it a good thing, but it is also appropriate to give the process priority for a certain time. With stronger cohesion, this attention to the process will undoubtedly enhance the team's task.

Steering a group is like navigating a sailboat

A well-suited comparison is that of a sailor who wants to go on an extensive trip alone. Of course, such a trip begins with choosing the destination. Then the sailor prepares himself by purchasing good equipment and navigation gear. Once the boat has set sail, something else comes into play – the natural forces at work on the ship – which the sailor wants to take advantage of as much as possible.

He cannot organize these forces, for they are alive and spontaneous. But he will have to do something with them. How does a sailor utilize these natural forces?

Anyone who has ever sailed knows that one rarely reaches the destination if the boat is surrendered to those natural forces. The wind drives the boat in only one direction until it ends up in shallow waters. The destination will not be reached either if the sailor only thinks of his goal without taking into account natural forces. For example, if the goal lies upwind, this sailor will try to sail upwind, obviously to no avail. Thus, a sailor is successful only when he knows where he wants to go and, at the same time, has knowledge of the natural forces and how to use them. That is precisely how influencing and steering a group works. It is knowing where you want to go and using the process dynamics of the group to do so. And because those processes are alive and unpredictable, it cannot be done other than through playful detours and in a spontaneous manner.

In other words, steering a therapy group is a playful art in which, as a group therapist, you flexibly shift your attention between reinforcing the task or confirming important processes, and connecting them. Nevertheless, some situations make it immediately clear when paying attention to the task is appropriate and when paying attention to the process takes priority.

Next, I list three typical group situations where paying attention to the task takes priority and how a group therapist can best do that. Afterward, I do the same with the processes: When is it useful to pay extra attention to processes, and how can you do that?

5.4.2   When is it useful or necessary to pay extra attention to the group task?

Educating and re-explaining the group task when ambiguity arises
In the previous chapter I said that 'organizational technique' is a continuous essential part of the group therapist's mindset and actions. The pitch at the start, about the goals, working method, and task of the therapy group, needs regular 'maintenance.' Group therapy is a complex form of treatment, often not clear for the participating clients. It is not a strange thought that clients have to *learn* to do group therapy. Regularly educating and explaining how group therapy works and what is expected of the participants increases the chances of success. This educating function can be

seen as a part of the group therapist's normal task and role, especially in the beginning period but also often later because of normal confusion or ambiguity. This is especially true for online group therapy in which this ambiguity is always greater. That is why it is good that the group therapist always has the task in mind, and some 'organizational mottos' ready to refresh the target group, the working method or the task. For example, 'Yes indeed, Joyce, reducing the effects of trauma, that's what this group is for.' Or 'Shall I explain again why we work here in an unstructured way, and not in a rotation system?' Or 'That's why, Ray and Christa, it's so helpful to read that information about autism in childhood beforehand.'

Re-explaining the working method and task

In the fifth session of an intensive interactional group psychotherapy for elderly clients with a personality disorder, it is still not clear to every member how it all works. Gene is talking about his sadness because of the breakup with his children. That's why he doesn't see his grandchildren anymore. He doesn't understand what happened that caused everyone to leave him: his wife, his children, and also some friends. The group members sympathize with Gene and try to cheer him up with advice and reassuring comments. It doesn't seem to help Gene very much, as his mood and feelings about himself are getting worse rather than better. He has tears in his eyes. The group therapist David intervenes: 'Who recognizes something in Gene's problem?' Sarah: 'Shouldn't we address and solve Gene's problem first, because he's in bad shape, David?' Group therapist: 'Of course, advice and solutions are sometimes very useful, Sarah, but the power of this group therapy lies mainly in the insight into yourself and how you interact with others.' Sarah: 'I don't get that, David, I thought that group therapy means that you are a bit of a therapist for each other, and help each other with tips and your own experiences.' David: 'Certainly the intention is that you learn from each other, but not so much by being each other's therapist but mainly by being yourself and responding honestly to each other and giving feedback about what you are experiencing with the other person at the moment so that you start to recognize your own patterns in the group.' Rachel: 'For me, it's very clear how things work here, David, and I think I can give Gene some feedback on how he comes across to me.' Group Therapist: 'Okay, Rachel, what do you want to say to Gene?' Rachel: 'I hope you don't find this too annoying Gene, but to me you sometimes seem a bit helpless, I mean I've seen you five times now and I only heard about . . . your weaknesses . . . where's your strength?' After some silence and reflection, Gene responds: 'Of course I've heard that before, my ex often blamed me for it. . . . But I don't understand why that happens, or what I'm doing wrong?' Group therapist: 'Don't try to judge it right away, Gene, it's brave that you recognize your pattern, and for those questions about how that came about, that's what this group therapy is for.'

Rewarding task behavior when the group therapy goes well

The second situation in which it can be fruitful to recall the task is when group members work very well on the group task. It is very stimulating for a therapy group to hear from the group therapist that they are working exactly as intended. It would be a waste if the group therapist let such a situation pass without acknowledging group members and the group. For example, he may turn to the group after a member has learned something important and say, 'What Christine has just experienced is what I told you at the start. That's what this group is all about.'

Acknowledgment of a group member working well on the task

In a group therapy for emotion regulation, Okan did the homework assignment remarkably well and experienced success. He proudly and contentedly tells the group how he was able to contain his anger during an argument with his girlfriend. The group therapist says: 'Okan, you have made it very clear to us that you are really getting the hang of applying the limiting technique. You even managed to control your emotions last week in a tough situation. Fantastic!' Okan looks pleased and somewhat embarrassed by the group therapist's response. The group therapist continues: 'The way Okan managed to control his emotions is what we want to achieve with this therapy for all of you.'

Restoring the task when it threatens to disappear:
the meta-conversation protocol

Sometimes the task is under pressure or even in danger of disappearing. It then becomes vital that the group therapist clarifies and emphasizes the task. He makes it clear in a directive way that the group members will have to take up the task again.

If that does not produce the desired result, the group therapist must apply a more rigorous approach. He must then halt task performance and explore with the group what is going on and the possible underlying cause. That cause may have something to do with the task organization. This is the case when the group and the group therapist have let the task slip. For example, the task may be unclear or too complex. Stagnation could also stem from the group process. For example, a new group member whose behavior evokes fear, conflicts, strong insecurity and anxiety, disruptive bonds, and so on. And of course, the behavior of the group therapist himself, or how he is perceived, can play a role in the stagnation of normal task behavior.

Such an intervention involves a meta-level talk; the group task and the group process temporarily become the main topic. We call this technique the *meta-conversation*. This is an interim evaluation talk − 'helicoptering' − on how the therapy group is functioning to reflect on the collaboration. How long the meta-conversation lasts depends on how complicated the task stagnation is. For example, it may take ten minutes or require several talks.

When the group therapist succeeds in working with the group to resolve the cause of the stagnation, he returns to the regular task. Sometimes with agreed adjustments or with an appointment for an evaluation moment to again reflect on how things are going.

A meta-conversation is always a confrontational intervention that group members sometimes experience as intense. The regular task is halted, so something must be going on. Quite often, group members feel that they might have done something wrong. It is important for the group therapist to correct this immediately by explaining that it is normal for a therapy group to self-examine in this way. The group therapist is clearly the initiator in this exercise; after all, the task, the group's raison d'être, is at stake. This could involve a meta-conversation focused on the therapy group as a whole, but attention may also be directed at an individual member or a couple or to the therapist's own behavior. A meta-conversation may be tough for the group therapist as well; it is daring to confront the group. The group therapist actively leads the group through such a reflective talk. The meta-conversation intervention works best when the group therapist carries it out step by step.

Table 5.1 Meta-conversation protocol for a therapy group.

Step	The interventions of the group therapist
1	Resolutely halt the task; communicate this clearly, pragmatically, and above all, nonjudgmentally.
2	Express concern about a negative aspect of the collaboration or the process.
3	Ask for recognition; make the group the owner of the problem.
4	Look for causes together with the group. Initiate a talk with an inquisitive, not-knowing, and questioning attitude. Take your time, do not jump to conclusions, and avoid solutions until it is clear what is going on.
5	Check when the possible cause becomes more clear.
6	Discuss a possible solution or change if needed.
7	Conclude and return to the actual task.

A step-by-step application of a meta-conversation in a therapy group

A therapy group for training in assertiveness is going well, except at one point. In the sessions, the members participate well in the role plays, give helpful feedback, and are always present. Only when it comes to practicing at home, they don't show up. The group therapist doesn't understand why, and has already explained a few times why 'practicing at home' is so important. The fourth meeting will start shortly, and when the group members have failed to do their homework again, the group therapist decides to have a meta-conversation.

Group therapist: 'Welcome to our fourth session of our assertiveness therapy group.' *After the announcements, the group therapist always starts with the homework.* Group therapist: 'How did the homework assignment go? Last session was about "standing up for your rights," and the homework assignment fit in with that. You would buy something in a store and return it the same day and ask for your money back. I'm very curious to see how that went. Who wants to tell about it?' *A great silence ensues, which May finally breaks.* May: 'I did buy something but didn't return it, because I could use the dog food for my puppy.' Group therapist: 'And how did the others fare?' Another long silence. Gerald: 'Sorry, I just forgot.' Jerry: 'I tried, but just before I entered the store, I turned around and went back.' When questioned further, it turned out that no one had completed the homework assignment. Group therapist: 'Then I suggest postponing today's topic for a while and discussing the homework aspect, because I don't think I understand what's going on. You are doing really very well in the sessions of this assertiveness training, only the homework assignment you can't manage, while that is an important step in this group therapy. I am curious if that is recognizable?' *Various group members nod in agreement.* Group therapist: 'Okay, so you noticed it as well. Does anyone know why this is happening?' George: 'I don't know exactly why, but it just doesn't work.' Group therapist: 'Is it clear George that that homework is important for the result of the group therapy?' George: 'Yes, that's clear to me, it's logical that you have to practice at home, but I find that difficult in one way or another.' Janet: *(to the group therapist)* 'I think the exercises are often too difficult . . . this one too . . . who is going to deliberately return something and ask for a refund, I just find that weird and therefore very difficult, I am embarrassed for the seller when I am back in the store like this.' *Other group members agree with what Janet says.* Group therapist: 'Okay, so you see the importance of practicing at home, but maybe I'm making the exercises too difficult?' *Various group members nod in agreement.* Group therapist: 'Okay, I am glad you told me, I wasn't aware of it, and of course that's not my intention. How can we make that homework more feasible?' In the conversation that follows, various suggestions are made, such as more concrete preparation during the group sessions, the possibility to carry out some assignments together, and to make the steps a bit smaller and easier. Group therapist: 'What good suggestions, let's try to use them in the homework preparation for the session next week.'

5.4.3   When is it useful or necessary to pay extra attention to the group process?

In Chapter 1, I described the group process as a great asset that every group therapist should cherish. Group processes are essential to group therapy, they can make or break its outcome, and thus, every group therapist must be able to handle them. Not surprisingly, there are ongoing moments in the life of a therapy group when focusing on the process should be paramount.

Exactly how the group therapist does that depends on *what* processes are at play. As I explained in Chapter 3, there are several processes. Here is the overview once again.

Table 5.2 Process structure with elements.

TASK	PROCESS
Task Structure	**Process Structure**
TARGET GROUP A selected group of people with a corresponding help request	**GROUP COHESION** A group's attachment network and its positive perception by the group members
GROUP GOALS and INDIVIDUAL GOALS What group members want to have achieved by the end of the group therapy	**INTERACTION and RELATIONSHIP PATTERNS** Interaction among group members lead to certain relationship patterns
THERAPEUTIC METHOD and WORKING METHOD Therapeutic method and the concrete procedure by which goals are pursued	**DEVELOPMENT STAGES** The group's course of development
THE GROUP MEMBERS' TASK The task actions that all group members are expected to perform	**NORMS and SOCIAL INFLUENCE** The emergence of group norms and a group culture
IMPLEMENTATION Organizing the group implementation, such as composition, duration, frequency, and the setting	**ROLES** The manifestation of roles among different group members
EVALUATION/RESULT How the outcome is evaluated or measured	**TERMINATION PROCESSES** The process of parting and participants detaching
AN APPROPRIATE NAME A clear and logical name	

Over the past 80 years, these processes have been discovered and described through extensive theoretical and experimental research in social psychology and group dynamics (Forsyth, 2017; Nijstad, 2009). It was established that they are universal; in other words, they occur spontaneously in any group regardless of the task. The group process begins with the forming of *cohesion*. The collaboration between group members becomes visible in recognizable *interaction* and *relationship patterns*. The development of the group becomes concrete in *phases*. Over time, the process becomes more regular and reflects a visible structure of *norms* and *roles*. And when the group or a group member stops, it is accompanied by a natural process of *termination* and *detachment*. These are the 'laws' of group dynamics (Dion, 2000; Forsyth, 2017; Nijstad, 2009). Each of these processes is unique in how it works and influences. We want to take advantage of those principles and specific knowledge of each process to help the group therapist understand exactly how to use the processes to steer the group. In Part 3 that follows, we will reflect on each process, and I will explain how the group therapist can use each process to steer the group.

Part 3

Steering and utilizing group processes in group therapy

Introduction

The practical manual

Part 3 deals with the steering and utilizing of group processes in group therapy. Group cohesion, interaction patterns, group development, group norms, roles, and termination processes are discussed sequentially, each topic in its own chapter. First, I describe the specific theory available on the process topic as concretely as possible, and then I translate that theory into practical and applicable knowledge. Each chapter includes a 'Practical Manual.' In it, I demonstrate how to steer and utilize each group process for the task of the therapy group.

The three basic techniques

For each process topic, we see how the group therapist can use the three basic techniques I introduced in Chapter 4 to lead the therapy group: *organization technique* at important organizational moments (at the beginning, for example) and the combination of *verbal techniques* and *relationship* or *attitude techniques* during the course of the group therapy. In each case, I summarize the most important technical actions in a table. In the text, I indicate the different techniques distinctively: the organization technique in plain letters, the verbal technique in *italics*, and the relevant relationship or attitude technique according to the Interpersonal Circle model in SMALL CAPITALS.

DOI: 10.4324/9781003368786-8

Chapter 6

Group cohesion

Attachment forces
in a therapy group

6.1 Introduction

Being able to utilize groups and navigate our way within them are evolutionarily acquired social abilities set in our DNA (Kameda and Tindale, in Schaller, 2006; Flores and Porges, in Marmarosh, 2018). The complex relational network between members that we now call group cohesion is perhaps the most amazing example of this. Cohesion is the most group-like subject that exists within the research domain of groups. Without unifying features – without cohesion – there is no group, just a separate collection of people (Bollen and Hoyle, 1990; Lewin, 1951/1997).

This chapter focuses on the topic of group cohesion and its usefulness within therapy groups.

The following topics are addressed:

- What is group cohesion
- The development of group cohesion
- Negative development of group cohesion
- Perceiving group cohesion
- The essential function of group cohesion for group therapy
- Practical Manual I: fostering group cohesion in a beginning therapy group
- Practical Manual II: utilizing group cohesion in an ongoing therapy group
- Exercises

6.2 What is group cohesion?

What is group cohesion?

Scholars are still debating what group cohesion is exactly, but everyone agrees that group cohesion is a relational phenomenon. Bollen and Hoyle (1990) speak of 'belongingness,' Burlingame et al. (2018) speak of 'relationship structure and relationship quality,' Billow (2003) calls it 'bonding,' Carron et al. (1985) and

DOI: 10.4324/9781003368786-9

Lott and Lott (1965) refer to it as 'sticking-together,' Lawler et al. (2014) calls it 'relational cohesion,' and Leszcz and Malat (2015) 'interpersonal belonging and acceptance.' It is, therefore, remarkable that one of the most important relational theories – Bowlby's attachment theory – has only recently appeared in group cohesion research (Rom and Mikulincer, 2003; Mikulincer and Shaver in Marmarosch, 2018; Bowlby, 1969). Based on a series of experiments, Mikulincer and his research group concluded that attachment theory adds value to understanding and explaining group cohesion. They discovered that just like an individual acts as an 'attachment figure,' so too can a group. When a group is sufficiently cohesive, it acts as a safe partner to connect with. Or, as Bowlby called it, a 'safe haven and secure base,' a place where members feel safe and accepted and have a sense of belonging. This attachment is accompanied by positive feelings, which makes sense as they involve existential human desires. In Chapter 1 I described how group processes cannot be separated from our fundamental desire for belonging and acceptance and our basic fear of being excluded (Baumeister and Leary, 1995; Williams, 2007). It is this relational acceptance and inclusion that members in a cohesive group often experience and express as their first and most important characteristic. They then say things like 'This is a good group because I can be myself here,' or 'I really want to commit to this group,' or 'I can trust everyone in this group, and that is what makes the people nice for me,' or 'I genuinely fit in, and that makes it a nice group.' By group cohesion, we mean the attachment network of a group and the positive perception of it by the members (Bollen and Hoyle, 1990; Rom and Mikulincer, 2003).

Where does the term 'cohesion' come from?

Pioneer Kurt Lewin (1951) was one of the first researchers to mention group cohesion. The emerging science of social psychology in the 1950s mirrored the natural sciences, and scholars liked to use terms from that domain for human behavior. The term 'cohesion' was adopted from physics and chemistry, which denotes bonding between similar molecules (Dion, 2000). This metaphor is apt because substantial binding forces also operate between people. And we also encounter such a comparison in social life. For example, we speak of 'good chemistry' between two people who get along exceptionally well.

How does group cohesion arise?

The emergence of group cohesion is a complex process between the individual members. A newly formed therapy group lacks cohesion. Such a group is a collection of individuals who do not yet know each other and thus have no bond. This situation is uncomfortable for each member. Each individual joins the group with his own desires in order to get something out of it but does not yet know whether he will succeed together with these strangers. This proximity may encourage attachment, but that attachment doesn't happen overnight. It always requires 'attachment labor.' One then has no choice but to investigate first whether those other group members are trustworthy enough to work with (Rom and Mikulincer, 2003).

Group members do this in two ways. First, they look for similarities among each other. Noticing that your neighbor in the therapy group suffers from the same problem as you creates a safe feeling and bonding. When various group members can sense wide familiarity, it provides an important basis for group bonding. The second way is to test the personal trustworthiness. Interpersonal trust is an essential part of the chain of rapprochement and attachment (Mikulincer, 1998; Bowlby, 1988). We see this probing in a beginning group through the elaborate ritual of 'sniffing out' each other. This involves questions and experiences such as 'Can I trust that person?' 'That woman does look sympathetic,' and 'How nice, that guy has the same hobby as me.' Familiarity and predictability are necessary ingredients for trusting one another and the group. If group members manage to experience sufficient interpersonal trust, the light for rapprochement is green. Members then dare to let others in, open up, and create the possibility for mutual acceptance. For the individual, this transformation is always stressful. Personality traits related to attachment history always play a role. Some people are very sociable and not afraid to attach themselves. Others have learned to be cautious around people and keep their distance much longer (Mikulincer et al., 2003). But even for people who are confident and sociable, it can be intimidating to place trust in an unfamiliar group of people and commit to that group. In this process, a gradual shift of attention takes place. This is a delicate process in which the individual member gradually invests his energy less in himself and more and more in the other group members (Lizardo, 2007). This transformation is indispensable for the creation of an effective group. People take an active interest in the other members and the group and engage more and more actively. People start seeing each other as collaborative partners, loyalty to the group develops, and sympathy toward some members arises (Lawler et al., 2002). Over time, this attachment spreads into the whole group, becoming more permanent and committed. And with this attachment network, group cohesion becomes a reality.

How does group cohesion work?

Cohesion always begins with something important that we have in common with our fellow group members that distinguishes us from others (Tajfel, 1971; Turner et al., 1994). For example, a common interest or goal, a shared belief, or a similar feature that makes us feel united and familiar. We saw previously that this similarity provides the safety that members need in order to dare trust each other and become attached.

Similarity and recognition are not the only sources of cohesion. Other features of a group can also promote it. For example, someone may become very attached to their Latin group because they can learn a lot about their biggest hobby: salsa dancing. In such a case, it is more about specific features, such as the group's purpose, that make a group attractive to an individual.

Group cohesion is thus a complex phenomenon with an individual and a collective aspect. Previously, social scientists believed that cohesion stemmed from just one defining factor. But nowadays, they view cohesion as a multidimensional phenomenon (Dion, 2000; Forsyth, 2021). By this, we mean that more factors determine cohesion. There are two main factors:

- Oneness, unity
- Attraction for the individual

Oneness is the attachment power that stems from feelings like 'belongingness,' 'feeling accepted,' 'solidarity,' and 'feeling united as one with each other.' It is the fundamental cohesion, the condition for both group efficacy and safety. It is the typical experience and perception on group level. For example, group members talk about 'the group where they truly belong,' 'the group that feels as one body' (Forsyth, 2021).

Attraction is more individual and specific in nature. It is the attraction that arises from the attractiveness of the group to the individual. This attraction occurs when the individual member is getting what he came for – when the group is able to satisfy specific individual interests or desires. For one member, the group is important because he likes people very much; for another, the group is valuable because it allows him to learn something fundamental. But this is not yet the whole picture. The complexity of group cohesion also extends to the relationships in which it arises. Whereas attachment theory describes attachment within a single relationship, the distinctive feature of group cohesion is that it involves multiple relationship formation; attachment always occurs in multiple relationships simultaneously. We distinguish three relationships in which people experience attachment power:

- Group member–the whole group
- Group member–group member
- Group member–group therapist

Table 6.1 shows us how six types of cohesion arise from the two main factors and the three relationships.

Table 6.1 Six types of cohesion.

The relationships	Type of attachment power	Type of group cohesion	The typical perception of a group member
Group member–the whole group	Attachment power in the group through the acceptance of an individual group member	Acceptance cohesion	'I've never felt more at home than in this group.' 'I feel accepted by you, which makes me feel safe.' 'I really feel like I fit in.'
	Attachment power of task, learning opportunities, and group performance	Task cohesion	'This is a wonderful group because here I can learn what I am looking for, namely, . . .'
	Attachment power of the group due to a solid group struc-ture and group boundary	Holding cohesion	'I feel safe in this group because everyone knows exactly what they must do and what others have to offer.'
	Attachment power of the identity and the typical features of the group	Social cohesion	'I'm proud of our group.'
Group member–group member	Attachment power between group members who like each other; experi-ence amicable feelings	Inter-personal cohesion	'I really like you.' 'I like you, too.'
Group member–group therapist	Attachment power through a shared positive experi-ence of the group therapist	Vertical cohesion	'We are lucky to have such a wonderful group therapist.'

We discuss the types of cohesion next.

1. Acceptance cohesion

Acceptance cohesion is the degree to which the individual group member feels he belongs to – is accepted by – the group, has attached himself to the group and group members, sees himself as a group member, and is loyal to the group. The feeling of being accepted by the other individual members is an important aspect of this. Acceptance cohesion is the most basic type of cohesion.

2. Task cohesion

Task cohesion is the degree of attractiveness of the task and goal of the group for the individual. This concerns the member's motivation to join a group. If the task and possible outcome are very interesting to a group member, it makes the group attractive, and the group member will want to attach himself to it. If the member sees that other group members have the same questions and are also there to find answers, then that will make it even more appealing.

Therefore, a therapy group with a clear task and carefully selected group members will quickly develop (task) cohesion (Podsakoff et al., 1997, cited in Nijstad, 2009, 6). An important aspect in this respect is what I call the 'jointness of the task.' In short, the more a group therapy method demands interactive collaboration (the 'jointness of the task'), the more it is likely that these collaborative relations become affective relations and let (task) cohesion come about (Thye et al., 2014).

3. Holding cohesion

Holding means safety because of a protective environment (Winnicott, 1986). The presence of holding cohesion is very important for group therapy, due to the safety associated with it. That sense of the group as a safe environment arises primarily because of a clear internal and external structure, for example, firm ground rules and boundaries. In Chapter 3, I pointed out the value of a clearly organized task for the group. That concreteness is essential for the execution of the task itself but also acts as a framework for process development. A clearly organized task not only directs the group therapy ('that's where we want to go'), but it also provides protection and footing: holding. The group therapist therefore has an influence on the development of holding cohesion. In a therapy group with holding cohesion, group members experience the group internally as a safe place with a clear group boundary that simultaneously offers protection from the outside world (Bowlby, 1969). The group therapist can also facilitate holding cohesion by thinking carefully about the implementation (the detailed organization of the group), such as the design of the therapy room, the circle of chairs, and so on.

This cohesion also occurs when the therapy group feels safe because the group therapist supports and embraces the whole group, so to speak. This unifying influence of the group therapist can be an important contribution to the holding cohesion. Think of a group therapist who sincerely praises the group after a heavy but productive session: 'It was tough, but you did very well today.' When this form of cohesion is prevalent, members begin to experience the group as a safe, protective circle.

4. Social cohesion

Social cohesion means the attachment associated with the attractiveness of group identity. It is the favorite group an individual likes to identify with because its values and typical characteristics appeal to them. We also call this cohesion *group pride* (Mullen and Copper, 1994).

We often encounter social cohesion in sports, politics, religion, or hobbies. It is the 'us versus them' cohesion of the soccer club, political party, or church, outwardly displayed cohesion associated with competitions with other groups or the emancipation of one's own group from the world around it.

This kind of cohesion usually does not play a significant role in therapy groups, but it is never absent. Social cohesion can also be functional in therapy groups for people with persistent illnesses or disabilities. In such groups, peer support is often an important part of the process. Social cohesion, pride, and standing strong together in corresponding problems are powerful therapeutic tools in those groups.

5. Interpersonal cohesion

Interpersonal cohesion is the degree to which group members individually like each other. It is normal for positive feelings to develop between group members over time (Lawler et al., 2014). This kind of cohesion is good for trust within the therapy group, and it creates solidarity and loyalty, which supports cooperation. However, if this becomes too prevalent, it can have adverse effects, as too much emphasis on friendship and contact will hinder the group task.

Hence, we often see that group agreements are made in therapy groups that discourage encounters outside the group.

6. Vertical cohesion

Vertical cohesion is the communally experienced attachment to the group therapist. This type of cohesion is especially important in the early stages of a group. After all, the group members are not yet attached to each other at that time because they barely know each other. The group therapist is then the most important source of safety. In a beginning group, there is a big need for this. This shared attachment to the group therapist creates a bond, which we call vertical cohesion.

Attachment to the group therapist is related to safety as well as positive feelings toward the group therapist. Vertical cohesion can become very powerful and be accompanied by feelings of admiration (positive transference), especially when the group therapist engages with the group positively and acceptingly. As the group develops, these feelings will decrease to normal proportions, and group members will then perceive the group therapist in a realistic way again. Vertical cohesion is then more or less replaced by horizontal cohesion – the cohesion between group members themselves.

Summary

- Group cohesion is the attachment network in a group and its positive perception by the members.
- Group cohesion is a multidimensional phenomenon: several distinct factors and types of attachment relationships determine cohesion.
- There are six types of cohesion: acceptance cohesion, task cohesion, holding cohesion, social cohesion, interpersonal cohesion, and vertical cohesion.

6.3   The development of group cohesion

The sequence of group cohesion types and formation of the workgroup

Group cohesion is not a stable, static state. Like any process it changes and develops gradually. In a newly established group or one where new members join at intervals, an initial group feeling usually develops fairly quickly. We can sometimes see the distinct moment when people experience and express cohesion for the first time.

> **The onset of cohesion**
>
> At an ongoing therapy group for women who have experienced sexual violence, two new members join simultaneously. In the first session, the group largely ignores the newcomers, but in the second session, they politely ask both members about their motives for joining. Joy opens up about her life immediately and, as a result, is positively rewarded and welcomed. But Brenda is more reserved and says she wants to wait and see how things go first.
>
> In the third and fourth sessions, they leave Brenda alone, but in the fifth session, the others again invite her to talk about why she wanted to join the group. They explain to her that the group is not about sharing the details of unpleasant experiences but mainly about being honest with each other in the present moment. Brenda then explains that she experiences her participation in the group as very stressful and that she always finds groups scary. Her openness about that is welcomed and rewarded, and a sense of relief spreads throughout the group. Everyone feels that Brenda now fits in just like Joy.

This initial cohesion changes and deepens over the course of the development of the group.[1] It starts with vertical cohesion. In the initial 'parallel' phase of a group, the group members do not yet have a bond with each other and seek support from the group therapist. She is then the main source of safety and attachment. If members feel safe with her, they will subsequently turn more toward fellow group members who are still unfamiliar to them. At this point, there is a big need to find safety in each other. In the following 'inclusion' phase, which is characterized by rapprochement and interpersonal 'testing,' cohesion develops in subgroups first. As Thye et al. (2014) discovered, cohesion development always runs bottom up, first in relations, then in subgroups, and at last in the whole group. Getting to know each other and creating safety and acceptance allows acceptance cohesion to grow. Based on that, task cohesion can also develop. Group members now want value for their money and try to form a basis with each other to move forward on the group goal. Task performance involves structure in group goals and the working method, which increases safety. Group members begin to experience a sense of shared safety and cohesion through the holding that the group provides. Over time, once the group has existed for a while, group members begin to get to know each other better on a personal level, and amicable feelings develop between certain group members, which leads to a more increased interpersonal cohesion. In the 'mutuality' phase, group cohesion is a group level structure that becomes more stable over time. If development proceeds normally, group cohesion will reach an optimum state for the relevant group. That stage of the workgroup is when cohesion provides sufficient safety, allowing group members to remain primarily engaged in working on the group task.

The development of cohesion in online group therapy

From the limited research so far, Marmarosh et al. (2024) draws the cautious conclusion that group cohesion in online group therapy is somewhat more difficult to achieve and may lag behind compared to that in face-to-face therapy groups. That's understandable. Previously, we saw that cohesion grows thanks to the cautious exploration and rapprochement that culminates in ever firmer and broader attachment between the group members. And it is precisely this interaction and cautious approach that is more difficult in online group therapy. And subgroup formation, the next intermediate step in the development of group cohesion (Levine, 1979: Lawler et al., 2014), is also more difficult in online group therapy. The participants only have to rely on limited images and sounds of each other in order to develop the needed interpersonal trust. This limited proximity makes attachment more difficult and keeping distance easier. Marmarosh sees an important task for the group therapist to explicitly foster group cohesion in online group therapy. The techniques in the Practice Manual of this chapter fit in perfectly with this.

Summary

- In therapy groups, cohesion increases rapidly in the beginning and then proceeds gradually.
- Cohesion develops in the following order: vertical cohesion, acceptance cohesion, task cohesion, holding cohesion, interpersonal cohesion.
- Each group has its own optimum level of cohesion.
- Cohesion in online group therapy is less obvious and needs some extra work from the group therapist to develop.

6.4   Negative development of group cohesion

Too little group cohesion

Organizational research pointed out that each type of group task comes with its own optimum level of group cohesion (Mullen and Copper, 1994). When we look at group therapy we can recognize that an educational therapy group needs less cohesion than, for example, an intensive interactional psychotherapy group where members encounter each other on a deep personal level.

Experience learns that group cohesion is never self-evident, and sometimes we see that group cohesion remains below the desired optimal level. Instead of a safe atmosphere and connection between the members, anxiety, distance, and isolation are in the foreground. At worst, we see a dramatic absence of cohesion, with destructive processes that make the group therapy task impossible, for example, intense conflict between group members, competing informal leaders, polarizing subgroups, and scapegoating, not to mention difficult characters. Group processes arise in the interaction between the individual participants with their character dynamics, and therapy groups are intended for difficult characters. Think of a group member with strong dominant traits, or a group member with a borderline personality disorder. Negative norms and roles may develop that amplify that decline. Being able to discuss and resolve conflicts can lead to increased cohesion, but there is always the risk that a conflict gets out of hand and becomes destructive. In that case, the forces driving the group apart have won over the cohesive forces (see also the troubleshooting guide).

A lack of group cohesion may be due to the task organization. An unclear task can seriously hinder cohesion development. Members who do not match each other or the group task disrupt the natural growth of cohesion. The selected target group also sometimes brings limited opportunities for cohesion. For example, clients with severe borderline or anxiety disorder do not bond as easily as people with mild neurotic issues.

The duration and rotation of group members are organization factors of great influence in this regard. If the composition of a therapy group changes too quickly, it will hinder cohesion formation. Because the development of group cohesion takes time, it cannot be established when a group is together for too short a time. Then, there are simply too few opportunities for group members to establish interpersonal relationships and bonding. An example of a unit in health care where this situation exists is a psychiatric emergency ward. Such a ward has a very unstable patient group. The arrival of patients is unpredictable because it depends on circumstances outside the group. In addition, it is a very heterogeneous group where careful selection and composition are not possible. As a result, a new group is actually created almost every day. Cohesion formation is practically impossible because the patients do not have the time to meet and bond. Also because the length of stay in a psychiatric emergency ward is unpredictable. Some patients stay for several months, and others leave after one day. Having some form of group therapy in such a ward is possible, but only if the group therapist compensates for the missing group cohesion by providing extra support, attention, and structure.

When it comes to clinical group therapy, it is even more complicated to maintain group cohesion. Clinical or part-time clinical units are complex organizations often designed for clients with severe pathology. Clinical group therapy, such as for addiction treatment, forensic care, or complex mental health patients, for example, works like a pressure cooker. When patients live together for 24 hours in a small, closed group therapy setting, it is always accompanied by intense group dynamics, with an additional risk of negative processes such as splitting and subgroup formation in the patient group as well as parallel in the team group. We sometimes see the emergence of a client group with an us-versus-them (the staff) mentality. The clients do not do what is expected (the task) but rather what is not allowed, such as drug use, sexual relations, and not showing up for therapy. It takes strong and sustained intervention at a ward level to limit and reverse such negative cohesion (Claassen and Leferink op Reinink, in NVGP, 2019).

Too much (of the wrong type of) group cohesion

Too much group cohesion is also possible. We know from Section 6.2 that cohesion begins with similarity. Similarities among group members are the basis for safety and efficacy. Group cohesion can contain too much similarity and develop into intolerant conformism. This is related to group norms. Cohesion is basically content neutral, but it reinforces the norms and opinions present in the group. Sometimes we see a group with strict norms and opinions that are reinforced by increasing cohesion. Rigid equality in thought and action then becomes the norm whereby individual deviations are considered 'wrong.' Imagine a group with a culture where everything must be done very seriously, humor is nonexistent, and members are not allowed to make any mistakes.

Contact between group members can also become too amicable and intense. Interpersonal cohesion prevails to such a degree that a 'sweet' group emerges.

Friendly feelings and contact then becomes the goal and overshadow the group task. Mutual confrontation is out of the question. For example, a therapy group whose members visit each other outside of therapy for socializing purposes has become very 'close,' which means that the task (confronting each other and learning more about oneself) will seriously suffer.

Summary

- Each group has its own optimum of cohesion.
- Cohesion is suboptimal at times, but too much (interpersonal) cohesion is also possible.
- Cohesion reinforces existing (negative or positive) group norms.

6.5   Perceiving group cohesion

In Chapter 3, I described that we perceive task and process via different receivers. The task mainly with our mind, the process – thus also cohesion – mainly with our senses. Group cohesion can be felt, heard, and seen. By listening to how group members talk about the group and picking up nonverbal cues of tone and behavior, we can perceive the degree of cohesion. If group cohesion is strong, group members talk about 'we' and 'our group' more than 'I.' There is a positive closeness with intensive interaction and eye contact between group members. The participants are also physically closer together.

However, if there is little group cohesion, the group members will hardly look at each other, behave in a noticeably more distant manner, and usually do not talk about 'we' and 'us.' The group feels unstable. To summarize, the degree of cohesion we perceive can thus vary. From an undifferentiated clump of group members to a fragmented bunch of loose individuals, with every variant in between.

Below examples of groups with much and little cohesion.

> **The nonverbal characteristics of a therapy group with much cohesion**
> The entire therapy group is already present when the group therapist enters the group room. The lively conversation, with the whole group sitting close together, goes on. After a 'good morning' from the group therapist the group turns to him and asks how he is doing. Group therapist: 'I am okay, thank you, . . . and I am curious what you are talking about, it sounded glad and enthusiastic. . . .' Aisha: 'Yes, we are, I have a new job, and Joa has a new boyfriend, so the group helps us get better, which makes us glad.' Joyful laughter from the others.

The nonverbal characteristics of a therapy group with little cohesion
The group supervisor of a department in youth care complains to his colleagues about one of the resident therapy groups. It is impossible to work with because there is no output. The participants are not working together, and no one addresses anyone else. The group members make no eye contact and stay silent. The tension during moments of silence is palpable.

A second aspect essential in perceiving cohesion is *what* we are looking at. Cohesion is a *collective* phenomenon (Carron et al., 1985). Sometimes group therapists find looking at the group as a *group* difficult. In their perception of group phenomena, they are biased toward the individual. Education and training in our Western culture are steeped in the belief that the individual is primary and independent (Goudsblom, 2000). Thus, our trusted measure of observation is looking at the individual. For a group therapist, it is critical that she not only look from an individual perspective but also learn to look from a *group-as-a-whole* perspective. By this, we mean that she is able to 'fade' the individuals into the background in order to thereby focus on what is happening simultaneously in the whole group, seeing the group as 'gestalt.' This not always easy, especially for novice group therapists, but can certainly be learned, by consciously practicing remote observation with the 'helicopter view.' Our group dynamics concepts are also helpful. Group concepts such as group cohesion, group norms, and group phases offer an interpretation scheme that helps to feel and see group-as-a-whole phenomena.

Summary

- We perceive cohesion with our senses.
- Perceiving cohesion means seeing the *gestalt* of the group.

6.6   The essential function of group cohesion for group therapy

Group cohesion, the individual member, and effective group therapy

The function of group cohesion for group therapy is difficult to overestimate. In this section, I explain the importance of group cohesion as a prerequisite for successful group therapy, and I describe how important group cohesion is as a therapeutic factor in its own right. And that while in the beginning of group therapy, group processes and group cohesion were viewed with doubt. Cohesion is a group phenomenon. Belonging to a group means togetherness and unity and conforming to it. This can clash with the intentions of group therapy, in which the aim is not to heal the group but to let the group members achieve their individual goals. For this reason, one of the first group therapists, Slavson (1964, 51–52), had a critical opinion about group dynamics and group cohesion. The equalizing dynamics of group processes would prevent the actual treatment of the individuals. Nowadays we know, from experience and through research, that successful group therapy is certainly possible and that it can be very effective for all of the participants, ensuring enough attention for individuals and individual differences (Burlingame and Strauss, 2021). How can we explain this? First, the phenomenon of cohesion itself already has a collective and an individual aspect. The task and holding cohesion provide the collective experience of belonging, within which the acceptance cohesion strongly focuses on the inclusion, acceptance, and development of the individual. Additionally, group norms and roles are highly helpful in this issue (Postmes and Jetten, 2006). Norms encompass views, opinions, and values. Thus, you have groups in which opinions emphasize the collective, for example, 'Together we are strong and fight cancer.' In other groups, such as therapy groups, opinions predominate that emphasize the importance and value of the individual. For example, 'Each individual is unique in this group, and that is why we can learn so much from each other.' Roles also help emphasize the individual by allowing each individual to step up to the plate and use their talent for the benefit of the group. I discuss this further in Chapters 9 ('Norms') and 10 ('Roles').

The double conditions of group cohesion for group therapy

Group cohesion is an essential condition for the functioning and survival of any group (Lawler et al., 2014; Rom and Mikulincer, 2003). It is a universal fact that people can work well with each other only after sufficient trust and mutual acceptance are established in the relationships. The same applies vice versa. Lawler et al. (2002) showed that business cooperation relationships always acquire affective characteristics over time. It does not matter whether the collaboration is of a business or friendly nature, whether a member joins voluntarily or on a mandatory basis; when people work together for a longer period, they cannot help but bond with each other personally. This fits well with attachment theory, which shows how proximity is always a stimulus for attachment (Bowlby, 1988; Flores and Porges, in Marmarosh, 2018).

This conditional function of cohesion is especially important for group therapy. The sensitive task of a therapy group, in which participants share extra vulnerable personal matters, requires a high degree of cohesive safety and acceptance. Although obvious, group therapists sometimes forget in the routine how exciting therapy groups are, and that cohesion is anything but self-evident. That is why it is so important to make the conditions for the *emergence* of cohesion optimal.

If we succeed in doing so, we will see this 'miracle,' the core of what this book is all about, namely, *Under favorable conditions, healthy group processes like cohesion develop naturally.* If the therapy group is well organized and led, with a concrete and subsequent task organization, an appropriate selection and composition, sufficient proximity (sufficient meetings with not too much time in between), then cohesion more or less arises automatically. Experienced group therapists know this and, like me, may be surprised again if they experience it. At a certain point, as a member and as a group therapist, you feel that the safe place arises, and you see how members show themselves to be vulnerable, reduce their fear and defenses, tolerate more arousal, make spontaneous contact, and respond honestly to others.

Other group dynamic processes help with this. Clear therapeutic group norms, in addition to the concrete task, give therapeutic direction to these cohesive processes. I will return to the importance of these therapeutic standards in Chapter 7. In conclusion, it is not possible to organize group cohesion, but it is possible to organize the conditions for its emergence.

Group cohesion as therapeutic factor

Traditionally, the group therapy domain has paid much attention to the importance of cohesion for therapeutic outcomes. In a meta-analysis, Burlingame et al. (2018) show a reliable moderate correlation between cohesion and therapy outcome in all types of group therapy. The researchers also looked at the effect of explicitly paying attention to cohesion. They found that in therapy groups where the therapist explicitly promoted interaction and cohesion, the relationship between cohesion and outcome was significantly stronger than in the groups without that specific attention. That makes group cohesion a therapeutic factor in itself, something that was mentioned by group therapy scholars as Yalom and Leszcz (Leszcz and Malat, 2015; Yalom and Leszcz, 2020). They describe how group cohesion is of therapeutic value specially for members with low self-esteem. Their conviction of not being accepted is so strong that they can't believe being accepted. Experiencing the unmistakable acceptance of a cohesive group is for such a client a moment of a corrective therapeutic experience. I elaborate on that in the practice manual of this chapter.

Summary

- In therapy groups, cohesion with a high 'individual content' is important.
- Cohesion in therapy groups is a therapeutic factor in its own right.

6.7   Practical Manual I: fostering group cohesion at the start and during the initial phase of a therapy group

6.7.1   Introduction

In Chapter 5, I explained that we cannot evoke group processes out of thin air, but we can steer them when they occur spontaneously. Likewise, we can steer the cohesion process when it begins to manifest. To do this, we use the three steering techniques: *organization technique, verbal technique,* and *relationship technique*. With a consistent task organization, we can optimize the conditions for the development of cohesion. Once the group is running, we steer cohesion development with a combination of the verbal and relationship techniques.

6.7.2   Fostering group cohesion when organizing the therapy group

In Chapter 3, I demonstrated how a well-organized task provides the necessary clarity that enables good process development and, thus, cohesion. The group therapist does this with organizational techniques. Beforehand, she determines the whole task side, as described in Chapter 3. That means a clear goal and an appropriate method and task. The following four conditions are especially important when it comes to fostering group cohesion:

1. *A clear definition of the target group and an appropriate selection of members:* members with a similar help request will recognize much in each other and will therefore quickly develop cohesion among themselves. Excessive differences in requests for help tend to alienate rather than create a bond.
2. *Influencing the 'jointness of the task':* before, I explained that Thye et al. (2014) found that the more a group therapy method demands interactive collaboration (the 'jointness of the task'), the more it is likely that these collaborative relations become affective relations and let (task) cohesion come about. A group therapist can take a close look at the working method and see if there are possibilities to intensify the interactive collaboration in the group, for example, by replacing certain individual working methods with a more interactive approach.
3. *The group size chosen:* we know that a group that is too large has limited interaction opportunities and thus hinders cohesion formation. The optimal size is determined by the group task.
4. *Duration and stability of the group:* because the development of group cohesion takes time, it cannot be established if a group is together for too short a time. Likewise, if a group changes members too quickly, it will

hinder cohesion formation. In both situations, there is simply too little stability and duration for group members to establish relationships and form attachments.

5. *Clear group rules:* clear group rules positively affect the formation of cohesion. They promote safe boundaries that foster the holding cohesion.

6.7.3   Fostering group cohesion in a beginning therapy group

The initial period of a therapy group – and in an ongoing group, the period after new members have joined the group – is a very suitable time for a group therapist to foster cohesion. At that moment, the group has not yet taken shape and can still be easily influenced. Moreover, group members have a great need for cohesion, for the necessary familiarity and safety to start engaging in the task. It is a prime moment for the group therapist to tap into that natural desire with her influencing skills. That begins at the start of the group.

6.7.3.1   Fostering group cohesion during the first session of a therapy group

The first session of a therapy group is a tense experience for group members. 'What is my impression of the other group members, and what will they think of me, how do I come across? How will I present myself? What is going to happen? What is the purpose? What will the others expect of me? Will I get along with the group therapist?' These are normal thoughts among members of a new group. It is precisely this tension that accentuates the need for cohesion. At the start, group members are mainly looking for similarities between each other. They attach themselves primarily to peers at first. The group therapist facilitates this recognition by regularly applying the *broadening* verbal technique.

Table 6.2 Fostering cohesion during the first session of a therapy group.

Verbal technique The group therapist focuses her attention on the other group members and promotes recognition of what a group member is presenting by *broadening*.	Relationship technique (attitude and tone) As the group therapist *broadens*, she demonstrates an active, accepting, and questioning attitude toward the group (HELPING/ COOPERATING).
Broadening example sentences: 'I wonder if anyone else recognizes that feeling Sandy has.' 'Lily, do you also recognize what Jamar just said?' 'Who else recognizes that?' 'Is Beyonce the only one curious about how things work around here?'	

The group therapist can help initiate group and cohesion formation during the first session by providing sufficient structure and information sharing. Structure and knowledge provide safety during an impalpable initial situation. And information can serve group members well to quickly see who is similar to them and who isn't. The group therapist can structure the first session using several steps.

1. Introduction

After a clear welcome from the group therapist, the first thing that should be addressed is the group members becoming acquainted with each other and the therapist. A comprehensive, serious introduction creates a sound basis for cohesion. Each group member is given the opportunity to introduce themselves, make his or her voice heard.

The question of how much structure the group therapist wants to apply at the introduction is best matched to the working method and group task. A therapy group with a structured task requires a structured introduction, and vice versa. From the first moment of interaction, the group therapist models the interaction. For example, she can provide less structure to a less fragile group by looking around openly each time and waiting to see who will introduce themselves next. With a more vulnerable target group, she can do just the opposite: emphasize a round of introductions by repeatedly looking at the next group member in the circle and inviting him or her by name.

In many therapy groups, an introduction means that all participants say their names, what they do in daily life, whether they have a partner and children, and anything else they might want to share about themselves. And, very importantly, what problems they face and what result they hope to achieve. The latter also sets a tone: 'We are here to work on a personal problem.' Depending on the task content and method of the group, the group therapist may add substantive questions, such as 'What do you expect to get from the group?' and 'What has been your experience so far with . . . (the central topic of the group)?' And if a group member doesn't want to answer or keep something to themselves, the group therapist will of course respect that. The group therapist immediately sets an important tone by clearly accepting each individual. She says, as it were, 'Each individual with their own uniqueness and background is important here.'

Naturally, the group therapist also introduces herself, even if she has met group members individually before. During the introduction, it is fitting and polite that the group therapist, like the group members, share what she thinks is relevant information about herself. In addition, she must introduce herself as a professional, for example, by sharing how long she has worked in the organization, what position she holds, what method and how many years of expertise she has and how effective she knows the group therapy is. This personal and professional information builds trust and makes attachment with the group therapist easier.

After a careful introduction of the group members, we often see the first tentative approaches between them; the personal information immediately provides clarity and recognition that lowers the threshold for rapprochement. These constitute the first step in the formation of cohesion.

2. The pitch: explaining group task and group rules

Because the start is such an enormously important and influential moment, a 'pitch' about what the group therapy is all about is very useful. In Chapter 3, 'Organizing a therapy group,' I wrote how important it is at the start of a therapy group to explain to clients what the corresponding problems are (the target group), what the therapist hopes to achieve with the group (the essential intent and goals of the group), the therapeutic method to be applied, what is expected of the client during the group therapy (the task), and what the group rules are. Not only does it help provide participants with the necessary information about what is expected of them in terms of the task, but due to its structure, it also promotes group cohesion.

3. The ritual start

Once the group has become sufficiently acquainted and everyone has received enough information, moving on to the real work and highlighting that moment is important. The group therapist can use that moment to give the group another cohesive push. This moment seals the cooperation toward a common goal. Like a coach giving his basketball team a pep talk before the game, the group therapist can give the group confidence at this moment by saying, 'I am confident that we will be successful!' or 'I hope for each of you that the group succeeds!' The group therapist can also take an alternative approach: 'We can talk at great length about how the group works, but let's get started and find out,' or 'Shall we get started?' Or 'I'm curious about what's going on right now.' Through this ritual, the group therapist signals a clear transition, on the one hand, but also shows confidence in the group and its successful outcome, on the other. Such a positive and powerful start full of hope and confidence has a very cohesion-fostering effect on group members.

6.7.3.2   Fostering group cohesion in the initial period of a therapy group

Fostering acceptance cohesion

As I explained in the definition of cohesion, 'acceptance attachment' is at its core. Group cohesion arises as a result of mutual acceptance. The initial phase of a group is an appropriate time to actively foster that acceptance. To this end, the group therapist can alternate between two techniques: *inviting with silence* and *mirroring with a questioning attitude*. I discuss both techniques.

1. Inviting with (giving space by) silence　In Chapter 5, I pointed out that *following* is the essence of influencing group processes. A following attitude then has more influence and 'power' than a leading attitude. As a group therapist, we must welcome the process, give it space, and then respond to it appropriately. Following practically means that in that initial phase of the group, the group therapist responds actively only *after* a group member has said or shown something. If the group therapist wants to foster cohesion formation in an incipient group, she should not constantly take the initiative but regularly allow the group to make the first move and patiently wait for that to happen.

This means that a group therapist in a beginning group remains silent at certain moments, giving group members space to provide input. Many beginning group therapists find being silent difficult. They would rather do something because that gives them a sense of control over the still unclear group situation. The danger of intervening too quickly is that the essential following attitude is replaced by a leading attitude. The group therapist then starts pulling the cart alone, making the group passive and preventing it from developing independent cooperation. Any group therapist cannot do without the application of silence. She will therefore have to learn the art of restraint. It will be helpful to realize that by doing *nothing*, she is also doing *something*.

Timing

How long do I stay silent? What can the group members do on their own? When should I intervene? All questions that every group therapist asks themselves regularly. Timing can be learned but not from a book. Timing is learned through experience. It is also a question of which style suits you. Some prefer to wait a little longer, others prefer to intervene a little sooner. Still, there are some general guidelines and rules. Situations in which intervention is always appropriate include the following:

1. If the group task is unclear or in danger of disappearing
2. If the group or a group member has worked very well
3. If the conversation pattern does not develop, a group member keeps repeating himself or herself, or development has clearly stagnated
4. If the tension among group members becomes too great
5. If silence prevails for a very long time

How can a group therapist who is quiet still be stimulating? By inter-preting silence as a *tool*. Applying silence, like the other techniques, is an influencing technique. I have named this the 'verbal' technique: *inviting with (giving space by) silence* (see Chapter 4). The group therapist is quiet, sits back, and observes the group ('monitoring') with a friendly attitude (COOPER-ATING). Her silence offers space and stimulates group members to engage; her friendly, nonverbal attitude acts as a benevolent invitation. With her silence, the group therapist implicitly gives the group members permission to start working independently, demonstrating confidence that the group will achieve results by itself. Over time, if all goes well, group members will begin to fill that space with their own initiative and input. That gives the group therapist the opportunity to apply the second technique, *actively fostering acceptance cohesion*.

2. Fostering acceptance cohesion with mirroring and a questioning attitude   When group members begin to react spontaneously, they will first direct their reactions to the group therapist. She is often the safest beacon in the beginning. The group members attach themselves to her and will start to experience the beginning of group safety through this shared attachment. The group therapist is at the center of that first, vertical, cohesion. It is often thought that she must be especially silent in the beginning to activate interaction among the group members. Silence is indeed a very important stimulus, as we have just learned. But the fact that vertical cohesion is so important in the beginning makes it a good trigger for activity. By being active in the beginning, the group therapist promotes cohesion rather than counteracts it. However, this does depend on *the manner in which* the group therapist is active. If she takes the initiative and interviews each individual group member at length or honors each question with an answer, she overshoots in her leading and active attitude. She then starts dragging the group while the group members sit back and do nothing. This will not promote cohesion among group members. The group therapist is much more effective in that initial phase if she is active in a *following* manner, by mainly responding to group members *after* they offer input. She can flexibly switch her attention from one group member to another each time after they talk about themselves. The group therapist is free to be active in this initial period, as long as she reacts in the following manner. One of the most powerful verbal techniques the group therapist can use in this case is *mirroring*. In Chapter 4, I explained that this technique consists of accurately reflecting what the individual participant has said. In doing so, the group therapist can choose to mirror either the *cognitive* or *emotional* content or both. And when the group member communicates with remarkable nonverbal cues, the group therapist can of course mirror this *behavior*. Very often, mirroring works even more powerfully if the group therapist says the name of the person she is mirroring.

Mirroring and the group as an information-processing system

The verbal technique of mirroring is a real 'power tool' for a group therapist, especially in a beginning group, but also on many occasions in an advanced group, especially combined with a questioning attitude, it not only promotes acceptance cohesion but also the processing of emotional and cognitive information. A group always functions as an information-processing system, and we see this in mirroring. Everything that the group therapist mirrors basically ends up in the middle of the group and serves as meaningful material that arouses attention. When the group is safe, the group members react intuitively to each other, also known as 'resonance' (Berk, 1992). As that material accumulates, group members automatically respond to it. Mirroring thus simultaneously promotes deeper reflection and thinking aloud about what is being said. Mirroring is also a powerful steering tool. In effect, the group therapist determines what she thinks is important to mirror and can thus steer the process.

Verbal techniques (verbal interaction) always involve a certain attitude (non-verbal interaction). Mirroring, especially in a beginning group, has an even greater cohesion-fostering effect if it is done in a *questioning* manner. This means a questioning sentence, in a questioning tone and attitude (COOPERATING). This questioning manner is usually experienced as respectful and also encourages further discussion and reflection. The model function of the group therapist also plays a role. Group members will adopt her listening behavior and attitude, making mutual acceptance palpable. Mirroring with a questioning attitude directly fosters the feeling of acceptance of the individual group member. And because more participants feel this way, this technique creates a generalizing effect, increasing acceptance cohesion throughout the group. Here are some example sentences of mirroring with a questioning attitude.

Example sentences of mirroring
'Do I understand you well, Tevin, that you had fun doing that exercise with Marian?'
'Mary, am I right in saying that you are very angry at me?'
'Daniel, is it true that you don't understand how this group would be helpful in dealing with your depression?'
'You look sad, Lloyd, am I right?'
'Denzel, do I understand correctly that you don't feel safe in this group yet?'

'Laura, did I hear you say that you find John's reaction useful?'
'Vernon, could it be that my explanation relieves you?'
'Do I feel it right that you are all very shocked?'

In a beginning group, the group therapist alternates the 'passive' technique of inviting with silence with the active verbal technique of mirroring in a questioning manner. Together, these techniques have a powerful cohesion-fostering effect, especially acceptance cohesion. In a beginning group, this is very important because attachment through mutual acceptance is a prerequisite for everything else in the group. Table 6.3 summarizes the combination of techniques through which the group therapist fosters acceptance cohesion.

Table 6.3 Fostering acceptance cohesion in a beginning therapy group.

Verbal technique	Relationship technique (attitude and tone)
The group therapist focuses her attention on a group member who presents something and questioningly *mirrors* his or her words as precisely as possible. The group therapist can choose to *mirror* mainly the emotional message, the cognitive message, or both alternately.	As the group therapist mirrors, she demonstrates an active, accepting, and questioning attitude toward the individual (COOPERATING/HELPING).
The group therapist alternates between this technique and allowing moments of silence *(inviting with silence)*.	The best thing for the group therapist to do when she is silent is to 'monitor,' lean back quietly, and look at the group in a friendly manner (COOPERATING).

Mirroring with a questioning attitude and giving space by silence
At the beginning of the second session of social skills therapy group, the group therapist asks the participants what they thought of the first session. A cautious response follows. Walter says that he still feels anxious about being in a group with strangers. Joshua says he is not looking forward to role-playing. The group therapist decides to use this moment for cohesion formation in this still-beginning group. She first mirrors the different feelings before moving on to the task at hand: 'Walter, do I understand correctly that you find it stressful to be here because you don't know the others yet?' Walter: 'Yes, I always have that with strangers. I clam up.' The group therapist: 'Aha . . . And you, Joshua? If I understand correctly, you

are dreading the role-playing? Is that correct?' Joshua: 'Yes, that's right. I'm afraid I might get it wrong.'

At this point, Ashley and Talisa nod in agreement. The group therapist joins that response and expands the conversation to group level. Once that is underway, the group therapist sits back, observing the group to see how the interaction progresses.

Fostering holding cohesion

Holding cohesion arises when, thanks to the concrete task structure and the protective behavior of the group therapist, group members experience the group as a safe place. In an ongoing group, *re-explaining* the group task and the group rules, for example, promotes holding cohesion. She also fosters holding cohesion if she compliments the whole group on the results they achieved from doing the work.

Because the group therapist has to contribute a lot when fostering holding cohesion, she typically uses more active verbal techniques, such as *explaining*, *convincing*, and *questioning*, interspersed with *mirroring* and *connecting*. The *broadening* verbal technique is also often helpful. For example, if a group member is brave enough to verbalize the group tension he is feeling, the group therapist will significantly foster cohesion if she uses a broadening question to invite the others into the conversation, such as 'I'm curious; are more of you experiencing a similar anxious feeling as Jack has about the group?' When fostering holding cohesion, the attitude is also often active: first, LEADING and when the conversation gets going, especially HELPING or COOPERATING. The form here is mainly that of group intervention, that is, directed at the whole group. It helps if the group therapist occasionally makes an embracing gesture with her arms. It is also helpful if the group then sits in the familiar circle setup. If holding cohesion is sufficiently present, group members will often experience the circle as a safe place.

Fostering holding cohesion by re-explaining the group rules

In his private practice, a psychiatrist is starting an educational group therapy for parents of children with a form of autism. He designed the group as carefully as possible and is looking forward to starting. During the first session, two of the eight participants are absent. One is ill, and there has been no communication from the other. When asked, it appears that the other member noted down an incorrect starting date. During the second session, two other participants could not attend because neither could find a babysitter for their children. It was only during the third session that everyone was able to attend.

The psychiatrist, now worried, takes ample time to discuss the importance of attendance with the group. He says with conviction: 'Without attendance, you will never be able to become a safe group, and then the group will not produce results. That seems like a waste of all your efforts.' He continues: 'What do you think about what I just said?' Shandra replies, 'I understand, but some matters are beyond our control, like when a babysitter suddenly calls in sick,' to which Jane replies: 'Well, I would like to say that I'm a bit fed up with how things are going right now. I must take leave to attend this group, so I expect everyone else to attend as well. Everyone knew the rules in advance.' The group therapist immediately responds, 'Thank you, Jane, that was very clear. So what you are saying is 'We agreed to be present. I take that into account, plan around it and rely on everyone else's attendance.' Jane: 'Yes, exactly!'

Fostering task cohesion

Task cohesion can also be a starting point for fostering cohesion in a beginning therapy group. Group members attend to learn or practice something, or to deepen their self-understanding. The task is the functional tool for doing so. A group task in which sufficient interaction is built in (the 'jointness of the task') already provides an important organizational basis for task cohesion.

Very soon after the group has started, group members will become curious and try to determine whether the task is yielding what they were told it would. The group therapist can share in this curiosity not only by re-explaining the task but also, for example, by *mirroring* group members' comments about it and *broadening* the conversation.

Once the group members figure out how to use the group and start cooperating with each other more while working together as a group, task cohesion will grow. The group therapist can contribute to this by using verbal techniques to repeatedly *explain* the task, *connect* group members to the task, *ask questions*, *broaden* the conversation about the task, and *mirror* and *reward* desired task behavior. In terms of relationship technique, the group therapist fosters task cohesion in the beginning the best with a mild leading position, consistent with a HELPING or LEADING attitude. Table 6.4 shows technical steps with which the group therapist fosters task cohesion.

Table 6.4 Fostering task cohesion in a beginning group.

Verbal technique	Relationship technique (attitude and tone)
The group therapist can foster task cohesion in many ways. Central to this is that the group therapist always links the input of group members to the group task. She can, in a questioning or stating manner: *Mirror* a group member's task behavior. Regularly *(re)explain* the task to the group. *Ask* a group member whether the task is clear. *Connect* group members to the task. *Broaden* the discussion about the task. Regularly *reward* task-oriented behavior.	The group therapist adopts an active helping and steering attitude (HELPING/LEADING).

Example sentences:
'Delon, is it true that you don't understand how this group can help you with your PTSD?' (*mirroring*)
'William, will you explain to the group what you have learned today?' (*questioning*)
'Do you know why Aaron and Barbara find the group's methods strange?' (*connecting*)
'Then why do you think you're here, George?' (*confronting*)
'Is Ricardo the only one with questions about today's assignment?' (*broadening*)
'Aha, you get it, Ali! You've figured out how things work around here. Great!' (*rewarding*)

Fostering cohesion anew in case of a changing composition of a therapy group

In Section 6.3 of this chapter, I described that the entry of new participants is also an important time to think about group cohesion. Changes in the composition always have an impact on a therapy group. All process phenomena that had a fixed structure – norms, roles, positions – are now affected. Cohesion will be absent for a short period and must be re-established after the arrival of those new group members. As with an entirely new group, the group therapist is free to lend a hand, first, by again giving a 'pitch' about the group goals and task, that will foster (holding) cohesion. Second, the group therapist can help the remaining old group open up. The remnant of the old group still has a partial cohesive structure but has to let the new members in, usually setting the stage. Sometimes, new group members have to 'wait in the waiting room' for a while; other times, they are hazed to a degree. But the old group cannot avoid letting in the newcomers, not least because after some time, they will begin to carve out their own position in the group. At that moment the group therapist can help the group, with its new composition, feel like a whole again, especially if the new entrant differs in characteristics from the existing group. Diversity can sometimes quickly lead to rejection, something every group therapist wants to avoid. In terms of organization, it is therefore wise to have not one but more newcomers join at the same time, if possible. To foster cohesion in this situation, she uses the techniques described previously (actively fostering acceptance cohesion and holding cohesion).

6.8   Practical Manual II: utilizing group cohesion in an ongoing therapy group

Attention shifts from cohesion formation to the task of the therapy group

In a beginning therapy group, group members are more concerned with each other and making the group safe and cohesive than with the task. Once group cohesiveness is at a working level that is optimal for that therapy group, the focus shifts from cohesiveness to task performance. At that point, we refer to the group as a *workgroup*. The preconditional work for cohesion development has been completed; the group therapist and group can begin to focus more and more on the task execution. Then, they will do three important things: first, utilize group cohesion for the therapeutic task by connecting the two; second, using cohesion as a therapeutic factor; and, third, restore cohesion when it is out of balance.

Utilizing group cohesion for the task of the therapy group

In Chapter 5, I demonstrated that the distinction between task and process orientation disappears at the *workgroup* stage. Everything is then naturally focused on the task, with the process playing a supporting role. When applied to cohesion, this means that the conditional safety and familiarity of attachment have been sufficiently established, whereby the group is free to engage in the task. Utilizing cohesion for the task then occurs naturally.

There are many moments during task performance when cohesion aspects such as a safe atmosphere, 'togetherness,' and a good task cooperation spontaneously arise with the group therapist or group members. If the group therapist intervenes, connecting task and cohesion is then often obvious. The group therapist does this connecting by referring to the task behavior along with the group cohesion behavior during the session and then highlighting the positive link between the two. See the following example.

Connecting group cohesion to the task

During the fourth session of a group therapy for adolescents with gender identity issues, the members suddenly share a lot of personal information. After a group member intensely talks about the lack of understanding about her feeling that she is living in the wrong body, members acknowledge this, followed by many emotional reactions. Feelings of anger and sadness are expressed. The group therapist says: 'Today, the level of safety was remarkable, wasn't it? You were able to share a lot with each other. And that is the intention behind this group.'

Cohesion as a therapeutic factor

Group cohesion as a therapeutic moment of its own is very useful. Cohesion/acceptance is one of the therapeutic factors listed in Chapter 1. The natural mutual acceptance of group cohesion embodies a strong therapeutic potential, especially for members with low self-esteem. Their conviction of not being accepted is so strong that they can't believe being accepted. Experiencing unmistakable acceptance is for such a client a moment of 'healthy confusion.' Yalom and Leszcz (2020) speak of a correctional emotional experience, clear helping new information, which can add to therapeutic growth (see Chapter 1). See the following example.

Table 6.5 Group cohesion as a therapeutic factor.

Verbal technique	Relationship technique (attitude and tone)
The group therapist uses *questioning, mirroring*, and *connecting* to facilitate realistic corrective feedback within the safe cohesive group environment.	For this situation, a HELPING attitude and tone fits best.

Cohesive acceptance as a therapeutic factor in a group therapy

In one of the meetings of an intensive interactional psychotherapy group for personality problems, Alicia angrily lashed out at Kane: 'I am fed up with you Kane, with your so-called jokes, which are no jokes because there is always criticism in it, like you said to Marjorie, '*in this dress you look like you are pregnant, Marjorie.*' That isn't funny at all, it's aggressive! So be honest and say your things open and direct if you don't like someone or something.' The whole group was surprised. Alicia was the most friendly person in the group; no one ever thought of her being angry at all. And, of course, also Alicia herself was surprised, even shocked. She sat in her chair, bent over and with her hands over her face. Alicia: 'I am sorry, Kane, for what I said,

I must have lost my mind . . . I feel so ashamed . . . I am sorry, people. This is not who I am, it won't happen again . . .' Group therapist: 'I see how shocked you are, Alicia, about your spontaneous reaction to Kane, but let's see how the others experience it?' Jasper: 'It is okay, Alicia, I think you show your strength, and that feels good, everyone has angry feelings, that's normal, it makes you more complete.' Charlene: 'I agree completely with what you said to Kane, I think it was strong and not bad at all; you are such a sweet person, Alicia, but maybe too sweet, this makes you more human.' Group therapist: 'How is that for you to hear Alicia?' Alicia: 'It is . . . it's so confusing, I think I am an aggressive monster, but I hear Charlene and Jasper say that it was okay, it makes me so confused, but maybe also there is a relief, a relief that I may stand up for myself.' (crying) Kane: 'Don't apologize to me, Alicia, I am the one who should apologize, because I think you were right with your honest reaction. Maybe strange for you, and even strange for myself, but your reaction was ok for me, even good. It felt like a limit, and safe limits are what I missed my whole life.' Alicia: 'Thank you, Kane . . . I feel confused and relieved.'

Restoring group cohesion

If group cohesion has developed optimally, it will become more solid as the group progresses. But, of course, something could always happen inside or outside the group that upsets the balance. For example, a member with a special role will leave, a group member may find himself in a crisis, group members may discover that they are falling in love with each other, or two group members may openly clash. These developments will reduce group cohesion, rendering the group very unsafe. Or the opposite may happen; the group becomes too comfortable or slips into conformity. The task is normative for appropriate cohesion and has an initial signaling function; it will begin to falter when cohesion is no longer appropriate. Then the group no longer functions as a *workgroup*.

When group cohesion is poor, the group therapist should not delay intervening too long. In most cases, she cannot restore cohesion immediately, simply because the cause of the loss of cohesion is unclear to the group members and group therapist. The group therapist must then apply the meta-conversation protocol (see Chapter 5). That is, temporarily pause the task and verify her impression of the task stagnation with the participants. If they share her concern, she can search for the underlying reason. That reason could be anything (see previously and Section 6.4). If the group therapist and group members succeed in identifying and discussing the cause of the lack of cohesion, the group will have made considerable progress. Sometimes, practical measures are necessary to restore cohesion. Perhaps the group therapist needs to adjust her own attitude, re-explain the group task and working methods very concretely, or even adjust them if necessary. In many cases, such a meta-intervention already has a cohesion-fostering effect, and the group therapist can quickly resume the task. She uses active verbal techniques for such an intervention, like *questioning*, *confronting*, and *exploring*, as well as *mirroring* and *connecting*. And because of the urgency, usually an active, LEADING, and HELPING attitude. Table 6.6 summarizes the technical steps the group therapist can take to restore cohesion.

Table 6.6 Restoring cohesion through meta-conversation.

Verbal technique	Relationship technique (attitude and tone)
The group therapist pauses the group task and uses *questioning, confronting, mirroring*, and *connecting* to try to discover why there is so little cohesion.	The group therapist adopts an active steering attitude. (LEADING/HELPING).

Restoring cohesion through meta-conversation

A therapy group for older people with social anxiety and a risk of growing lonely that, until recently, was running well is now stagnating. The group therapist notices this from the restrained atmosphere. People hardly interact, whereas before, they did. The group also no longer feels safe as a whole. During a session, when another icy silence ensues after Charlie bravely spoke about his fear but also his longing for contact, the group therapist decides to pause the task. 'Thank you, Charlie. You've told something very important. It's a pity you didn't get more reactions. That seems to be the case more often lately. Do you get that impression, too?' Everyone is silent and looks at the group therapist. 'Well,' the group therapist says, 'this is exactly what I mean. I am doing all the work. When we are discussing a topic, there is no response, no conversation, just like now, even though that is the intention. Why is that?' Mark replies: 'The atmosphere hasn't been the same since Lisa left.' 'Since Lisa left?' the group therapist asks. Mark: 'Yes. Lisa was very supportive.' Donna says: 'I think Lisa was like a therapist. She always asked everyone something, which was kind of nice.' Linda adds: 'I find it often difficult how to speak about myself and how to react to others in the group. I'm always afraid of saying something stupid, Lisa helped us with that.'

Group therapist: 'Okay, I am glad you said this about Lisa and her helping role. Do I understand you well that the biggest fear of all of you is that you say something that will be criticized by me or by the others?'

Mark: 'Yes, that's true for me.' Most other group members nod in agreement. Group therapist: 'Is that a real threat, did I or other members react very critically?' Donna: 'No, no one did, but this anxiety is there anyway.' Group therapist: 'Maybe we can trust each other and take a risk of talking about ourselves, and react acknowledging each other, how would that be?' Mark replies: 'I think that's a good idea, and I would actually like to say something about what Charlie had just told us.' Group therapist: 'Okay, let's continue and I look forward to hearing your reaction, Mark.'

Inhibiting or redirecting excessive group cohesion

Excessive group cohesion involves too much or the wrong kind of involvement, more than is good for the task at hand. We saw in Section 6.4 that a group could slip into extreme conformity or too much intimacy. What can the group therapist do to stop or redirect this development? In all these cases, it is helpful to recall the task because if group cohesion has become too intense, the task will suffer. In addition to the task, undesirable group norms always come into play. Norms can be very strict or very 'sweet,' and group cohesion always reinforces existing norms. Discussing and testing these norms against the task provides input to normalize cohesion again. Sometimes it involves persistent patterns, which have become a culture. Then a steering attitude (LEADING) is needed to *confront* the group with the nonfunctional state of affairs and to *convince* them to break those patterns. A meta-conversation intervention (see Chapter 5) is often necessary in such a situation. Table 6.7 summarizes the technical steps the group leader can follow to inhibit cohesion.

Table 6.7 Inhibiting excessive group cohesion.

Verbal technique	Relationship technique (attitude and tone)
The group therapist *inhibits* excessive cohesive behavior and suggests an alternative solution (*advising*).	For this situation, a friendly but cordial attitude and tone fit best (HELPING/LEADING).

A problem for the group therapist to redirect excessive cohesion

A very cohesive atmosphere and helping culture has developed in an online psychotherapy group for people with neurotic personality problems. Everyone always feels great compassion for everyone else, to the point where they only support each other and never offer any criticism. Moreover, this culture results in one group member being the center of attention in every session and for a very long time. Donald is going through a tough period because his girlfriend has just left him. In the previous session, he had already drawn a lot of attention to his relationship problems and the sadness they evoke in him. And today, again, he does not want to pay attention to anything else. The group is so compassionate toward him that they lavish him with that attention. The group therapist decides to intervene, as she foresees the session once again being devoted entirely to Donald and not to the underlying reasons for everyone's neurotic problems. 'Donald, I want to stop you for a moment. I understand that you are consumed with the breakup of your relationship, and I understand how sad and angry that makes you. But that feeling is a part of the process, I think. There is no medicine or trick to make it go away. Are you open to broadening your experience a bit and looking at intimate relationships together, how to deal with them, and what they mean in your life?' Donald: 'Well, I don't really know what's best for me right now.' Group therapist: 'Does anyone else recognize the questions and problems Donald is talking about, problems or experiences related to intimacy, as well as standing up for yourself in your relationship? Or whatever comes to mind.' Lizzy: 'What are you doing? We were dealing with Donald, and he is still very sad. Right, Donald?' Donald: 'Yes. I don't know how to deal with this rotten feeling.' Ann: 'I totally understand how desperate that makes you feel, Donald; you can call me anytime you feel like you can't cope anymore.' The group therapist slumps back in her chair, feeling helpless, not sure what steps she should take next.

Group members may take advantage of the overly intense group cohesion to pursue personal contacts outside the group. This is good in some types of therapy groups, such as support groups for persistent problems, but often not fruitful for other therapy groups. Then the group therapist must first redirect the focus back onto the task and *convince* group members that mutual contact outside the group is detrimental, as they undermine the task. Repeating and re-explaining the group rule 'The group as workplace' could prove helpful (see Chapter 3). If that does not work satisfactorily, the group therapist should *explore* in a meta-conversation with the group what the underlying reason for the outside contacts is in order to then restore the task.

Exercises

Observation exercise – 'cohesion in your therapy group' for students in a group therapy training:

1. How do you experience (feel) the cohesion in your therapy group?
2. What do you see? Do people sit close together? Do they look at each other? Do they speak of 'we'?
3. What kind of group cohesion do you see in the group you lead?
4. Which group members are attached to one another? Based on what?

5. How does cohesion feel like here, in this training group, and what do you recognize it by?

Tool training – 'fostering cohesion in a beginning group' for students in a group therapy training:

1. The students are role-playing a social skills group therapy that has just started. The introduction has just taken place, and the group therapist takes a moment to ask how everyone is doing, what it is like to take such a social skills group therapy, and whether they find it very stressful or hardly feel stressed at all.
2. Each student acts as the group therapist for five minutes.
3. The practicing group therapist is instructed to only practice *mirroring* in a questioning manner, alternating this *inviting (giving space by) with silence*, and not to worry about the overall process. What is important here is that during the mirroring, the practicing group therapist calls the name of the person being mirrored. Each practicing group therapist deals with two or three interventions.
4. After five minutes, the trainer interrupts the role-play, and there is an opportunity for feedback from the role-playing group members on the *mirroring*, the *inviting with silence*, the questioning attitude, and the naming by the practicing group therapist.
5. After about five minutes of feedback, the next student continues as group therapist.
6. The role-play carries on. The member role-players are asked to play their roles in such a way that the practicing group therapist is given enough material to try out the skills.

Note

1 In this section we refer to the names of the distinct phases we discuss later in Chapter 8, 'Group development.'

Chapter 7

Interaction lines and relationship patterns in a therapy group

7.1 Introduction

In Chapter 2, I explained what interaction is and how we can use the Interpersonal Circle model to understand it. This chapter is about why interaction is so essential in group therapy, how interaction works, and how we can use it in practice.

The following topics are covered:
- The importance of interaction in group therapy
- Perceiving interaction in a therapy group
- Interaction lines and relationship patterns as important therapeutic material for group therapy
- Practical Manual: steering and utilizing interaction in a therapy group

7.2 The importance of interaction in group therapy

In Chapter 2, I defined interaction as behavior in one person that evokes behavior in another and vice versa. When people come together in a group with a purpose, interaction comes naturally. Interaction always takes place simultaneously in two ways – with words (verbal) and with behavior, posture, and tone (nonverbal) – and is expressed in countless ways (Bales, 1950). Some examples: a group member poses a question to which another member responds, a group member laughs in response and the other group members laugh along, a group member demonstratively leans back in his chair after the group therapist ignores his message, and a sad story of a group member evokes sadness in another group member thanks to resonance. In each case, there is an interpersonal action and reaction that goes hand in hand. A group therapist can take advantage of this natural interaction dynamic by giving it space and then directing it.

DOI: 10.4324/9781003368786-10

Interaction and communication

Although they come from different theoretical perspectives, interaction and communication concepts overlap. 'Communication' comes from information theory, meaning the transfer of information between the sender and the receiver (Shanon and Weaver, 1964). It is not surprising that 'communication' has been incorporated into domains of psychology and health care because information transfer is crucial in human contact. Likewise, it is impossible to imagine our therapy groups without the exchange of information.

As with the interaction concept, communication theory also distinguishes between the verbal and nonverbal aspects (Watzlawick, 1973). In communication theory, the verbal element is referred to as 'content' (the substantive meaning of the words), and the nonverbal element is referred to as the 'relation' or 'relationship definition.' In this chapter, I interpret the concept of interaction broadly and include all features of the communication concept. For clarity, I use the term 'interaction' for all human interactions in this book.

There are several reasons why interaction is so important for group therapy. First of all, interaction is the members' 'basic activity' for the group therapeutic task and therefore an essential prerequisite for a good outcome. As we know, group therapy works thanks to 'learning from each other.' Whether a group therapist works with a protocolized method or an in open interactional way, different forms of interaction are always needed for the group therapy task to be fruitful. In a protocoled group therapy, for example, it is necessary for the group members to do an exercise or role-play and discuss it with each other, while in an open interactional method, interpersonal feedback is needed for the working method. The therapeutic experiences that group members need occur in these interactions. Task interaction is so essential that if she stays away or is skinny, the group therapist should be worried.

Interaction is not only the vehicle for task-based learning experiences but also the 'engine' and 'lubricant' for the development of group processes. Without interactions between participants, group processes cannot develop. For example, in the previous chapter, I demonstrated how indispensable interaction is for the development of cohesion.

Finally, interaction is also the most important tool for the group therapist himself. *Verbal techniques* and *relationship techniques*, discussed earlier, are *interactional* techniques. By inserting oneself into group interactions and steering them in the right direction, the group therapist can actively promote purposeful learning experiences and process development. Enough reasons to put interaction high on the list of important topics.

Summary

- Interaction is interpersonal action and reaction, behavior in one person that evokes behavior in another and vice versa.
- Interaction is verbal and nonverbal.
- Interaction is the basis for task-oriented work in a therapy group: learning from each other.
- Interaction is the 'engine' and 'lubricant' for group processes.
- Interaction is also the group therapist's primary work tool.

7.3   Perceiving interaction in a therapy group

How do we perceive interaction?

Interaction always takes place through both words and behavior. Nonverbal behavior, our body language, features a wealth of expression possibilities. It includes behavior such as external appearance, posture, (hand) gestures, facial expression, eye contact, and tone of voice (Mehrabian, 1972). Although there are no precise figures, the nonverbal aspect is considerable, possibly as high as 33 percent (Markus, 2021). Despite the large nonverbal interaction aspect, its importance should not be exaggerated (Lapakko, 2007). Language remains indispensable for information transfer and leadership within our therapy groups.

We observe these two interaction aspects in different ways. We observe the verbal part of the interaction with our mind, the nonverbal part with our senses, our feelings. This sensory perception is especially important because the nonverbal aspect during interaction is extensive. We *see* the interaction between two group members and *hear* the emotional charge in the verbal exchange. If the interaction is accompanied by a great deal of excitement, we sometimes *smell* the physiological reactions. And when allowed to touch, we can *feel* the physical tension. In order to pick up on these interaction signals, which can sometimes be very subtle, the group therapist must use all his senses and take his own emotional signals, his feelings, as a source of information seriously.

In addition to his own feelings and emotional perception, the group therapist has another valuable antenna at his disposal: the group members. They are far more involved in the group than he is and often see the subtle interactions of their fellow group members sooner. If the group therapist sees and trusts the participants as fellow observers, he can make use of this important observational resource.

The best observers are usually the quieter group members. Their calm attitude and often somewhat peripheral position make them the natural observers of the therapy group. As a result, often they are able to observe what is happening during the interactions objectively and adequately. It is not uncommon for a group therapist to be surprised by group members' attentiveness and detailed, accurate observations.

Perceiving interaction through a fellow group member

An outpatient mental health youth department has a protocol-based therapy group for adolescents with anxiety and shyness. The meetings are characterized by inhibition and silence. The group members avoid eye contact and barely react to each other spontaneously. Dylan is one of the shyest boys in the group, but he already dares to participate in an eye contact exercise. The group therapist asks Dylan to indicate on a scale of 1 to 10 how much tension he felt during the eye contact exercise with Robert. Dylan answers: 'Well, 3 or 4 maybe. I didn't really feel much tension or anything.' 'And what did you notice about Dylan, Xander?' the group therapist then asks. 'I think Dylan was pretty comfortable with it.' He then sees Mary frowning at Dylan and asks: 'What are you looking at, Mary?' She replies: 'I see sweat beads on his forehead, so I think you were a little tenser than a 3, Dylan!' Dylan responds: 'Well, um, I don't know. Maybe. But honestly, I don't really pay that much attention to it.'

We automatically and naturally use our feelings to observe in daily life. Using our feelings as a professional instrument to observe occurs less naturally. For the novice group therapist, the disarray of interactions that a therapy group displays is often difficult to grasp. In this situation, it is not unusual to see the group therapist fall back on the certainty of intellectual information, such as knowledge. Consider a group member who constantly reacts in a mildly irritated way to everyone while saying very sensible things in terms of content. The group therapist, who observes only with his mind, hears the content message but misses the irritated emotional undertone of the interaction. In this case, the mind is thus insufficiently helpful because interactions are mainly detected through feelings. Therefore, you need to trust your sensory information to observe the interaction.

Different observational perspectives

Observing, and observing learning group members, is an ongoing task of any group therapist. There is no group therapy method which goes without observing and reflecting by the members. And for the group therapist himself, steering a therapy group is impossible without the 'helicopter view,' the skill of observing.

Group phenomena can be observed from three perspectives. First, we can take the group as a whole as our perspective; we then turn our focus to phenomena that affect the entire group. We discussed this perspective in Chapter 6 because cohesion is a typical group-as-a-whole phenomenon. A second focus we can adopt is the individual perspective; when we look at a group from that perspective, we pay special attention to the phenomena belonging to each individual group member. However, the third perspective from which we can observe group phenomena, namely the *interactional perspective*, is relevant to this chapter. This perspective means that we focus on the interaction between two group members. We explain this shortly.

When observing the interaction, what we look at is important. Because we are so used to looking at the individual, observing through the interactional perspective does not come easily to us (Goudsblom, 2000). We are quick to look within the group members, whereas we should look *between* the group members when they interact. By that, we mean that the group therapist is able to let the individuals 'fade' to focus on the *relationship* between two or more individuals.

An example. Suppose two group members are constantly talking to each other but keep not understanding each other. The group therapist can then focus on one member and watch how that person becomes angrier each time. But he can also take a step back and focus on both group members together, thus on their miscommunication. Then, for example, the group therapist might notice how both group members are not listening to each other and are only sending and not receiving. He can use the IPC model to score the interaction (both members interact from a LEADING position, for example) and thus understand it even better.

Alternating between observational perspectives

A group therapist must be able to alternate between observational perspectives with ease. Occasionally, the important thing is what is going on with an individual, and he then focuses on what is happening inside that individual. If the others react to this, he may choose to fade the individual to the background and bring the interactional side to the forefront. If appropriate, he may also shift the focus to the group level. We call this *alternating between observational perspectives*.

The position the group therapist takes can help with his alternating observations. He must dare to play with distance in his position and literally, with his chair a bit more inside or outside the group. The metaphor of the 'swimming pool' from Chapter 5 (Figure 5.1) helps with this. Quietly observing from the periphery of the group (sitting on the edge of the pool), the group therapist has a good view of the group as a whole. To feel what is going on with and between the individual members, he has to move closer to them (get off the edge and jump into the pool). A group therapist who can do this feels what is going on and sees opportunities to use the different perspectives as starting points for his actions.

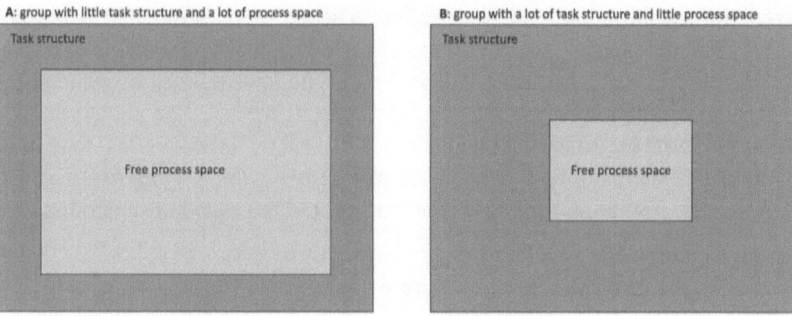

Figure 7.1 The 'swimming pool.' Figure by the author

Alternating between observational perspectives is not only an observational quality but also a technical tool. Each observational perspective corresponds to a focused verbal technique: the group-as-a-whole perspective fits the group intervention, the individual perspective fits the individual-oriented intervention, and the interactional perspective fits the interaction-oriented intervention. His feelings will help the group therapist choose on what level to interfere. When there is much energy in or with an individual member, the group therapist may choose for an individual intervention, when the energy is collective (for example, the whole group looks very confused) the group therapist can choose for a group intervention, and when an interaction 'line' between two members is 'hot' then an interactional intervention may be fruitful.

Sometimes it is the task that determines the intervention strategy. For example, a group therapist may opt for an interaction-oriented intervention because he wants to stimulate task feedback. If he wants to clarify a task topic, he does so in a group-oriented way.

Switching from an interactional to an individual observational perspective

In a therapy group for patients with unexplained pain, Wayne and Abigail repeatedly clash in vain. Wayne is highly annoyed with Abigail because she does not take the therapy group very seriously, whereas he considers the group very important. Discovering that his neck problems, which he has had for years, are caused by the tension from all his pent-up anger was an enormous eye-opener. Abigail's resistive attitude annoys him immensely; she trivializes the group. She is convinced that they will find a physical cause for her severe headaches one day. She, in turn, is highly annoyed with Wayne, who obediently does what the group therapist asks.

When they once again get stuck in an argument, the group therapist intervenes. He starts his intervention with the interactional perspective and then switches to the individual perspective to see if there is more to be gained: 'Wayne and Abigail, stop for a moment, please. That you are able to engage each other in battle is clear by now, but do you have an idea of what all that arguing says about you? About you as a person, Wayne? And about you, Abigail?' After some silence, Abigail says: 'I can't accept the fact that none of the specialist examinations I've had have turned up anything. I am extremely disappointed. It's hard for me to accept that it could be related to something else.'

Perceiving the task and process side of the interaction

In Chapter 3, I explained how useful it is when a group therapist knows how to distinguish between task and the process during group collaboration. This also applies to the interaction associated with the task or the process. Because the task is the starting point for the group, the task side of the interaction – task interaction for short – is often the first thing we focus on. We see how group members work together and do the things that the task dictates, such as discussing a homework assignment, giving each other feedback, or exchanging opinions.

Seeing and recognizing the task interaction is essential for the group therapist. The task interaction is the most concrete translation of the group task and thus a benchmark for group functioning. Are the group members doing what they are supposed to do? Therefore, in Chapter 3, I described how important it is for the group therapist when organizing a therapy group to describe the task interactions accurately and to explain to new group members what task interactions he expects of them. Here, the *concreteness* in the description of the expected task interaction is not solely important but also its *comprehensiveness*. Often, several interactions are expected, and it is good to describe and explain them all. For example, in a therapy group for clients who suffer from depression, members are expected to practice, among others, these interactions: analyze what's behind the depressive mood and choose a focus, listen and react to each other, give personal feedback and support to each other. In a social skills therapy group these interactions are expected: discuss homework, participate in role-play, give feedback about the role-play. If these interactions are lacking, the group therapist knows that there is uncertainty about or resistance to the task at hand.

Besides the task side, every interaction also has a process side, namely, the characteristic way the group members carry out the task interaction with each other. That unique way of interacting stems from the persons themselves, from their characters. When a therapy group has existed for a longer time, members dare to be themselves more. Then the personal tone in the group interactions will be more obvious in recognizable behavior. For example, the provocative jokes between two group members while working together may become noticeable, the commanding tone in which one group member always approaches others, or the witty way in which someone always says things. We then sense that such an interaction style is unrelated to the task but rather to the person.

This personal side to task performance (the process side) is part of the job and is usually enjoyable. It allows for personal spontaneity and involvement and adds color to the group therapy work.

In some therapy groups these personal interaction styles are precisely important because focusing on it *is* the task of that group. That's the case in therapy groups for personality disorders, where clients want to get insight into their personal interaction patterns in order to change them.

A fierce conflict that completely displaces the task

Two female clients clashed fiercely at an unexpected moment in one of my psychotherapy groups for personality disorders. One of them, let's name her Chiara, just recently joined the group but had already started opening up more and more. Chiara received a lot of appreciation and confirmation for this from the other group members.

One woman, whom I shall call Susan, remained silent, so conspicuous that I asked her what she thought of it. She did not address her answer to me but to Chiara instead and ruthlessly berated her. She could not see anything good about Chiara: she was fake, sneaky, a suck-up, and so on. Before I could intervene, Chiara replied. Susan was no good either. She was a know-it-all, arrogant, and so on. The conflict quickly escalated. It evoked so much fear in the group that a group member asked: 'Willem, will you please put a stop to this?' And I did because this interaction was no longer constructive.

The sudden ferocity surprised me so much that I revisited this issue the next session. It turned out then that the two women knew each other from a training course a year earlier, during which a fierce personal feud had developed. When Chiara entered the group, they did not mention that they were acquainted. Together with the group I tried to find out the source of their conflict, but that proved after some sessions so difficult that their joint presence in the group became intolerable. I then found another group for Chiara (the last to enter), in which she continued her therapy.

7.4   Interaction lines and relationship patterns as important therapeutic material for group therapy

Recognizing the first signs of interaction: seeing interaction lines in the therapy group

When interaction is initiated, the group therapist can sense after some time between which members the interaction is taking place. He can see and sense the involvement and reciprocal reactions to one another through tentative signals, negative or positive. Examples of negative signals are not looking at each other, exchanging nasty looks, sighing demonstratively, mockingly staring when the other speaks, and maintaining distance. Examples of positive signals are always responding affirmatively to each other, having regular eye contact, smiling at each other, and regularly sitting next to and close to each other.

When these positive or negative signals become strong enough, the group therapist begins to sense the interaction tension between certain group members as if a *connecting line* is forming between them. Thus, in a new group, the interaction can grow from very tentative nonverbal cues between certain group members to more verbal affirmations and then to multiple consecutive verbal and nonverbal responses to each other. 'Seeing' the incipient interaction lines is useful for the group therapist as they are the starting point for fostering group interaction.

The group therapist can map out the interaction lines he observed after a group session and can thus gain insight into the group's nascent interactional field. In social psychology, such a graphic representation of interaction lines is called a sociogram.[1] It can be an overall impression of a group session or represent a specific moment of interaction. Figure 7.2 shows an example of such a retrospective representation. The group is shown as a circle of group members. Interaction arrows have been drawn between the group members. These indicate who interacted with whom. Each arrow indicates the direction of the interaction. An arrow toward the center of the group means that that group member has primarily addressed the entire group.

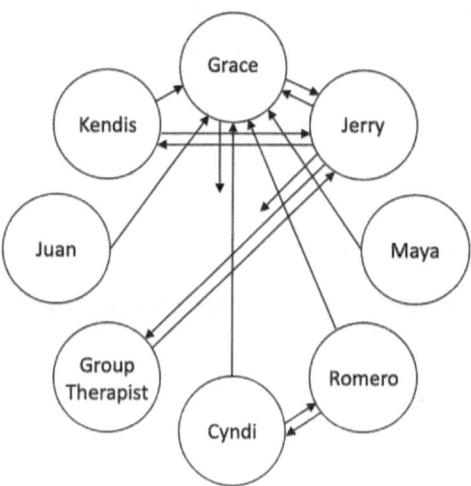

Figure 7.2 A sociogram representing interaction lines in a group session. Figure by author.

The overall retrospective impression of the interaction lines ('sociogram') in session three of a group therapy for work-related mental disorders

A therapy group for health care professionals with depression and 'burnout' symptoms meets ten times, and members discuss themes, do assignments, and have group discussions. When a thematic discussion on stress management is scheduled in the third session, the interaction lines begin to crystallize.

As usual, Grace speaks first and explains to the group how she deals with stress. All of the group members respond to her story, and some get a response back from Grace, especially Jerry. In Figure 7.2, we see an arrow from Grace to the group and arrows from the group members to her. There are two arrows between Jerry and Grace, one in each direction.

As the session progresses, the group's attention shifts to Jerry, who shares his experience with a mindfulness method. This leads to quite a discussion with Kendis, who makes it clear to Jerry that mindfulness is not for him. In the sociogram, we see an arrow from Jerry to the group and two arrows between Jerry and Kendis, one in each direction.

Romero and Cyndi do not actively participate in the conversation but only occasionally whisper to each other. We see two arrows between Romero and Cyndi in each direction in the sociogram.

The group therapist mainly interacted with Jerry during the session. In the sociogram, we see lines back and forth between the group therapist and Jerry.

Although such a sociogram is only a sum of successive interactions, it proves to be a valuable tool for group therapists to gain insight into the developing interaction structure in a group.

Relationship patterns among group members and their importance for group therapy

As we saw in the example, the cautious interaction lines are often a precursor to a more recognizable interaction structure. When interaction patterns between group members or members and the group repeat themselves and become increasingly recognizable, we refer to them as *relationship patterns*. Those repeating relationship positions and patterns are important therapeutic material in most therapy groups, because they incorporate the problems clients seek help for. Take someone who suffers because of his constant quarrels, rivalry, and poor functioning in his job; after some time he will show the same behavior in the therapy group, and the members and group therapist will recognize it, analyze it, and help the member with finding ways to adopt more rewarding interactive behavior.

An extra strong relationship pattern will emerge if there is a corresponding relationship definition. For example, the helping and the needy group members find each other. This way, an increasingly clear giver–helper relationship emerges between the two. The interaction positions have a mutually affirming effect, causing this relationship pattern to become stronger and stronger. The positions of the individuals within those relationship patterns are recognizable and predictable and provide learning materials for more people at the same time.

Sometimes it is the group task and content, which is the main trigger of the interaction. Take a group session where several members recognize themselves in an important experience or topic. Those members will respond to each other with interest and in-depth questions. In another therapy session, for example, members have intense interactions because they're debating their different opinions about an experience or topic.

As the therapy group and its relationships develop, we begin to see that they not only consist of horizontal but also of vertical relationships. The group members of a beginning group adopt a follower-like attitude toward the group therapist. Later, in the group development, we see how group members with dominant personalities start to manifest themselves. Among the group members, relationships develop between leaders and followers. Some group members clearly call the shots, while others comply and follow.

The IPC model is the best tool for mapping and understanding relationship patterns because of its interactional principles. An example: if a group member is used to behaving helplessly (Under), that behavior in the group will trigger helper behavior (Above). Someone in the group whose predisposition is to help (Above) will have difficulty resisting that trigger. The two are likely to find each other. If this continues for a period of time, a relationship pattern visible to everyone emerges. Another example: a group member is used to being very critical of others (Distant/Counter). This behavior evokes the same (Distant/Counter) behavior from other members. The group member who naturally has a hostile attitude (Distant/Counter) will feel the trigger more. The chances are that these two will also find each other and develop a solid relationship pattern, but in this case, conflict will dominate.

Interaction thus begins with individual interaction positions finding and confirming each other in a mutually affirming relationship pattern. We can use the IPC to track down those relationship patterns, dissect them, and thereby begin to recognize and understand them.

We do this as follows. We have a printed copy of the IPC at hand. When we want to dissect an interaction pattern, we start by looking at the individual interaction position of the two group members. We 'score' the behavior of both group members in the IPC by assessing which behavioral variant (LEADING, COOPERATING, WITHDRAWN, etc.) the behavior of both group members fits. We write the first name of both group members in the appropriate behavioral variant. By placing the name within the behavioral variant in the precise spot, we can indicate the strength of the behavior. With the IPC, a place closer to the outer edge of the model means that the behavior is strong and inadequate. A place more toward the middle means that the behavior is mild and adequate. Now we have the IPC in front of us with names in two sections. By applying the principles behind IPC, we can often quickly understand why the two group members found each other during the interaction. For example, when we see that the name of the first group member is in behavioral variant DEPENDENT (Under behavior) and the second in behavioral variant LEADING (Above behavior), it is easy to understand the strong relationship between a group member with pronounced dependent behavior and a group member with a strong directing attitude. We can use the same method to score and examine more interactions in a group session. When appropriate to the task we not only use this information for observation purposes but can share this with the group members for therapeutic use. An example follows.

A strong relationship pattern in a therapy group session

For an educational therapy group for depressed widows, the group therapist chooses a current topic of concern for each meeting in consultation with the group. After a short introduction by one of the group members, the main part of the meeting consists of exchanging personal experiences around the topic. Michelle, originally a French teacher, dominates the group and tends to lecture the others. They are constantly impressed by Michelle, with her academic training, French words, and directing attitude. They fall silent and apparently do not dare to stand up to her. The group therapist tries to stimulate the submissive members to stand up for themselves and to put their opinions forward. But the relationship between Michelle and the group seems unwavering. Michelle calls the shots; the others follow. Until another meeting where the topic is power and oppression. Michelle has prepared the topic and gives a short introduction. The group discussion that follows gets off to a good start, partly because Michelle keeps to the background as the introducer. But she cannot keep this up for long. When, after a while, she broadly expresses how powerless and oppressed she has been all her life, Ronnel snaps. She confronts Michelle in an angry tone about the discrepancy between her self-description and her behavior in the group. Others agree with Ronnel. Even the usually silent Amy contributes by expressing her annoyance toward Michelle, who is completely perplexed and taken aback. It seems that she did not expect this at all. The group therapist helps her to understand the feedback. Michelle indicates that she is not able to participate at the moment and withdraws, sitting in the group silently. She only feels comfortable saying something at the end of the session again. She indicates that the feedback has hit her like a ton of bricks and that she wants to revisit this issue in the next session.

Interaction lines and relationship patterns in online group therapy

Interaction, interaction lines and relationship patterns are just as important in online group therapy as they are in face-to-face group therapy. Only, you can't see them, especially not the incipient interaction lines. With the people in the cubes on

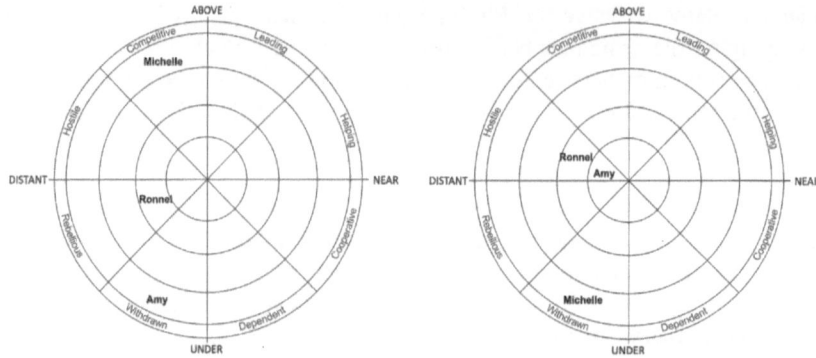

Figure 7.3 IPCs with the interaction positions before (left) the fierce confrontation with Michelle, and during the fierce (right) confrontation with Michelle. Figure by author.

the screen, you can never know who is looking at whom or who is looking away from whom. That is why a sociogram of the interaction lines is also difficult. This is possibly the biggest flaw of online group therapy, even though interaction is so important. Fortunately, the group therapist can compensate for this deficiency to some extent. Here, too, this compensation comes down to what Weinberg (2024) calls 'presence,' a combination of an active present and a helping attitude and technique, with which in this case the group therapist actively detects and names the interaction. I will come back to this in concrete terms in the Practical Manual.

Summary

- We observe interaction in the group with our senses, feelings.
- There are three observational perspectives that a group therapist can alternate between: looking at the individual, seeing the group as a whole, or shifting the focus to an interaction.
- The interaction between group members has a task-oriented and a process-oriented side.
- The start of interaction in a group is reflected through emerging interaction lines.
- Interaction develops over the course of the group and then becomes more structured.
- Interaction in an advanced group expresses itself in clearly visible, repeating relationship patterns, which is useful information for group therapy.
- In online group therapy, interaction lines are not observable. Relationship patterns can become apparent over time.

7.5   Practical Manual: steering and utilizing interaction in a therapy group

7.5.1   Facilitating interaction, before and at the beginning of a therapy group

Interaction comes spontaneously. Nevertheless, the group therapist can facilitate the interaction in advance, namely by taking into account the 'jointness of the task,' as described in the previous chapter (Thye et al., 2014). The more interaction is built into the working method, the better it is for the process development, both of the interaction itself and of cohesion.

After the group has started the group therapist can stimulate spontaneous growth and the use of the interaction in different ways.

7.5.2   Inserting

Interaction is the group therapist's basic work tool. Every group therapist wants to steer the spontaneous interactions (and, with it, the group) in the desired direction. How can he steer the interaction? First, he has to 'break into' the interaction between the group members, try to get in among them. He does this by *inserting* himself, that is, mixing in with the group members. The group therapist is able to do this because of his double role. He is not only a group leader but also a participant and a player in the interactional field. This allows him to enter the interactional field via the participant role and steer the interaction between the group members in the desired direction from within.

Of course, every intervention is an interruption of the interaction between the group members.

A technique that works well for this is when the group leader 'asks permission to enter.' This is mostly done with a literal question but is also possible by pronouncing a group member's name in a questioning manner and waiting for the consenting response for a moment. When inserting, the verbal technique of *asking* with a COOPERATING attitude is generally appropriate. The group therapist uses the question to slow down the interaction and create an opening to insert.

Insertion by the group therapist

A therapy group for clients with autism has been discussing the theme 'isolation or contact.' One group member, Jaden, is talking a lot. The group therapist notices that more and more group members are disengaging nonverbally. The group therapist decides to intervene. Group therapist: 'Can I interject for a moment, Jaden?' There is silence for a moment.

Jaden: 'Um . . . of course.'

Group therapist: 'Are you guys still able to follow the conversation?'

Irene: 'Ahh, finally someone who dares to say it. I lost track half an hour ago!'

Insertion by the group therapist

In a veteran's therapy group on trauma, a heated discussion ensues, with Kenneth unexpectedly suggesting that he wants to quit because he doesn't find the group helpful. Group therapist: 'Kenneth?' Kenneth: 'Uhm . . . Yes?' Group therapist: 'Did I understand you correctly? Do you want to quit this group?' Kenneth: 'No, I don't . . . I didn't mean it that way because . . .'

7.5.3   Fostering interaction in a therapy group

Facilitate the emergence of interaction in advance

Interaction is so important that the group therapist should feel free to facilitate it. This can already be done before the group starts. The clearer the task organization, the easier the process, including interaction, can be. Explaining that interaction is a necessary activity of the group members, and explaining what interaction precisely is expected, quickly lowers the threshold for interactive contact.

Initiating interaction with a group invitation

When a therapy group meets for the first time, it is quite normal for group members to take little initiative and wait to see what will happen. The group therapist, as the formal leader, must take the lead. He can welcome the group members, introduce them to each other, and clarify the purpose of the group task while explaining what interactions are expected of them.

Once all that is done, the moment arrives when the group members have to get to work and take the initiative. Whether it is a protocol task or a free group conversation the group members must get going and interact with each other. How do you get a group of strangers to talk to each other at that moment? As a group therapist, how do you get the interaction started?

Fortunately, the group therapist can help by using the *group invitation technique*. He uses this to invite the therapy group in a resolute tone of voice with a simple but clear sentence that has four characteristics:

• The sentence emphasizes a transition
• The sentence places the responsibility on the group

- The sentence is always a group intervention (the individual form does not work because it encourages interaction with the group therapist rather than between group members)
- In addition to the verbal technique, the group therapist directs this transition moment with his attitude. During the pronouncement of the group invitation, he makes an open gesture with his arms toward the group (like he is putting something down with the group), then sits back noticeably, remains silent, and avoids any gazes directed at him during the silence by briefly looking elsewhere, for example, looking outside or at his satchel on the floor. Everyone then feels that it is the group's turn, and it usually doesn't take long before a group member breaks the silence.

This effective technique for getting the therapy group talking can also be used during many other moments in a group, for example, when a group is evaluating an exercise or end result, needs to make a joint decision, or after the group therapist has just explained a new part of a task. Table 7.1 provides a summary of this technique and some examples.

Table 7.1 Initiate interaction with a group invitation.

Verbal technique	Relationship technique (attitude and tone)
The group therapist collectively invites the group with one statement or a question (always with a group intervention).	To exert his influence, the group therapist voices the group invitation in a resolute tone of voice (LEADING/HELPING), after which he noticeably leans back in his chair, remains silent, and looks away for a moment (avoiding intense eye contact with the group).
A few examples of a group invitation: 'I'm curious to know what's on your minds right now.' 'I've been talking long enough; it's your turn now.' 'We could talk about what it would be like for a long time, but I think you should go ahead and try it out.' 'What do you think about how this group is doing right now?' 'I'm wondering what you thought of this exercise.' 'I'm curious about whether this meeting provided any benefit.' 'How can you resolve this?'	

Fostering interaction in a beginning group
When interaction begins, some stimulation from the group therapist could be beneficial. It is common for group members to initially be hesitant about interacting with each other and focus primarily on the group therapist. In a beginning therapy group, group members naturally expect the interaction to take place

primarily between them and the group therapist. This expectation is related to the image of group leaders and caregivers as authorities.

To replace this expectation with an image of interpersonal conversation, the group therapist must do two seemingly contradictory things: first, react modestly to the group members' individual appeals, and then actively help foster the interaction between the group members. The *type* of activity of the group therapist makes the difference here. If he honors each individual member's appeal personally, the group therapist fosters group dependency rather than spontaneous interaction among group members. Therefore, the group therapist would serve the group better by not answering every question immediately, ignoring the dependent appeals of individual members, and directing his gaze toward the other group members. Because group members will often follow that gaze, and as a result, he will naturally turn their attention to each other as well.

If the group therapist does want to give the group members attention, he can best do that by focusing on the interaction *between* the members themselves, thus deliberately using the interactional-observational perspective.

Every cautious attempt by a group member to interact with another group member is an opportunity for the group therapist to engage. We then speak of an incipient interaction line, as discussed in Section 7.4. This interaction line is the group therapist's starting point for fostering interaction. The most important technique he could then use, is the *connecting* verbal technique.

The importance of connecting

Interaction is the source of the work done in a group. Therefore, it is not surprising that 'connecting' is one of the most effective verbal techniques. I am not the first to concretely describe this interaction-facilitating intervention. Yalom and Leszcz (2020) describe how interactional stimulation can be achieved by asking a question about a group member via another group member – 'via the side' – and group therapist Ormont (1990) calls his interaction-promoting intervention beautifully 'bridging.' In system therapy, making a connection between three people is called a 'triadic intervention' (Hoijtink, 2001).

Since the group therapist may take on an active role, a HELPING posture will work best. The essence of the *connecting* technique is that he reinforces the interaction line by calling the sender by name, calling the receiver by name, and repeating the message from the sender to the receiver (usually in a questioning manner).

In doing so, the group therapist draws a line from the sender to the receiver with his hand in the air. He thereby emphasizes the line of interaction he considers important – draws it across, as it were. Almost always, the interaction between the mentioned persons then continues, and that is exactly the intention. A simpler form of connecting is what is called 'the question via the side.' In this case, the group therapist asks a question to group member B about group member A (see the following examples). Despite the active technique and attitude of the group therapist, these combination techniques actually encourage interaction among group members.

Example sentences – connecting

'Joshua, are you actually saying to Mira, "The way you treat Sebastian makes me angry!"?' (the group therapist draws a line from Joshua to Mira)

'Lebron, is your message to Suzan maybe "I find it much more pleasant to work with you when you act like this!"?' (the group therapist draws a line from Lebron to Suzan)

'Are you asking me to do something about that, Ruth?' (the group therapist draws a line from Ruth to himself)

'Amanda, say it to Donald . . . ' (the group therapist draws a line to Donald)

'You're nodding, Sarah. What do you want to tell Carol and Peter with your nodding?' (the group therapist draws a line from Sarah to Carol and Peter)

'Khalid, how do you think Rosy views John?' (connecting triadically)

'What do you guys think of Mary's story?' (via the side)

'Steven, do you have any idea what is going on in Amanda's head?' (via the side)

'Is Roger's proposal a good idea? What do you think?' (via the side)

In combination, the group therapist's silence is also a valuable stimulus to provoke interaction between the group members. For this purpose, the group therapist uses the *giving space (inviting) with silence* technique. This silence is meant to create space and to invite interaction. The silence increases the tension, which a group member will break after a while. A waiting attitude is best suited to such a silence as a relationship technique, that is, COOPERATING and, in the meantime, looking around (monitoring).

This combination of techniques greatly enhances the spontaneous interaction between the group members, and it contributes to the group members' feeling that they can and may co-manage within the group and thus to the development of an independent group. Table 7.2 summarizes the technique combinations with which the group therapist fosters interaction.

Table 7.2 Fostering interaction in a beginning group.

Verbal technique	Relationship technique (attitude and tone)
The group therapist *ignores* individual appeals by looking at other members and redirecting the interaction that way.	A HELPING attitude is appropriate for this technique.
The group therapist *connects* by calling the sender by name, calling the receiver by name, and repeating the message from sender to receiver (usually questioningly). At the same time, he draws a line in the air from sender to receiver.	Monitoring (look around calmly during the silence)
The group therapist alternates between the preceding technique and *inviting with silence*.	

Connect and establish interaction lines

In a student therapy group to strengthen self-esteem and self-compassion, Christopher and Donna are regularly at each other's throats.

Group therapist: 'If I understand correctly, Christopher, you are telling Donna (in a HELPING tone and drawing a line from Christopher to Donna) that her behavior just now really puzzles you?' 'That's correct,' says Christopher. Donna: 'Well, then, I'd like to know what you don't understand, Chrissie . . . I thought I made myself clear to you.' Christopher: 'You, clear? Well, not to me. I really don't understand your reaction at all.'

During the ensuing tense silence, the group therapist looks at the group. Kyan has a pensive look on his face and breaks the silence: 'I don't like your bickering; it distracts from what we are doing here: learning to become stronger within ourselves. I think you prefer arguing instead of focusing on that.'

The group therapist immediately adds: 'Kyan, are you in fact telling Christopher and Donna (in a HELPING tone and drawing a line from Kyan to Christopher and Donna): 'You are arguing so that you don't have to focus on yourselves and not on the task for which each of you are here?' Kyan: 'That's exactly what I mean.' Donna: 'But Kyan, you also argue with Christopher sometimes, don't you?' The group therapist jumps in: 'Donna, can you relate to what Kyan said about preferring to argue rather than focus on yourself?' Donna: 'I don't know. I do know that I often have disagreements, but I've never looked at it from that point of view.'

Connecting in online group therapy
Because beginning interaction lines are never visible in online group therapy, the group therapist has to actively think aloud about them, and then connect the people involved. An online group therapist is not completely devoid of interactional information. In addition to verbal information, he sees facial expressions, some body language, and he hears the tone in which the message is communicated.

> **Connecting in online group therapy**
> Group therapist: 'Rochelle, do I see and hear correctly that you are irritated?' Rochelle: 'Ehh, yes that could well be the case.' Group therapist: 'Does that have to do with what Johanna just said, about her complaints that keep happening?' Rochelle: 'That's exactly right.' Group therapist: 'Do I understand correctly that you say to Johanna, "I feel annoyed Johanna when you talk about your complaints like that"?' Rochelle: 'Indeed, and . . . I say to you Johanna, I can't take your complaining anymore, will that never stop?'

7.5.4   Utilizing interaction for group therapy

Utilizing interaction for the task
After a while, attention to the task will increase when the therapy group gets a sense of what the task is all about and that they can achieve results. This is the perfect time for the group therapist to focus interaction on the task. It depends on the type of group therapy what the main task interaction of the members is. The chosen therapeutic method is of course very decisive in this respect. In a protocol-working group therapy, members are, for example, expected to discuss the experiences of the assignments, homework, or exercises with one another; in an intensive interactional psychotherapy group, giving each other feedback is one of the main tasks. The group therapist connects the spontaneous interactions that always arise to the task. Fostering task interaction involves multiple verbal techniques, such as *asking and explaining* and *connecting and mirroring*. Given that the task is never up for discussion, the group therapist will take a somewhat directive stance (HELPING/LEADING) in promoting task interaction.

Table 7.3 Utilizing interaction for the task.

Verbal technique	Relationship technique (attitude and tone)
The group therapist *asks* group members about the task, *explains* the task, and *connects* group members to each other and the task.	When it comes to the task, the group therapist usually assumes a responsible attitude (LEADING/HELPING).

Example sentences of *connecting* to the task:
'Talisa, could you explain how we do things to the new group members?'
'Lisa, I get the impression that the group task is as vague for you as for Roger. Is that right?'
'Kenneth, does your silence have something to do with the exercise you just did and the feedback you got from Paul?'
'What do you think of Roger's helping thoughts? Do you have questions, or advice for Roger?'
Group therapist: 'I want to ask you something, Sarah, is that okay?' Sarah: 'Hmm . . . okay.' Group therapist: 'Is the way you hide yourself in the group not precisely the problem you came here for?' Sarah: 'Yes . . . I am shy in every group, and now I am also very shy in this group . . . it is terrible, and . . . I . . .' (starts to cry).

Utilizing interaction by strengthening task interaction

A social skills group therapy has lost its 'spirit' a bit. The group members obediently carry out group tasks, such as role-plays and homework assignments. But they avoid giving each other feedback, which is an important part of the task. The group therapist interrupts the training: 'People, I want to discuss how the training is progressing. I am very satisfied with how you practice here and do the homework assignments. But I notice that you are not giving each other feedback. Do you agree?' Silence . . . 'Shall I explain again why the feedback is so important?' Ron: 'Yes, please, because sometimes I don't quite understand what you expect from us.'

Interaction as a therapeutic tool: feedback

As I made clear at the beginning of this chapter, interaction in our therapy groups is always accompanied by information exchange. We call this purposeful form of interaction and information exchange feedback. By feedback, we mean that one participant provides another participant with concrete and objective information on how his or her behavior is perceived, understood, and experienced (Remmerswaal, 2015).

Feedback regularly occurs automatically in therapy groups because it is a natural consequence of interaction. However, feedback is also sometimes used in a purposeful way, for instance, as a therapeutic tool. In many therapy groups, such as social skills group therapy or a psychotherapy group, interpersonal feedback is an integral part of the therapeutic task. According to Yalom and Leszcz

(2020), interaction and interpersonal feedback form the core of the group therapy method. If a therapy group is safe enough, participants will give each other feedback about how their behavior comes across to each other, how they experience each other, or how they think about each other. This can provide new information members learn from. For example, a group member gets feedback about her maladaptive interaction pattern she repeats in the group, or a member in a self-image group may hear for the first time that he comes across as friendlier than he thinks. If that member hears that more often, then that new information can have a therapeutic effect, such as causing him to adjust his self-image positively. And this is where the big advantage of group therapy counts: feedback is more easily believed in group therapy because group members are more likely to accept something from each other as human and hands-on experts than from a professional group therapist. Not surprisingly, feedback is one of the therapeutic factors I described in Chapter 1.

In addition to being part of the working method in group therapy, feedback also lends itself well as an evaluation tool. The purpose of feedback, as accurate feedback as possible, makes the tool suitable for evaluation or measurement moments of a group therapy (Koementas-de Vos et al., 2018). It can be task-oriented feedback, that is, when evaluating therapy goals, but it can also be interpersonal feedback. It is always important to let the interactive feedback take place as objectively and safely as possible. The rules of the game and practical implementation for this are described in Chapter 11, 'Termination.'

A table that is helpful in understanding interaction, feedback, and new information is the so-called Johari window (Remmerswaal, 2015). That table (see Table 7.4) is based on two principles: first, the distinction between how someone sees himself and how someone is seen by the other; second, the distinction between known and unknown behavior. This creates four quadrants, each with its own characteristics. Quadrant A describes *visible behavior*, behavior that is familiar to someone themselves and known to the other, for example, Mike's humor and jokes that everyone experiences and that Mike is also aware of himself. Quadrant B describes 'blind spot' behavior, behavior that a person is unaware of but that others notice. Sometimes the 'habitual attitude' I mentioned in Chapter 2 also falls under this category. This typical personal habitual behavior is often so familiar (ego-syntonic) that the person is not aware of himself, while others do see it. For example, Mike's nervous side, which others notice by his fidgeting and rapid speech. This behavior is Mike's blind spot: he doesn't fully realize it himself. Quadrant C describes *hidden behavior (feelings, thoughts)* that a person knows about themselves but that the other person does not see, for example, Mike's secret, which is his positive feelings for Sharon. Finally, quadrant D describes *unknown* behavior, behavior that is unknown, both to someone themselves and to the other, for example, Mike's unconscious feelings of failure and inadequacy, which neither he nor the other are aware of. Behavior in quadrant D is unknown, thus hypothetical.

The Johari window shows many ways in which new personal information can emerge in the interaction and thus how tremendously instructive interaction and feedback can be in group therapy. For example, feedback from the other group members about Mike's nervous behavior can be so convincing that he begins to recognize this behavior, thus reducing his blind spot. When Mike overcomes his shyness and confesses that he likes Sharon, it is new information for the group. Finally, someone may discover something completely new about themselves; for example, Mike becomes aware of his insecurity, which he was not aware of before.

Table 7.4 The Johari window.

	Known to myself	Unknown to myself
Known to the other	A Visible behavior	B Blind Spot
Unknown to the other	C Private/secret	D Unknown/unconsciously

With permission adapted from Remmerswaal J (2015) *Group Dynamics: An introduction.* Amsterdam: Boom Nelissen.

Feedback as part of the working method in a therapy group
In an interactional psychotherapy group there are some irritations now and then, but Thomas is convinced that he never feels any anger. He thinks he does not have that feeling. Nancy reacts: 'Then you should look in the mirror more often Thomas.' Thomas: 'Why, Nancy?' Nancy: 'Well . . . when you react to others in the group I think I see irritation in your eyes?' Thomas: 'Irritation in my eyes? I don't understand that at all?' Emily: 'I often hear irritation in your voice, Thomas, so you're human too, like all of us.'

Rebooting stalled interaction
Interaction is a reciprocal process between the group members. Sometimes we see how the interaction between the group members falters, has completely stagnated, or only flows in one direction. The group therapist can then *connect* the group members in a more powerful way or – in the case of one-sided interaction – *broaden* the scope. If, for example, group member Jamar keeps on speaking and the others just listen, the group therapist can break this pattern with the *broadening* intervention: 'Are there others who have experienced something similar to what Jamar experienced?' This verbal technique breaks one-way interaction and broadens it so that more people will participate in the conversation. If the faltering, stagnation, or one-sidedness persists, it would be best for the group therapist first to investigate and discuss what the cause might be. This could be, for example, a lack of clarity about the task or group members being afraid to connect more with each other.

It can also be that a group member tells something unusual or exceptional, which decreases understanding and interaction and leaves him or her isolated. In that case, the *de-isolation* verbal technique is the best way to get the interaction going again. By clarifying, discussing, and correcting the underlying reasons, sufficient space is often created for the interaction process to start flowing again. As this is about breaking a one-sided interaction pattern, the group therapist adopts a firm attitude when *broadening* or *de-isolating* the conversation: usually HELPING, occasionally even LEADING, but always in a questioning manner. Table 7.5 summarizes these technique combinations.

Table 7.5 Broadening one-sided interaction.

Verbal technique	Relationship technique (attitude and tone)
The group therapist *asks* others for recognition by *broadening* or *de-isolating*.	To break one-sided interaction, a firm and helping attitude is needed (HELPING/LEADING).
Example sentences – *broaden*: 'Do others also experience that tension before role-playing?' 'How do you experience that?' Example sentences – *de-isolate*: 'Do any of you sometimes experience the same as what Carl is telling us now?' 'Is Roxanne the only one who sees it that way?' 'Can any of you imagine feeling the way Rachel does?'	

Broadening one-sided interaction

In a support therapy group for parents with children born with Down syndrome, everyone repeatedly focuses on Becky. After the birth of her mentally challenged son, she was depressed for some time. She is now getting back on her feet but is still vulnerable and afraid that the depression might return. The group members are concerned and keep giving her tips and advice.

When the group therapist notices that she is overloaded with all this help, he intervenes (in a helpful tone): 'You have made yourself very clear, Becky. But I'm curious whether Becky is the only one who is sometimes gloomy or worries about herself and her child?' It is silent for a moment, but then Jessica answers: 'Actually, I have exactly the same thing as Becky. Maybe not the same depression as you had a month ago, but I worry a lot and often feel guilty.' Mark replies, 'I lie awake a lot because of it.' As several people talk about their sad feelings, the group therapist notices Becky looking surprised about the many others who can identify with her.

Using interaction strategically in fixed relationship patterns
It regularly occurs that a group member or a group becomes stuck in their own attitude and behavior. Such a fixed position is usually not very fruitful for the therapy group because it easily affirms relationship patterns that increase the inflexibility throughout the group. In such a situation, the group therapist can influence the relationship pattern by first realizing the relationship position of the particular group member or of the group in the IPC model. He then 'strategically' chooses the relationship position that does not confirm the attitude of the group member or group. Table 7.6 shows two examples of this strategic technique whereby the group therapist does not confirm the fixed relationship pattern.

Table 7.6 Influencing a fixed relationship.

Adopting a strategic behavior position to influence fixated behavior

Tip	Example
Do not react irritated (what is evoked) to an angry group member, but use a friendly disarming attitude and tone to maintain the relationship.	'You sound very angry, Richard. Sorry if I hurt your feelings. That wasn't my intention' (COOPERATING/HELPING)
Do not help or advise (what is evoked) a very dependent group member, but use a dependent position and tone yourself	'I don't have a ready solution on how to help you with that right now' (DEPENDENT)

7.5.5   Slowing down the interaction in a therapy group

Sometimes, the interaction does not flow the way you want it to. For example, interaction can take a wrong turn when group members discuss topics or do things that do not belong in the group at all. For example, a group member in a trauma therapy group shares extensively her trauma experiences in great detail, while the rule is to only mention the trauma in general terms, because of the risk of re-traumatization. In such a situation, the group therapist can best draw attention to the task again and explain to the group members once more what exactly is the purpose and the working method of the therapy group. This will often provide enough structure to stop unwanted interaction.

Other times, there might be too much (of the wrong) interaction, for example, nicknaming or blaming each other. The group therapist then has to intervene in a structuralizing way and slow down or stop the overstimulated interaction. He can reduce the excess interaction to a manageable level by using *structuring* and *limiting* verbal techniques. Agreed group rules, norms, and 'commonsense' standards are often useful criteria for the undesirable behavior. Shifting the focus to the more observant participants will result in tranquility and a detached, observing attitude in the group. This way, he helps to make strong emotions manageable again and helps the group refocus on the task at hand. The group therapist must be clear and directive and combine *structuring* verbal techniques with a firm LEADING attitude.

A tricky form of overly intense interaction is when two group members become intensely conflicted. I explain how the group therapist can manage such a conflict step by step in the troubleshooting guide at the back of the book. Table 7.7 summarizes the combination of techniques the group therapist can use to *limit* and *structure* the inappropriate interaction.

Table 7.7 Limiting and structuralizing overly intensive interaction.

Verbal technique In the case of inappropriate interaction, *explain* the task again and verbalize which behavior is inappropriate and must stop Get violent interaction to stop by setting clear boundaries (*limiting*) and then *inviting* an observing group member to participate	Relationship technique (attitude and tone) The group therapist maintains control with a directive attitude (LEADING).
Example sentences – *limit* and *structure*: 'Hang on, Matthew . . .' (in a soft tone and with a small nonverbal signal) 'Wait a minute, David. Let's finish this topic first . . .' 'Hey, Steven! You are rambling on.' 'We have to stop.' 'That's enough, Marian! We agreed not to discuss things like that here.' 'Stop, everyone. I'll explain to you how we can achieve more results from our working method.'	

Structuring and limiting interaction

A conflict in a protocolized therapy group for veterans with PTSS between Roy and Arkan is seriously escalating. Their conflict, a rivalry about who is the worst combat victim, is getting personal and running out of hand. When the two begin to call each other names, the group therapist intervenes: 'Hey, guys. I want you to stop this.' Once things have calmed down (in an energetically leading tone): 'Okay, what is your opinion, Megan? You've been quietly watching for a while.'

Exercises

Exercise: 'seeing interaction lines' for students in a group therapy training

1. Hand out the IPC model on paper with the description of the behavioral variants.
2. Ask a number of students to form an inner circle.

3. Assign a partner to each student in the inner circle. The partners form the outer circle.
4. The inner circle students each choose a random behavioral position from the IPC (leading, dependent, and so on) and discuss the corresponding behavior with their partner.
5. The inner circle students role-play a topic for about ten minutes (e.g., a press forum discussing cuts in health care or a group of politicians debating the usefulness of our monarchy), during which they emphatically display (especially nonverbally) the behavior chosen from the IPC.
6. The partners in the outer circle have a dual observation task: they write down which behavioral positions from the IPC they recognize in the various players. Additionally, they draw on paper the sociogram of interaction lines that they see developing between the role players.
7. Without discussion, the same inner and outer circle repeat exactly the same thing, only from newly chosen behavioral positions from IPC model.
8. In the post-discussion, all the participants exchange their observations of the recognized positions and examine how the interaction lines and patterns of the two role-plays differ. The players can share what differences they experienced in the two role-plays and which interactions they could feel in the first and second role-play.

Tool training: 'foster interaction with the connecting verbal technique' for students in a group therapy training

1. The students role-play a therapy group for people suffering from burnout. They role-play different health care professionals who have all stopped working due to their burnout. They all have personal problems such as not being able to say no, demanding too much of themselves, and wanting to do their best. Because of these pitfalls, they have become stuck in their work, resulting in burnout. The fictional burnout group has 20 meetings, and meeting four is now underway. The topic of the day is, Is the role in which you got stuck at work also recognizable in this burnout group?
2. Each student (or, if there is not enough time, a pair) acts as a group therapist for five minutes.
3. The practicing group therapist is instructed to only practice *connecting* verbal techniques (see Section 7.5.3) and not concern himself with the process. This involves two or three interventions.
4. After five minutes, the trainer interrupts the role-play, and the role-playing group members can give the practicing group therapist feedback on the *connecting* verbal technique. It is essential to note whether the practicing group therapist, repeating the message from A to B, called the names when connecting and used his arm(s) to indicate the line between interactors.

5. After about five minutes of feedback, the next student proceeds to play the role of a group therapist.
6. The role-play carries on. The member role-players are asked to play in such a way that the practicing group therapist is given sufficient material to try out the skills.

Note

1 The sociogram and its associated branch of science, sociometry, were conceived by group dynamics pioneer Jacob Moreno (1941).

Chapter 8

Group development in a therapy group

8.1 Introduction

This chapter focuses on the theoretical and practical knowledge about group development. This knowledge can help the group therapist discern whether the behavior in the therapy group says something about the participants individually or whether the behavior is related to the development of the group. Moreover, knowledge about group development provides tools to tailor interventions explicitly to the group's current development level (Robbertz and Wolters, in NVGP, 2019). The following topics are discussed:

- What is group development?
- Group development sources
- Recognizing group development: the Levine model
- Development stagnation
- Practical Manual: steering and utilizing group development in a therapy group

8.2 What is group development?

Anyone who has dealt with a group for some time knows from experience that there is never a standstill, but always movement. Old behaviors give way to new ones. Eventually, the group members we initially like become less interesting to us. Things that are important in the beginning disappear from the agenda after a while. At the same time, we experience how things in such a group become stable and structured. The uncertain probing at the start gives way to typical interaction patterns and fixed habits. Over time, the atmosphere in the group becomes more predictable and stable. What we are dealing with is what we call the *development of and in groups* or, in short, *group development*. With this, we mean the development of the group and the self-development of group members, which becomes visible in a group's changing phases, interaction patterns, and group dynamic structures (cohesion, norms, and roles; Forsyth, 2017; Nijstad, 2009). Group development is

DOI: 10.4324/9781003368786-11

universal for all groups, from soccer teams to charity societies and from book clubs to our therapy groups.

8.3 Group development sources

As I explained in Chapter 1, groups and group dynamics cannot be separated from our human nature and evolutionary origins. That is particularly applicable to group development. The formation and development of groups is originally a natural process that serves the function of the group as instrument for our (survival) goals (Brewer and Caporael, 2006; Dawkins, 2009; Durkin, 1981). By keeping evolution in mind, we can better understand and explain human group development and its sources.

Group development is a natural process

Development is a natural process that occurs spontaneously. Under ideal environmental conditions, a tree grows naturally, and a baby learns by itself how to crawl. It is the same with a group of people. If we have done the proper preparation and there are no hindering factors present during the group, a group will develop automatically and naturally. Development is locked into the group, in a manner of speaking.

However, because development is standard, we worry when it stagnates. The development of a group can stagnate, just like a toddler whose development progresses slower than naturally expected. For example, a therapy group may remain unusually inhibited and silent or display a persistent agitated atmosphere. That never simply happens; there are always reasons. We will return to this later on in this chapter.

Group and individual development go hand in hand

According to Levine (1979, 70),

> Social development is recapitulated in the course of therapy groups in two major ways. First, each and every member recapitulates his social development in the process of becoming an integral member of the group. Second, therapy group development itself parallels the ontogenetic development of individuals.

Group development in itself stimulates individual growth (Erikson, 1968; Schroder and Harvey, 1963, in Levine, 1979, 70). The broadening of possibilities and movement within the group stirs things up in individual group members and stimulates curiosity, discovery, and learning. Consider the sheer amount of cognitive and emotional information created during the development of a therapy group of eight participants.

Group development follows the laws of evolutionary theory: differentiation and integration

As evolutionary theory shows, all life develops from a state of simplicity and becomes more complex (Brewer and Caporael, 2006; Dawkins, 2009). This development involves two aspects. On the one hand, it is a *differentiation* process: the developing organism develops new functions and skills each time. On the other hand, these new functions within the organism become more and more structured and coordinated: the process of *integration*. Differentiation and integration characterize the development of plants, animals, and humans (Schroder and Harvey, 1963 in Levine, 1979, 70).

This development from simple to complex is also seen in natural social systems (Durkin, 1981). An ant colony initially forms only a small hill with two entrances but could develop into a sizable mountain with dozens of entrances wherein thousands of ants work together highly efficiently – integration – according to a complex division of tasks – differentiation (Wilson, 1975, in Goldsmidt, 2022).

It works the same way in human groups. The first group phenomena are simple: the interaction flows individually from each group member to the group therapist. Later, we observe a much more varied pattern in which some group members interact more than others. In short, group members start to do more, develop more of their own initiatives, take on new roles, and agree on new norms. So here, too, we see differentiation. At the same time, as a group develops, the patterns of interaction, norms, and roles become more established. This is the process of integration.

Group development progresses from dependent to independent

Life develops not only from simple to complex but also from small too big. Again, this applies to plants, animals, and humans. As babies, we depend on our caretakers because we cannot do many things yet, but as adults, we have so much skill, knowledge, and experience that we can manage just fine. We are independent (Erikson, 1968; Levine, 1979).

We see a similar development occurring in (therapy) groups. At the start, group members feel insecure. Consequently, they often adopt a dependent attitude toward the group therapist, conforming to her expectations. This solution is initially safe but becomes uncomfortable in the long run. Group members want to develop and spread their wings. Thus, the interaction toward the group therapist decreases while it increases between group members. The group therapist is needed less and less; the group has become independent. Such group development promotes individual development toward independence among group members.

Collaboration and interaction: the facilitating and stimulating factors for group development

Previously, in Chapter 6 on 'Cohesion' and Chapter 7 on 'Interaction' I mentioned the great importance of the 'jointness of the task principle' of Thye et al. (2014). In short, the more a group therapy method demands interactive collaboration (the 'jointness of the task'), the more it is likely that these collaborative relations become affective relations, that is, let cohesion come about.

Closely related is the older 'Interaction principle' of Homans (1966), which says that within a group that meets sufficiently, the participants will gradually start liking each other more and, therefore, want to get together more often. That will result in them enjoying each other's company even more and also wanting to meet more often.

These theories have implications for the organization of our therapy groups, which we elaborate on in the Practice Manual later in this chapter.

Each group develops a task-oriented cooperative structure

In Chapter 3, I described that a group always has a functional basis. That functional basis, the task and goals of a group, also provoke development (Tuckman, 1965). To execute the task well, a group typically develops a task-oriented cooperative structure. Once this has been established, a *workgroup* is formed. The *workgroup* is the mature stage of the group. The point at which the workgroup stage arises during group development is not the same in every group. Not every group's development can progress equally far; that impacts the phase the *workgroup* is at. Levine (1979) does not see the workgroup as a development phase itself. According to him, a workgroup can form during any phase.

Group development progresses and declines

Besides a group's natural *progression*, it also undergoes a natural *decline*. Like plants, animals, and individual humans, groups have an arc of life. First, development progresses until it reaches the mature stage. Then, after a certain amount of time, it regresses and comes to an end (Tuckman, 1965). In our therapy groups, that inevitable end of group life typically constitutes the end of treatment. It involves a process of evaluating, letting go, and separating. This phase of group development is often underestimated, but it is almost as important as the progression of development. In this chapter, I only discuss the development progression; the natural decline is discussed in Chapter 11.

Summary

- Group development is a natural development process of the group and group members, which becomes visible in the changing phases, interaction patterns, and group dynamic structures (cohesion, norms, and roles) of the group.
- Group development follows the laws of evolutionary theory: differentiation and integration and from dependent to independent.
- A working method with much interaction stimulates group development
- Group development stimulates individual learning.
- Every group develops a task-oriented cooperative structure.

Besides a group's natural progression, it also undergoes natural decline.

8.4   Recognizing group development: Levine's model

Theories on group development

Over the past decades, social scientists have developed several models to illustrate group development (Kuypers, 1986; Levine, 1979; Robbertz and Wolters, in NVGP, 2019). These models have many similarities: aspects like group formation, conflict, personal closeness, and separation are reflected as laws in almost every model, albeit using their own terms. But there are also differences. The distinction between *sequential* and *recurrent* development is an important factor in these models. Some authors see group development as a succession of clearly recognizable phases, hereby assuming a learning process in which a new phase can only begin when the previous one has been fully mastered (Kuypers, 1986). Other authors describe group development as a cyclical, repeating phenomenon with important themes recurring at a deeper level each time. A classic phase model is that of Bennis and Shepard (1956). The successive phases in this model are dependency, resistance, proximity, and termination, with each phase presenting a dilemma that must be resolved through compromise so that the next phase can commence. Tuckman's (1965) model is another frequently cited phase model with the terms: forming, storming, norming, performing, and adjourning (stopping). Unlike the other theorists, Tuckman explicitly includes the task aspect of a group (performing) as a developmental aspect.

The model developed by Schutz (1985), in which the themes of inclusion, control, and affection are repeated and deepened over and over again, is a well-known example of recurrent development. Whitaker and Lieberman (1964) also view group development as a cyclical deepening of essential interpersonal themes.

There exists no scientific validation about any model, or which model is the best. The complexity of the group development phenomenon and the many factors involved play a role in this (Dion, 2000). Scientific evidence of the development of distinct aspects, such as the change of interaction patterns and processes like cohesion, norms, and roles, has been found (Kuypers, 1986; Nijstad, 2009).

Group therapist Baruch Levine maintains a distinct position in this chorus of scholars. Levine (1979) developed his own integral model in which he ingeniously combined the major views on group development at the time. He combines sequential and cyclical development, clarifying how one phase can move on to the next. Cyclical development takes place in recurring thematic crises. Levine draws extensively on the knowledge of group dynamics and therefore ties in well with the contents of this book. His model describes the change processes of interaction, cohesion, norms, and roles, precisely the changes for which evidence has been found. For these reasons, Levine's model is the chosen model on group development of this book.

Levine's model: development phases and development crises

The *phase* and *crisis* concepts are central to his theory of group development. First, I discuss the development phase concept and then address the development crisis concept.

We define a development phase as *a relatively stable period of group functioning distinguished by a particular interaction structure*. The principles of development that I described at the beginning of this chapter are easily recognizable in the development throughout the phases. The interaction structure shows us that interaction with the group therapist decreases while it increases between group members. This reflects the development from dependent to independent. We can also see that the interaction structure changes from simple to complex. The interaction lines not only increase in number, but the interaction structure as such also becomes more complex.

Thereby, we will see that group dynamics phenomena, such as cohesion, norms, and roles, change along with the development of the phase. In each phase, these group dynamic phenomena have certain typical characteristics. Collectively, they form the group dynamic structure typical for that phase. Each phase is a leap forward, a developmental step upward.

1.   The parallel phase
The name of this phase stems from the dominant interaction pattern in the initial phase. All group members are equally related, in a *parallel* manner, to the group therapist. During the uncertain beginning of the group, members virtually do not interact with each other yet but do interact with the group therapist. The interaction is then almost exclusively between each individual group member and the

group therapist. The group members expect clarity and safety from her; she is the first person they bond with. Hence, she occupies a very central position in the group field. The scarce interactions between the members are mainly meant to see with whom they share similarities or have differences.

Therefore, the only cohesion that grows during this parallel phase is vertical cohesion, the attachment around the group therapist. Hardly any group norms exist during this phase because group members mainly adapt their behavior to what they assume the group therapist expects of them. Also, group members have not yet taken on group roles; they still occupy the familiar roles they use in their home situation.

2.   The inclusion phase

In this second phase, the *inclusion phase*, a group begins to take shape. This phase owes its name to the process of being *included, belonging*. As said before, inclusion is such a central human need that we always see this happen in group development. The group as a whole is not yet safe enough, so members first create subgroups to belong to. Subgroups of equals emerge naturally in terms of views on task and cooperation. Increasing intimacy develops within the subgroups. However, some distance and sometimes a power struggle exists between the subgroups, which could affect the future direction of the overall group. In this phase, the group therapist is no longer the central figure around whom all interaction revolves but still occupies a central position in the interactional field – she has contact with every subgroup and all singletons. With this inclusion phase as a necessary intermediate step, Levine had foresight. Later Thye et al. (2014) demonstrated that cohesion (group) development always runs bottom up, first in relations, then in subgroups, and at last in the whole group.

In terms of cohesion, the inclusion phase is primarily about acceptance and belonging. Acceptance and inclusion manifest themselves mainly in the subgroups and not yet in the whole group. Each subgroup consists of kindred spirits, the like-minded people with whom you belong. During this phase, small subcultures with unique subgroup norms cautiously emerge within the subgroups. One should not expect the whole group to agree on group norms during this phase because the different subgroups with their unique norms are still very significant. Therefore, group norms are by no means stable during the inclusion phase; they are still being negotiated. Likewise, the roles of the various group members have not yet been confirmed. As such, no crystallized division of roles in which everyone's place in the group is more or less clear has yet been established. In this phase, group members are still experimenting with roles. If certain roles do not seem to appeal to the other group members – because they do not lead to what this phase is all about, namely, *inclusion* in the group – they just as easily discard the roles and try out other roles. Besides seeking acceptance (inclusion), this phase allows participants to experiment with their behavior and position.

This necessary phase of subgrouping is more difficult in online group therapy, and that slows down group development in those therapy groups. There are certainly subgroups of like-minded people, but they cannot have informal contact from the sidelines as they can with the face-to-face therapy group, for example, in the waiting room or when leaving. Everything is collective on the screen. Some online group therapists therefore use the breakout room function to consciously create moments with subgroups to foster trust and development. See the following example.

The importance of subgroups in group development
In an online course on group dynamics, the topic 'Group Development' raised the question of how the course group itself had developed up to that point. After some discussion, the participants found out that there was no mutuality phase and possibly no inclusion phase. Because of the rather heterogeneous composition, cohesion formation was quite inhibited. During that conversation, we discovered something important: the usefulness of natural subgroup formation during coffee and break times. These cannot form during an online course, and this group regretted not having that opportunity. For me, this is proof that small groups of like-minded people are an essential phase in the development of a course, or therapy group.

3. The mutuality phase
If the group is able to do so, group interaction can develop into a completely open and reciprocal interaction structure. Anyone can interact with anyone. In the mutuality phase, group members have figured out among themselves what the essential group tasks are and how much personal contact and openness are required. It creates an extensive network of relationships in which everyone can be themselves and realistically work together on the task.

The group therapist no longer occupies a central position but instead moves to the periphery of the group. She is no longer needed in that central position due to the group's high level of independence. However, the group therapist still interacts with each group member and the group as a whole during this phase. Cohesion concerns the whole group. The norms are realistic and supportive of the task; roles are flexible and can be personalized.

4. The termination phase
In this phase, group members conclude their contact with each other and the group. They pause to evaluate the results, consider what they need after the group has terminated, and say goodbye to each other. The reverse process of attachment, *detachment*, occurs in this phase. Group cohesion decreases. Singletons and fleeting subgroups reappear. The intensity of the interaction lessens, and

the energy is directed toward group members' affairs outside the group. I return to this phase in detail in Chapter 11.

Levine's model: the development crises

In Levine's theory on group development, the development crisis is the second fundamental concept. Within his theory, a crisis is *a relatively unsettled period in which group members are focused on one specific development theme.* Levine distinguishes three different crises that all revolve around a universal human development theme: the *authority* crisis, the *intimacy* crisis, and the *separation* crisis. These crises also have a facilitating function in the transition from one phase to the next, but more on that later.

An *authority crisis* can occur when a group faces dilemmas regarding leadership and authority. An *intimacy crisis* can occur when a group suddenly faces issues or experiences dealing with closeness and personal openness. Similarly, a group may face experiences related to parting or loss, which will evoke a *separation crisis.*

Incidentally, it is important to know that a crisis does not always exist when authority, personal experience, or emotional loss are involved. We speak of a crisis only when the issue becomes so prominent that the whole group has to deal with it, meaning they must find a modus vivendi within the group before it can resume its normal course.

In group development, crises are *recurrent* (except in a new group – more on this later). This is in contrast to phases, which are *sequential.* A crisis can occur at any point in a group's existence and could recur. Each recurrence means that the associated theme is revisited and explored deeper.

According to Levine, crises are periods of *emotional conflict* around a central theme, when a *desire* and a *fear* clash. Group development may be an evolution-based natural process, but that does not mean that it is always a piece of cake for the individual members. Like more authors (Kuypers, 1986), Levine sees development as a dialectical process between two forces that must reach a synthesis, a solution. In any development crisis, that contradiction between desire and fear must be resolved with compromise.

Take, for example, the emotional conflict of the development theme, authority. It is quite normal for group members, in the course of their development within the group, to want to behave more freely and independently toward the group therapist. Yet they struggle to accomplish this. In fact, this desire for development simultaneously evokes fear: fear of displeasing the group therapist, sometimes even fear of being punished by the group therapist for 'unfaithful' behavior, but also fear of the responsibility inherent in the desired autonomy. Can we live up to this autonomy? What if we fail as a group? Each crisis comes with its own emotional conflict about the associated theme to which one seeks a solution together.

An intimacy crisis involves emotional conflict concerning the desire for greater familiarity and closeness in group members' interpersonal contact and the anxiety that this desire evokes. An intimacy crisis can arise, for example, as a result of confrontational feedback from one group member to another or when a group member suddenly shares a very profound life experience with the group. Such a personal interaction or profound experience forces group members to reflect on how they want to deal with closeness and intimacy. The better group members get to know each other, the stronger the desire for closeness (Homans, 1966). But this desired rapprochement evokes fear at the same time. For example, fear that the rapprochement will be oppressive or that more intimacy evokes feelings of shame or the fear of a loss of individuality and identity. It sometimes happens that a group member is very vulnerable and open too early in the development, for example, talks extensively about sexual problems, or confesses very honestly that he has committed a lot of shoplifting. If the group is not yet ready for this, then after such an outpouring there is often a painful defensive silence that often leads to shame for the person who brings it in.

A separation crisis occurs when themes such as stopping, parting, and loss become foregrounded in the group, such as when a beloved group member ends her group therapy or when participants suddenly realize there are only two sessions left. The imminent termination of the group evokes fear in group members that they might lose their safe place. Conversely, the desire arises to be able to let go, to be independent.

Both desire and fear represent an interest to group members. Responding to the *desires* in these conflicts means giving development opportunities a chance. Accommodating the *fears* means providing safety and security. This conflict of interest causes tension, for which group members seek a solution together. Finding a solution often takes time because group members must collectively find an acceptable compromise between this desire and anxiety.

If the solution is more responsive to the desire, we speak of an *enabling* solution.[1] Such a solution provides space for group development, leading to the deepening of interpersonal relationships and maturation in individuals. An enabling solution to an authority crisis, for example, means more daring and a freer attitude toward authority and, thus, more group autonomy.

If the solution responds more to fear, we refer to it as a *restrictive* solution. This solution gives the development limited space and primarily maintains the safe status quo. For example, a restrictive solution to an intimacy crisis results in caution with closeness and personal openness.

Regardless of whether an enabling or restrictive solution is chosen, they both have significant consequences for the further development of the group. In effect, agreed-upon group solutions become the group's opinions and norms regarding these important themes, thus determining the space for further deepening of the group therapy.

Development in a new group

The development in an entirely new group follows Levine's phases with a striking transitional function for the crises. A new group begins in the parallel phase. This progresses to the inclusion phase and successively to the mutuality and termination phases. Each phase has a relatively stable duration and structure. According to Levine's theory, the transitions between these individual relatively stable phases are triggered by the three crises discussed. These emotionally charged moments of instability bring about the disturbance of the balance needed to move the group to the next phase. The word 'crisis' here does not have a negative meaning but a positive one instead: a balance disruption that brings about change. During a crisis, the group becomes momentarily unstable, so to speak, after which a new structure becomes possible. A crisis is thus the impetus for development within a group and ensures the transition to the next, more mature phase.

The authority crisis appears as the first crisis at the end of the parallel phase. In this phase, group members make themselves dependent on the group therapist, but in the authority crisis, the relationship with her is challenged. The group members decide together how much autonomy they consider desirable in the relationship with the group therapist. The moment this is agreed upon, the authority crisis is resolved. Once the relationship with the group therapist – the *vertical* relationship – has become clear, attention shifts to the *horizontal* relationships – the cooperation among group members.

The authority crisis provides the transition from the parallel phase to the inclusion phase. In this phase, group members 'stick and lump together' into alternating subgroups. At this point, they are busy exploring and testing who they want and do not want to get closer to. At the end of the inclusion phase, the intimacy crisis occurs. In this crisis, group members agree over time on the degree of closeness they feel is appropriate for the entire group. The intimacy crisis acts as a transition from the inclusion phase to the mutuality phase, in which intensive mutual contact between all group members is possible.

The separation crisis occurs when the time has come for the group members to go their separate ways. In a closed and limited group, this becomes very apparent toward the end of the group. Realization of the imminent parting evokes not only separation anxiety but also the desire to dare to say goodbye and be independent. The separation crisis, and its resolution, act as a transition from the mutuality phase to the termination phase, the final phase in which the group can realistically deal with parting and ending.

It is important in the development of a new group that crises be resolved in the most enabling manner possible. With not too much fear and a helping therapist, members will more easily take a risk to go for an enabling solution. An enabling-resolved *authority* crisis promotes group member autonomy and group independence, while an enabling resolved *intimacy* crisis promotes openness and spontaneity of interactions among group members. These benefit (creative) cooperation among group members, which in turn benefits task performance. In the Practice Manual, I show how the group therapist can steer these influential moments for group development.

Table 8.1 Development in a new group.

Phase 1		Phase 2		Phase 3		Phase 4
	Transitional crisis 1		Transitional crisis 2		Transitional crisis 3	
Parallel phase	Authority crisis	Inclusion phase	Intimacy crisis	Mutual-ity phase	Separation crisis	Termina-tion phase

This development model may give the impression that development is incomplete until the mutuality phase has been reached. That is not entirely correct, as not every therapy group can reach or needs that phase. The *workgroup*, the phase in which the group functions optimally for task performance, can also occur in the inclusion phase or even as early as the parallel phase. Only in a limited number of therapy groups does the *workgroup* occur at the mutuality phase level. There are several reasons for this.

First, some target groups involve limited development opportunities. For example, adolescents with psychotic disorders have limited development opportunities regarding interaction and social contact. Groups for these patients will usually continue to function in the parallel phase. This is fine because you should not want or expect more from such groups: these groups naturally continue to require a great deal of guidance from the group therapist than what other groups do.

Second, external organizational factors affect the possibilities for group development. It is evident that a long-term group with a fixed composition will show more development than a group that ends quickly or in which the composition changes frequently. For example, a group in a psychiatric crisis unit will always remain in the parallel phase since the composition changes almost every day and, thus, in effect, is a new group every time.

Finally, the task required of the group also affects the development phase yet to be achieved. A group focused on education about a disease does not require much mutual personal interaction for task performance. As a result, the *workgroup* will function well in the parallel or inclusion phase and will not need to develop more.

Experiencing 'textbook' group development

Some years ago, I was affiliated with general practitioner training in the capacity of a behavioral scientist. The two-year training program consisted of an individual internship and an extensive education program. Each group had its weekly education day. The group was explicitly applied as a learning environment for that weekly education day.

Because the group and the safety within were considered to be of such importance, much attention was paid to group formation at the start of the training. Each new group of general practitioners in training initially went on retreat to a formation center for an introductory week to help the group develop into a safe tool. It was my job as a behavioral scientist to guide that process.

During those introductory weeks, all phases and crises transpired: the dependent and uncertain beginning of the parallel phase, my 'dethroning' during the authority crisis, the 'sticking together and lumping' of the subgroups during the inclusion phase and, without fail, an intimacy crisis at the end of the introductory week. This revealed the conflict between group members who wanted more personal exchange and the more 'businesslike' members, who believed that this was not a therapy group but a course group instead. Each group came up with its own compromise for this field of tension. A significant event concerning an individual group member was often decisive in this regard. When a group member broke the spell with a personal confession about his professional experiences, it often provided an extensive solution to the intimacy crisis. Other participants also became personal, thus establishing the 'personal' culture of the group. But the solution could also tilt in the opposite direction if, for example, a dominant group member strongly emphasized the importance of personal boundaries. At that point, that culture would subsequently become firmly established.

Development in an open, ongoing therapy group

Levine's development model described here evolved from observing closed groups with fixed compositions and a limited duration. Such groups usually show 'textbook' group development. Within the group therapy domain, we often encounter closed therapy groups such as a social skills therapy group or an educational therapy group. The phases and crises described in this chapter can often be easily recognized therein. But many therapy groups have been organized in an open and ongoing manner. The question then is, What does group development look like in an open group where the composition changes over time?

Typically, group development in an open group is less evident. Much depends on the duration and participant turnover of the group. After all, development needs time and stability. A long-term therapy group, in which new members join only occasionally, has sufficient stability for development. At most, the group will briefly regress to a previous phase when a new group member joins. If, due to certain circumstances, half of the group members are replaced at once, this will have a greater impact, and the group will regress further. In this case, we can say that a new group has been formed.

According to the strength of the group culture and the degree of autonomy of the remaining old group members, the therapy group will then resume development more quickly or more slowly. A group that changes frequently will always remain in the early stages of group development.

8.5   Development stagnation

Group development is a natural process. If the circumstances are favorable (clear task organization, good group selection and composition, and sufficient cohesion), the development will start automatically. Development is normal, but stagnation is not. However, it does happen that a therapy group's development stagnates.

Stagnation occurs when the therapy group remains stuck in a certain development phase when it could actually be moving forward. What we notice then is that the group structure does not change. The patterns repeat themselves; they start to bounce around. An important indicator is that attention to the task weakens and is drawn to the stagnant process development. As a result, group members lose motivation. Over time, a stagnant group will show typical symptoms, such as poor attendance and declining attachment and loyalty. Because group members are capable of more, there will almost certainly be dissatisfaction in the group. After all, group members' self-development is being hindered. As we have seen in earlier chapters, a group therapist perceives group processes not with reason but with her feelings and senses. The same applies to stagnant group development. Sometimes the stagnation is not immediately visible because it occurs below the surface. That is why it is important that the group therapist always has her 'feeling radar' turned on and dares to trust her intuition. If what is happening in the group feels off, it will be wise to take that indicator seriously and for her to first investigate what might be going on and then explore it together with the group.

The causes of group development stagnation may vary. One possible cause may be the group task. Often something is wrong with the logical structure of the task organization. For example, a group may stagnate because the group task does not sufficiently match the target group, or it turns out to be too difficult. Another vulnerable point is the selection and composition of the group. If the group members' help request varies too much, resulting in insufficient recognition, it can cause stagnation. Another possible cause of stagnation is the too frequent changing of group members, resulting in a lack of safety.

Something can also occur in the group process that has a blocking effect. For example, it may come to light over time that some group members, although they fit well within the target group, do not like each other. The resulting personal animosity and conflicts can increasingly paralyze a group. Severe psychopathology in vulnerable and complex personalities, scapegoating, secret alliances, passivity, or resistance in the group: such process phenomena can also block group development. All attention is then drawn to these process phenomena.

The severity of stagnation in a group can vary. A low degree of stagnation will allow the group therapist to discuss it with the group in a meta-conversation with not too much difficulty (see Chapter 5). In retrospect, such an exercise is often perceived as instructive, as the group succeeded in solving a problem together. The stagnation can also take on a much more severe form resulting in a negative development. Then, the destructive and disintegrating processes are so strong that the group can easily fall apart. The group therapist must then pull out all the stops to reverse the negative process. Experience shows that this does not always work. Sometimes, the reality is that a group will fall apart or must be disbanded in order to limit the damage to group members.

Summary

- Levine's model has four sequential phases: the *parallel phase*, the *inclusion phase*, the *mutuality phase*, and the *termination phase*, and three recurring crises: the *authority crisis*, the *intimacy crisis*, and the *separation crisis.*
- The crises are the engine of development for groups and group members; they provide the transition from one phase to the next. The recurring crises ensure deepening of the authority, intimacy, and separation themes.
- Each of the phases has its own distinctive group dynamic structure.
- In a closed group, phases and crises are often more observable than in an open group.
- The *workgroup* can occur during any phase, depending on the target group.
- Group development can stagnate during any of the phases due to a variety of reasons.
- In online therapy groups, group development is slower, partly because natural subgroups are more difficult to form.

8.6   Practical Manual: steering and utilizing group development in a therapy group

8.6.1   Introduction

Under favorable conditions, group development occurs naturally. The group therapist can co-steer that natural process before and during the group. To do so, she uses the now familiar three techniques: organization techniques, verbal techniques, and relationship techniques.

Shortly, I discuss all the phases and crises and show the techniques the group therapist can use. The group therapist has the most influence at the beginning because group development is still open. She can facilitate group development, especially during the *parallel phase* and *authority crisis*. Therefore, I pay extra attention to that phase and crisis. Finally, I address how the group therapist can influence stagnant development of a group.

8.6.2   Fostering group development in advance

The group therapist has a big potential to create (organize) favorable conditions for group development. Group development is one of the group dynamic processes, and is related to the other group dynamic processes. Cohesion and interaction are the key factors to take into account. The prior organizational conditions for group development are exactly the same as those for promoting cohesion (and interaction). Let me list them again:

- A clear task organization with concrete goals appropriate to the target group
- Especially important in the task organization: enough collaboration and interaction in the working method (the 'jointness' of the task). I mentioned these conditions for cohesion and interaction development previously (see the 'joint task' principle of Thye et al., and Homans's Interaction principles in Section 8.3 of this chapter)
- The proper composition of the therapy group
- An adequate group size
- Duration and stability of the group
- Clear group rules

This means that when organizing the group, the group therapist should use a working method with a lot of interactive collaboration, schedule the sessions with short intervals in between, avoid changing group members too soon, organize a sufficient number of sessions to allow group members adequate time to attach to each other. The exact tailoring of these points depends on the target group and the group task.

8.6.3   *Fostering the development of an ongoing therapy group*

Parallel phase
In the parallel phase, group members are all focused on the group therapist, and there is no group structure as yet. Group members have a great need for clarity and safety, for a sense of belonging. Everything is still open, and the group therapist has a lot of influence. That is why this initial phase is so suitable for promoting development. The onset of group development coincides with cohesion development. The first cohesion that occurs revolves around the group therapist, which corresponds to the parallel relationship structure in this first phase. When it comes to promoting group development at the beginning, the same applies as when promoting cohesion at the start of a group.

In summary, the group therapist can foster group development in the parallel phase in two ways: first, by regularly (especially in the very beginning) explaining the task with a 'pitch' and connecting it to what group members contribute and, second, by fostering group dynamic processes, the spontaneous feelings and thoughts of group members, by welcoming them and, when appropriate, connecting them to the group task. I briefly explain both of these technical actions.

Explaining the task and connecting it to what concerns group members
Group members attend because of the task. The task is an important anchor in the ambiguity that often prevails at the start of a group. Therefore, in the parallel phase, it is developmentally beneficial to explain the task regularly and connect it to the spontaneous feelings and thoughts (group dynamic processes) that group members put forward (in the following example, the group therapist connects a group member's spontaneously introduced experience to the task). She explains the task using the *explaining* and *connecting* verbal techniques. Because the group therapist initiates this explanation to group members, she does so with a somewhat directive attitude (HELPING). Table 8.2 summarizes this technique and illustrates it with an example.

Table 8.2 Fostering group development in parallel phase I.

Verbal technique	Relationship technique (attitude and tone)
The group therapist *explains* the task at appropriate times. At other times, she *connects* the task and the thoughts or feelings group members express.	As the group therapist explains the task, she demonstrates an active and helping attitude (HELPING).

Explaining the task and connecting it with the members' experiences

In the third session of an emotion regulation group therapy, Kimberly says she still does not quite understand the objective. The group therapist welcomes the question and then explains the purpose and task again. Group therapist: 'It is quite normal that the way we work here is not immediately clear to you, Kimberly. It takes a while to get the hang of group therapy. The most important goal of this group is that you learn to better control your emotions when they get out of hand but also understand them and learn to effectively express them. From you as participants, I expect that you share moments when your emotions were not under control but also that you read the information we hand out at home and do the exercises we prepare in each session. All with the aim of learning to handle your emotions better.' Kimberly: 'Okay, I figured it was something like that, but I wasn't sure. Thank you for explaining it again.'

Foster group dynamic processes, spontaneous feelings, and thoughts by welcoming them

Because group members are very uncertain in the beginning about their place in the group (do I belong? Am I out of place here? Am I the only one without a partner?), *acceptance* (as I called it in Chapter 6), is the most important development aspect for the group therapist to promote. Since the group therapist is the primary source in the parallel phase, that acceptance must primarily come from her. The group therapist accepts the group members by inviting them by *giving space with silence* and by *mirroring* their verbal messages in a questioning manner at appropriate times. In doing so, she may readily sound convincing and express a helping attitude (HELPING/COOPERATING). This is done exactly the same way as promoting cohesion in a beginning group. Table 8.3 summarizes this technique and is illustrated with an example.

Table 8.3 Fostering group development in parallel phase II.

Verbal technique	Relationship technique (attitude and tone)
The group therapist focuses her attention on a group member who presents something and questioningly *mirrors* their words as precisely as possible. The group therapist alternates the aforementioned technique with *giving space with silence*.	As the group therapist mirrors, she demonstrates a persuasive and accepting attitude toward the individual (HELPING/COOPERATING). The best thing for the group therapist to do when she is silent is to lean back quietly and look at the group (monitor) in a friendly manner (COOPERATING).

Mirroring with a questioning attitude and giving space with silence

At the beginning of the second session of a structured therapy group for traumatized refugees, living in the Netherlands for several years, the group therapist asks the participants what they thought of the first session. She receives a few cautious reactions. Aleksandr says he still feels anxious about being in a group with strangers. Musa says he is not looking forward to the sessions to come because of the trauma story of Tatiana in the first session. He experienced flashbacks of his own brutal experiences from the time he lived in Syria. The group therapist realizes the delicacy and vulnerability of this group and the importance of safety and cohesion. She mirrors the different feelings: 'Aleksandr, am I correct in saying that you feel anxious because you don't know the others yet?' Aleksandr: 'Yes, I always have that with strangers. I clam up.' Group therapist: 'Right, and you, Musa? You are not looking forward to the coming sessions because Tatiana's sad story overwhelmed you too much. Is that correct?' Musa: 'Yes, that's right. I was very anxious and upset after the first meeting.'

Anna: 'I was shocked too, but if we can't tell our story here, where can we?' Group therapist: 'Do I understand correctly Anna, that you think it's important that we have to give your trauma experiences a place here, because it can't be done anywhere else?' Anna: 'Yes exactly, and that's what this group is for?' Group therapist: 'And because you believe that this group is meant for that.' Anna: 'Definitely.' Elena: 'But I also understand Musa, it can be so intense that we are traumatized again, you (she looks at the therapist) call that the 'window of tolerance.' Group therapist: 'Do I understand you correctly Elena, that you think it is wise to build in safety in our exchange so that we stay within our 'window of tolerance'?'

Then the group talks about the rules of the game in order to be able to talk about each other's experiences but also to take each other's 'window of tolerance' into account.

Authority crisis

Crises are the engine of development. They are short-lived periods of emotional conflict that, if resolved through enabling, provide an impetus for deepening and unfolding. In a beginning group, crises also function as transitional moments between phases. The solutions to the crises have far-reaching consequences for the group's further development. They become the group norm about the corresponding issue. An enabling solution provides many development opportunities, while a restrictive solution does not. So crises are vital moments for group development and, therefore, important starting points for the group therapist to apply influence. She can help the group extensively resolve the crises. 'Pushing' a group toward an enabling solution is not the most effective technique here. The group therapist will have to take into account the group members' fears and will be more successful if she manages to reduce them.

In the authority crisis, the group therapist's activity is especially important, because it pertains to her position. If she manages not to react defensively, this crisis can be a very influential moment for her in the group's development. Of course that's a challenge. When the group members' desire for autonomy emerges at the end of the parallel phase, it clashes with the (perceived) position of the group therapist up to that point. In the group members' perception, the group therapist is the absolute authority. But from the moment they desire more independence, they feel like that authority is holding them back. Some group members rebel against the group therapist in an effort to break free from her reins. Others are disappointed in the group therapist because she has not lived up to their expectations. For these group members, the group therapist has fallen off her throne. Reason enough to challenge, criticize, undermine, or strip the group therapist of her power. This takes courage and bravery on both sides. Group members find it very daunting to attack authority. The group therapist, in turn, needs resilience to endure the criticism and to react appropriately.

The most natural response that group members' behaviors evoke in the group therapist is to get defensive or even counterattack (IPC: Distant/Counter evokes Distant/Counter). These responses backfire. They lead either to a fruitless power struggle between the group and the therapist or to the startled withdrawal of group members. The members subsequently do not dare stick their necks out again and prefer to huddle together in an underground resistance alliance or a position of docile dependency. In this case, the group and group therapist have resolved the authority crisis restrictively. As a result, the group therapist has an unpleasant group to work with.

How can the group therapist approach and handle the 'mutiny' so that an enabling resolution becomes possible? First, it is important for her to realize that group members' critical expressions and attitudes come from an authority crisis. And that this is a healthy rebellion that leads to emancipation and autonomy and, thus, to a much more pleasant cooperation. The group therapist should not take such messages literally but regard them as a *developmental phenomenon*. The authority crisis can be seen as transference from the group to the therapist, who is experienced as a strict mother or father. This realization helps put the overly critical messages into perspective. Subsequently, it is important that the group therapist can suppress her natural tendency to defend herself and instead allow the criticism, help to clarify it, and take the *message* from the group members seriously.

Out of fear, group members do not always address authority directly. Therefore, they often indirectly criticize the group therapist, for example, by complaining about the group's methods not helping or by disqualifying bosses in general. It helps when the group therapist regularly, actively, and openly seeks out criticism meant for her ('Are you perhaps referring to me?' 'Isn't that message actually meant for me?'). Naturally, this is not easy, but every group therapist can learn this by daring to do it. It is precisely then that group members feel their essential message has been heard and recognized. That is the moment when they floor and dethrone the group leader. The very act of listening to and openly acknowledging the affect, the anger, and the dissatisfaction about her functioning (incidentally, this is not the same as agreeing with everything the critical group members say) contributes to the creation of an enabling resolution of the authority crisis.

How can the group therapist use the technique in this regard? If the group therapist wants to welcome group criticism, the best thing she can do is *mirror* all those messages, especially the angry or rebellious feelings in them. If group members address a direct or indirect message to the group therapist, she can then name this line of interaction with the *connecting* verbal technique and thus interact with the group members. Because an authority crisis is a moment of heightened emotional tension in the group, such an episode requires an active attitude on the part of the group therapist. By doing so, she demonstrates that she can handle this relational situation and stand up to scrutiny, which reduces anxiety. Because the group therapist is under attack as an authority, an overly directive attitude will not be appropriate. A clear Under attitude (COOPERATING) fits best.

Furthermore, as a group therapist during an authority crisis, it is important to not get 'floored' completely and to stand firm as a participant. She does not have to accept too much abusive or unfair criticism, for example. The group members need some authority they can challenge. As mentioned, hearing and understanding criticism is different from agreeing with group members.

When the peak of the authority crisis is over, more space is sometimes created to realistically consider the group's criticism. Sometimes the group may have a point, or perhaps they would like to do things a little differently than what the group therapist is used to. Then the therapist can accommodate the group, for example, by adjusting the working method. The group members experience this as 'sharing the power.' In essence, an authority crisis is about expressing anger and being heard. The group therapist does not always have to make genuine concessions. Usually, the criticism disappears before the next session, and the group's attention has shifted from the group therapist to the group members among themselves. The group therapist notices this due to the completely different atmosphere. The group increasingly takes the lead, which indicates that the group has resolved the authority crisis and moved into the inclusion phase. Table 8.4 illustrates a summary of this technique and provides an example.

Table 8.4 Fostering group development during an authority crisis.

Verbal technique	Relationship technique (attitude and tone)
The group therapist affirmatively *mirrors* the group members' direct or indirect critical statements, specially the affects. The group therapist draws the criticism to herself with the verbal technique of *connecting*.	In handling the crisis and facing the rebellious group members openly, an active, accommodating attitude is appropriate (COOPERATING).

Confirming criticism through mirroring and connecting it to yourself as group therapist

During the fourth session of a protocolized group therapy for people with a borderline personality disorder, the group therapist is waiting until everybody is present. Normally she starts at the usual starting time, but in this case she waits because it seems like a bad habit is emerging. In the first three meetings there were always two or three members more than ten minutes late. When everybody has arrived she decides to discuss the late arrival. 'What strikes me is that people are always late, and that makes me concerned about our cooperation. Do you recognize that?' the group therapist asks. Joshua replies, 'To be honest, I really have no use for this therapy at all!' Betty concurs with him: 'I feel the same way. I've had group therapy like this before, but that was much harder; we were forced to confront our issues. But that doesn't happen here at all.' Group therapist: 'Betty, do you think I am being too cautious, that I should be tougher on you?' Betty: 'Well, I'm sorry, but I think you are much too soft.' Group therapist: 'What do the others think of the therapy? And my approach? Do you think I am too soft? Should I be tougher?' Lisa: 'I get a lot out of it, but I find some exercises too slow as well. You could speed things up a bit as far as I'm concerned.' Kevin (smirking): 'I think you are still old school with your soft approach.' 'She can't help it,' says Emily, laughing. 'Because she is often late herself.' Group Therapist: 'That last comment is incorrect, Emily, I am on time every session. But the message I am getting from you is that you are not satisfied with the working method, that it could be tougher, and that I should confront you more. Well, I'll think about that and revisit the issue at our next session.'

The next session. Group therapist: 'I thought about our last session and plan to use a different approach with you and . . . ' Joshua interrupts her: 'Do we really have to talk about our last session again? I totally have other things on my mind because I had a rough week and would like to talk about that.' 'What happened, Joshua?' Lisa asks. Joshua: 'Actually, what happened is pretty good too. I finally told my boss what I thought of his attitude, and he took me seriously!' 'Good on you, Joshua,' says Jeff. 'I have a boss like that, too, and I . . .'

We do not always see such an evident authority crisis as the one previously. An authority crisis – like any crisis – can also occur quite unobtrusively. Sometimes an authority crisis is nothing more than a critical remark about the group task. Other times, as in the previous example, it can become quite a spectacle.

The inclusion phase
In this phase, group members take the time and effort to really get to know each other. Because safety has not yet been established in the whole group, a few subgroups form initially – small groups of like-minded people with the same opinions and experiences. The main feature of this phase (beyond the subgroup formation) is intensive interactive activities. After all, participants want to get to know and figure out each other. With about eight group members, this is a challenging interactive task. They discuss and negotiate task performance and how group members would want to cooperate during the process.

During this phase, it is evident that fostering interaction aids group development. During the inclusion phase, the group therapist functions as an 'interaction helper.' She is also a 'translator' of messages between subgroups and among group members. She applies interactive verbal techniques, especially *connecting*, but also *broadening, questioning, exploring*, and *deepening*. Because the group members are still cautious in approaching each other, an active, supportive attitude is appropriate in this phase (HELPING).

Intimacy crisis
If the inclusion is successful, at some point, the question, 'How personally and intimately should and do we want to work together in this group?' arises. Not all therapy groups will reach such an intimacy crisis. It requires maturation and a not too vulnerable personality of the individual group members. Not all clients have these characteristics. When an intimacy crisis does occur, we see vigorous discussions and negotiations, often between two parties or their spokespersons. One party's view is that it doesn't all have to be so personal; the other finds it enjoyable and necessary to become more personal about oneself.

In this crisis, the group therapist does not have to be as active as during the authority crisis. The group members can and do a lot independently and want to resolve it themselves. Therefore, it is imperative that the group therapist initially leaves her own opinion or desire out of the discussion. The group members are independent enough to figure it out for themselves. So how can the group therapist help? By *mirroring, connecting*, and *helping* to clarify the interaction – nothing more. It requires a more supportive attitude (COOPERATING).

A time when the group therapist does need to be proactive is when a restrictive solution threatens to arise, which will not be beneficial to the performance of the group task. For example, if in a recently started intensive interactional group psychotherapy, an intimacy crisis is resolved by concluding that mutual criticism does not suit the group, this will not benefit the task performance. Because in such a therapy group, critical openness is necessary for the group members' learning process. The task cannot be accomplished without this. At such a time, the group therapist must be alert and intervene before the decision-making process is complete. She must prevent such an undesirable resolution by blocking the decision-making process and making it negotiable. The group therapist then steers the verbal interaction in the group with a series of investigative and confrontational verbal techniques, such as *questioning, exploring, explaining, confronting*, and *convincing*. A directive attitude is necessary given the importance of and need for active direction (LEADING).

An intimacy crisis or too early intimacy

In a new group therapy for young adolescents with gender identity issues, an inhibited atmosphere prevails. A number of participants are still struggling with their sexual identity, while others feel more secure about their transition. Because of the uncertainty and shame, the participants often keep their worries and questions to themselves. Recently, Kim joined, a vibrant transgender who recently embraced a female identity. She is on the waiting list for gender surgery that she is very dreading about. She often suffers from depressive and anxious moments, but sometimes she is very spontaneous and open. In one of the sessions, she talks extensively and in detail about a sexual adventure with a woman that makes her doubt her transition again. She is curious about how the others deal with sex, but she doesn't get an answer to that question. The group is startled by her intimate questions and withdraws. The group therapist tries to keep the conversation about intimacy on the table, and to discuss the fear of it. Group therapist: 'You are very clear about your experiences, Kim, and about the search for yourself. Apparently, your sexual adventure has raised a lot of questions for you this week, and that's why you would like it if others would also share their experience with intimacy, is that right?' Kim: 'Yes, indeed, that's why we're in this group, isn't it?' Group therapist: 'Certainly, but I also see that a number of people are startled by your invitation. . . . May I ask what scares you so much?' Rachel: 'I just find it difficult to talk about those things, maybe because I still have doubts, but also because it's so close, I'm ashamed of myself.' (looks down) Group therapist: 'How good Rachel that you dare to share how scary it is to talk about these things . . . What's that like for the others?' In the following sessions the group opens up slowly, step by step.

Mutuality phase

A group in this phase has a high degree of independence and internal freedom. The group therapist can leave a lot to the group. Relationships and interactions have a degree of reciprocity and mutual affirmation that feels special to many group members. For a lot of clients, the corresponding safety, closeness, and belonging is quite unique. It creates many opportunities for group members to have new learning experiences. The group therapist will focus on task performance with group members during this phase. She can make use of all verbal techniques in the process. Because the group possesses a high degree of independence and cooperation, the group therapist will often use cooperative techniques such as *connecting, broadening*, and *deepening* and show a HELPING/COOPERATING attitude.

As I wrote earlier in this chapter, not every therapy group must or can reach this stage. For some target groups, the extensive openness and closeness is too delicate. One should always take into account the window of tolerance of the clients. For example, a group therapy for people with severe PTSS symptoms will be overloaded with too much closeness and proximity. With those target groups, the group therapist must continue providing more structure for the group task. Her attitude will continue to be more guiding and directive. She will have to accept that the inclusion phase, with occasional interpersonal closeness, is best suited.

I discuss the next crisis, the separation crisis, and the group's final phase, the termination phase, separately in Chapter 11.

8.6.4   Eliminating development stagnation in a therapy group

If the therapy group remains stuck in a particular development phase when it should be able to move forward, stagnation has occurred. What we observe then is that the group structure does not change. Patterns continue to repeat themselves. Because group members are capable of more, dissatisfaction will arise in the group. After all, the participants are inhibited in their own development. An important indicator here is that attention to the task weakens and is drawn to the stagnant process development. What can the group therapist do to eliminate the stagnation?

She can apply the same recipe as when dealing with poor cohesion formation (see Chapter 6). First, she can make an effort to stimulate the group again to get it going. If that fails, she should halt the task and initiate a meta-conversation (see Chapter 5). That means halting the task temporarily and discussing the identified developmental stagnation with group members. If they share her concern, the underlying reasons can be explored together. Those reasons can be anything, as we saw in Section 8.5.

The group therapist uses active verbal techniques for this intervention, such as *questioning*, *confronting*, and *exploring* but also *mirroring* and *connecting* techniques. Because of the urgency – after all, the group therapist does not want the stagnation to continue for too long – she usually shows an active LEADING and HELPING attitude in the process.

Explore and eliminate stagnation

In one of my newly started therapy groups, a very evident stagnation soon occurred. I felt the stagnation. The group felt 'distant,' closed, and inhibited, and I struggled to connect with group members. After renewed explanations of the group task and inviting and encouraging participation had no effect, I halted the task and shared and discussed my impression with the group. The following happened.

Lanelle (fictitious names): 'I recognize what you are saying, Willem. I feel like I have to tread very carefully.' 'I feel like that, too,' Michael adds. And more people appear to be experiencing that feeling of having to be cautious. 'Why do you think this is happening?' I ask. Becky replies: 'I think you are the reason, Willem. You once said that the intention was not to criticize, which has made me very cautious. In fact, sometimes I do feel critical or dissatisfied about how things are going here.'

A sense of surprise overwhelms me, which I immediately share: 'Did I say that? Where did you get that from, Becky?' It turns out that Becky is not the only one who has taken my explanation of the group rule 'respect each other as individuals' as a prohibition against criticism. After I explained that I did not mean it that way and that criticism, also of me as group therapist, is perfectly normal, I observed noticeable relief wash over the group. Subsequently, several critical comments about the therapy come to light, which are taken seriously and discussed. After that, the stagnation was eliminated, and the group progressed much better.

Note

1 The concepts *enabling* or *restrictive* solution we find in Levine's theory implicitly but not explicitly. This terminology originates from the Focal Conflict Theory by Whitaker and Lieberman (1964), also a dialectical model of group development.

Chapter 9

Group norms and social influence in a therapy group

9.1 Introduction

In Part 3, I follow the development of the therapy group. I first focused on cohesion and interaction, in which group formation is paramount. The previous chapter focused on group development. I demonstrated how, in the course of development, group dynamics become structured. The longer a group exists, the more regular and predictable the group processes become. Together with the task organization, those group processes ensure the functioning and survival of the group. Norms and roles are the most important parts of that group dynamic structure. This chapter deals with norms and their function in a therapy group.

The following topics are covered:

- Group norms
- The function of group norms in group therapy
- The origin and development of group norms: social influence and group culture
- Norms in a therapy group: collective structure and individual space
- The special nature and vulnerability of therapeutic norms
- Practical Manual: utilizing group norms in a therapy group
- Exercises

9.2 Group norms

What are group norms?

When we observe a therapy group, we see that members' reactions toward one another are usually not neutral. Some things they say to each other are rejected, while other expressions are welcomed. Sometimes, the whole group enthusiastically agrees on a particular opinion, but at other times, they fervently negotiate on what is considered proper or improper behavior. If we broaden our view, we will see differences between the groups. Behavior that one therapy group does

DOI: 10.4324/9781003368786-12

not condone might be considered acceptable by another group. For example, in one group, it's okay to be a few minutes late, while another group makes a big fuss about it. Interaction between group members is subject to various informal rules. In group dynamics, we call this phenomenon *group norms*.

A group norm is a common opinion of what is considered appropriate and inappropriate behavior in a particular group situation (Hoijtink, 2001). This view is always accompanied by an underlying reason why this behavior is or is not considered desirable. We call that reason the *content* of a norm. For example, the group norm of calling each other by their first name has as its underlying reason the idea that, when doing so, it promotes mutual familiarity. When discussing the desirability of certain behaviors, we must broadly interpret the term 'behavior.' A group norm guides not only concrete behaviors but, as social psychologist Festinger (1950) observed back then, also beliefs, opinions, and views. The norm in a male therapy group, for example, may be 'men are strong; they do not show feelings because that is a sign of weakness.'

The appropriate norm behavior is rewarded by the group with positive attention to the person in question or with appreciation for their point of view or feelings. This is done openly but often also in various subtle, nonverbal ways. For example, a group member who acts very cooperatively in the group will usually receive positive appreciation, that is, through friendly responses, lots of eye contact, and affirmative nods.

The group punishes inappropriate behavior with sanctions such as disapproval, ignoring, loss of status, and exclusion. For example, in most groups, making fun of someone with a disability is simply *not done*. A group member who engages in such behavior can expect to be openly and severely rebuked. A group norm is a *shared* opinion, a collective structure at *group level*. A group norm exists when the entire group (or a large majority) supports it. If a group therapist wants to deal with a group norm, he will have to engage and influence the whole group. Group norms also have consequences at the individual level. Namely, they can make a group member stop certain (deviant) behavior or – conversely – make a group member conform to desired behavior (Schachter, 1951, in Nijstad, 2009, 24–25).

A prescriptive behavioral norm

In a forensic psychiatric clinic, a group patient examines the background of each person's offense behavior in the offense scenario therapy group. The task of that group is to identify for each member the reasons why they committed the crime: what emotions and circumstances triggered them and could possibly pose a risk of future recurrence. Tyler hates this group therapy because it is very confrontational. While everyone else has already opened up, Tyler has managed to avoid his turn until now.

However, the group no longer accepts this. The group reacts very strongly when it appears Tyler has forgotten his scenario for the umpteenth time. 'What are you even doing here, man?' Mark angrily asks. After many group members had joined in with Mark, Christofer tells Tyler in a somewhat friendlier tone, 'Just *do* it, Tyler. It's honestly not that bad, you'll see. We all have to deal with it, and so do you. So go get your thing and read it!' 'Okay, okay,' Tyler says and meekly walks to his room to fetch his offense scenario script.

Explicit and implicit group norms

Some group norms, including their underlying reasons, are discussed openly in the group. We call these *explicit* norms. Other norms – with possibly an equally strong influence – are more hidden in the group's everyday habits. We call those *implicit* norms.

An implicit norm is like an iceberg – most of it is hidden below the surface and thus cannot be observed. The behavior is visible and familiar to everyone, but the underlying reason has often become submerged. Implicit norms can also be called habitual behavior. Group members become aware of them only when that habitual behavior is addressed. For example, consider a group of colleagues at the hospital who, after work, see each other in the gym. They always have coffee together before the workout, until a new group member suggests to drink coffee not before but after the meeting because it's not very pleasant to exercise with coffee in your stomach. A discussion ensues, and group members then realize that 'coffee before' has become a habit, an implicit norm that had established itself at some point. Further in this chapter, I will show how the group therapist can use the difference between implicit and explicit norms when influencing group norms.

Group norms and group rules

Norms are different from rules. Rules are the *formal* work agreements in a group. They are part of the task organization, in which they are usually set out in writing. The intricate cooperation in a group cannot function without rules. For example, most therapy groups have formal rules about confidentiality, arriving on time, or doing homework as part of the task. The group therapist who takes his group task seriously does his best to establish those rules as norms. But that is by no means a given. As we all know, groups do not always follow rules. A rule is imposed or agreed upon in advance and *may or may not* become a group norm. In contrast, a group norm develops spontaneously. A group therapist can never impose a norm. However, he can deem a particular norm desirable and try to convince the group of its importance. Ultimately, with their mutual dynamics, the group members determine which behavior becomes a norm.

It often happens that spontaneously developing norms become distinguishable from official group rules, resulting in group members experiencing norm conflicts. Take, for example, an addiction clinic where some residents secretly consume alcohol at night. During the day, all the residents who know about the secret will feel the tension of the norm conflict.

9.3   The function of group norms in a therapy group

Norms, the shared beliefs about what is considered appropriate behavior, arise because groups need a 'group standard' (Festinger, 1950). In other words, a certain equality of thought and action to function. We can understand this by realizing that groups have an evolutionary origin. Clear and predictable behavior in our human history increased the survival rate of the group, and that still holds true today. Take a dramatic group situation. It is a known fact that a group that unexpectedly finds itself in life-threatening circumstances will quickly agree on what to do to survive. For example, in the early days of the dangerous COVID-19 crisis, we saw that the social-distancing rule proposed by the government quickly became the 'norm.'

Even under less extreme circumstances, norms have the function of ensuring group purpose and group survival. Cartwright and Zander (1968, in Hoijtink, 2001), divide that functionality into the following five sub-functions:

Group norms foster group task performance

The main function of group norms is that they keep the group on task by rewarding desired task behavior. An intensive interactional psychotherapy group in which the task of 'giving each other honest feedback' has genuinely become a norm is more likely to produce results than a similar therapy group in which that norm is absent. Because they are so essential, each group therapist will use his influence to allow task-oriented norms to develop.

Group norms ensure the preservation of the group

Another important key function of group norms is that they support the conditions for group functioning. Take, for example, attendance. Being present and arriving on time seems to be simple and obvious agreements, but those behaviors are often not the norm in a therapy group. Everyone has experienced groups where some members regularly arrive late. That could be a sign that 'arriving on time' has not become the norm, which can cause more and more members to come late. A group therapist who has experienced groups with many absences knows how it can undermine the task and atmosphere of the group. Of course, a member may be unable to attend occasionally, but the group therapist must be vigilant of regular occurrences of absence. If he senses that an increase in absence is becoming a habit, he should actively challenge that norm in a meta-conversation, remember the group of their attendance commitment, and explain and convince the members about the importance of attendance.

In addition to attendance, safety is an important condition for the functioning of a therapy group. Therefore, it is desirable that group norms such as respect for each group member as a person and for their privacy are established. Because these are such vital group conditions, many groups agree on them in advance to be group *rules*, hoping they will become group *norms*.

Group norms provide clarity about appropriate behavior

Norms, by definition, lead to standardization, which is useful for routine social situations. You then don't have to agree anew each time on 'how we will behave.' In this kind of situation, norms provide the codes of conduct and etiquette about what is and is not appropriate. Every group has a unique set of norms; these are not yet clear to a new group member. It usually does not take long before a new member realizes that he or she is doing something that is inappropriate. Suppose a group has a habit (norm) of dressing neatly, even in hot weather; typically, a newcomer who shows up wearing flip-flops and shorts on a warm summer day will not do so again.

Group norms help interpret social reality

Norms provide a framework for interpreting social reality. Group members regularly experience situations inside or outside the therapy group that are unclear and open to multiple interpretations. In these kinds of situations, they use the opinions and impressions of others as guidelines to form their own view of reality. In a therapy group, this aspect of norms can help in the process of the therapeutic corrective experience (Yalom and Leszcz, 2020). If the majority of group members convincingly approve or disapprove of certain feelings, beliefs or behaviors, then that norm becomes the consensus in that group. Yalom and Leszcz (2020) call it consensual validation. For example, a client may be afraid of their own feelings or needs, but sharing and feedback can make those feelings more acceptable. Consider the following conversation in a therapy group: Cindy: 'I find it very hard to admit, but I am sometimes jealous of other people, even here. It makes me feel very bad.' Jonas: 'Who are you jealous of here, Cindy?' Cindy: 'Well, I'm ashamed to admit this, but I'm sometimes jealous of you, Mandy, because you have such a lovely relationship, and it's just not in the cards for me.' 'Well, it's not that big of an issue, Cindy,' Jonas says. 'Everyone is jealous sometimes, and everyone wants a wonderful relationship, right?' Mandy: 'I don't mind that you are a bit jealous of me, Cindy. I do understand, and I hope you will also experience such a nice relationship.' Cindy: 'Wow! So you don't think it's crazy or mean that I have these feelings?' Mandy: 'No, I think it's healthy because having a good relationship is normal and a basic need, and it's sad when that doesn't work out for you.'

Group norms create group identity

In the chapter on cohesion, I wrote that people derive their identity largely from the characteristics of the groups to which they belong. By identifying with the group, we outwardly show who we are, our social identity. Norms foster that group identity (social cohesion) by reinforcing typical collective group characteristics and related values. Often it is pleasant for group members to experience this 'social togetherness' of the therapy group.

Summary

- Group *rules* are the formal rules set out in the task; group *norms* are the informal agreements between group members.
- Group norms reflect beliefs about what is considered appropriate or inappropriate behavior or opinions within a group.
- Group norms always contain an underlying and substantive reason for that approval or rejection.
- Explicit norms are discussed openly in the group.
- Implicit norms are hidden within habitual behavior.
- Group norms foster the function and survival of the group; they provide group identity and serve as a benchmark for the interpretation of social reality for the individual group members.

9.4   Origin and development of group norms: social influence and group culture

How group norms work: social influence

I explained previously that a group needs unity for its functioning and that norms make an important stabilizing contribution to this (Festinger's 'group standard'). It is impossible for a group to become effective if the members have completely different opinions about what the intention is, how they interact with each other, and what is really important. This uniformity and predictability of behavior and opinions foster safety in human relations. Clarity about desired behavior makes it easier to behave as such and win the group's acceptance. It is thus normal for members of a beginning therapy group to be preoccupied with finding a common vision of what is desirable in this group in terms of behavior and opinions. This search for unity among group members, which always involves opinion formation, debate, mutual influence, and negotiation, is what we call *social influence* (Barron, 2004; Crano, 2000).

Social influence

Two classic experiments demonstrated for the first time how strongly people in a group are influenced by each other. Sherif (1936, in Nijstad, 2009, 31–32) showed how group members adjusted their opinions in a situation that could not be clearly interpreted. In his experiment, several members were asked to estimate how far a stationary point of light moves in a completely dark room (it appears as if a stationary light is then moving). Individually, the estimates varied significantly. When members were then asked to determine an estimate together, a mutually agreed upon distance gradually emerged, a standard to which everyone conformed.

Asch (1952, in Nijstad, 2009, 31–33) did a similar experiment but in a clearly interpretable situation. He had group members take turns comparing the length of a standard line to three clearly unequal lines (the standard line was as long as the middle one of the three unequal lines) aloud. The first few members in the circle were actually co-workers who intentionally gave wrong answers. More than a third of the subjects gave the same wrong answer. People in a group appear to regularly adapt to each other, even against their better judgment.

Social influence is nothing more than a relational influencing game between members of a group. It is a process of assimilation and conforming, which does not mean that 'sameness' always results. Sometimes, a majority wants to push a particular opinion against the will of a minority, but if that minority sticks to its argument, it can also be influential. We will see that the outcome of an influence game is often an agreement with nuances, a compromise. An influencing game of social influence plays out in any beginning group, and its outcome becomes the shared norms of the group. Norms then monitor agreed-upon opinions and behaviors.

How exactly does this social influence play out in the interactions between members?

This interactional influence can occur in two ways: first, by convincing and changing the other person's opinion. We call this *informational* social influence. The second is, by rewarding or punishing the other, for example, by ignoring, excluding, or positively enticing the other to embrace group norms. We call this *normative* social influence. The social influence mechanism is not only effective between members but can also be applied by any group therapist. Leadership is a form of social influence, as I described in Chapter 4. The distinction between informational and normative social influence is an important starting point for guiding a therapy group. A group therapist can influence behavior, in this case, normative behavior, by convincing group members of his views or sanctioning them where necessary. I discuss this further in the Practice Manual at the end of this chapter.

Social influence at the start of a group therapy

A newly started therapy group for adolescents has yet to develop. At the first meeting, one of the young people talks extensively about his problems. But in the meantime, the other members have questions. Can I also tell my own story immediately, or does the therapist or group think that is a bad idea? Will my input be taken seriously? Can I contradict the other person in the conversation? Who decides how things go here? Beneath the surface of task behavior, the influence game of social influence plays out, as it should in any beginning group. Informally and formally, the social rules, the norms that structure cooperation, gradually emerge.

How group norms arise and develop

Norms always have content; they concern an *opinion* of what is appropriate behavior. But where does this content come from? The task and process of a group produce those opinions. For example, the opinions in a group in geriatric care will be influenced by that group's task, such as its vision regarding the treatment of the frail and elderly. But the content of the norms is also colored by the process side, by the people themselves. In a group, all members' personal backgrounds, such as their beliefs, habits, and culture, are thrown into the mix, and the first group norms arise out of this 'melting pot.' A beginning therapy group with many spontaneous personalities starts with different norms than a new group with many inhibited ones.

After that initial start, we see existing norms change and new norms emerge. In the previous chapter, I explained how new norms arise through the development of the group and group members. These norms are the product of the developmental crises (authority, intimacy, and separation crises) that occur regularly in the course of every therapy group. In each developmental crisis, there is an emotional conflict between desires and fears regarding the developmental theme. For example, a social skills therapy group may debate the (intimacy) theme of 'openly giving each other feedback.' Some group members find more openness desirable because it can actually be of great benefit, while others believe that more mutual openness is undesirable and not necessary for the skill training. A group always negotiates a solution to such a contradiction. If the solution mainly takes into account the fear, we call it a restrictive solution. If desire is the primary consideration, we call it an enabling solution. This is when we can see the 'mechanism' of social influence at work. By debating and negotiating with each other, group members form their opinions on these issues and try to reach a compromise with each other. This compromise becomes the group norm regarding the topic. That norm may be restrictive in nature, or it may be more expansive with respect to the topic. In the previous example of a social skills group, the following compromise (read: norm) may result: 'more openness to each other suits the goals of this group; let's give each other clearer feedback but only if someone asks for it.'

This creates specific norms for all kinds of themes that are discussed during group interactions. Group members in fact determine the group norms. This does not mean that the group therapist cannot influence this. The group therapist ensures that he participates in the discussion during the meeting. He can, if desired, intervene in the debate and try to steer the norms in the desired direction, but he cannot impose them.

The nature of the norms corresponds to the development stage in which they arise. There is a great need for clarity in the uncertain beginning of the parallel phase. Therefore, simple, straightforward norms quickly arise during the first meeting, establishing rules and guidelines to provide clarity and security. For example, if group members introduce themselves to each other in a circle during the first meeting, the order in the circle often also remains the starting point for how they take their seats and talk to each other in the second meeting (following the same 'order' in the circle). As the group develops further and members begin to feel more secure and uninhibited, those kinds of strict initial norms become uncomfortable. They cease to be functional and are abandoned.

The *inclusion phase* is a typical experimentation phase. We can see this in the norms: new norms are tested without hesitation and are just as easily discarded if the group disapproves of them. For example, a group may have the norm that making jokes about each other is acceptable for a while until some group members get fed up with it, and the norm of 'roasting each other' disappears again.

In the *mutuality phase*, norms become more stable and tolerant. In terms of content, norms change to the extent that individuals can distinguish themselves more. For example, a typical group norm from this phase is that you are free to disagree, as long as you respect each other's opinions.

Group culture

In a longer-running group, norms acquire a distinctive structure and character for that group during the stable phase of the workgroup. We call this *group culture*: a coherent system of forms embedded in the life and history of the group. In the next section, I elaborate further on the concept of group culture.

Summary

- Group norms arise naturally; they are part of group development and become visible in the group structure.
- Norms arise from the restrictive or enabling solutions of substantive debates among group members regarding important emotional group themes.
- Social influence determines the norms that arise.
- Social influence occurs through convincing (informational social influence) and punishment and reward (normative social influence).
- Some norms are quickly abandoned because they are no longer functional; other norms grow into firm ground rules for how group members think and act.
- In a longer-running group, a coherent system of norms arises, providing the group history and identity: group culture.

9.5 Group norms in a therapy group

Norms: collective structure and individual space

Norms align group members in their thinking and actions. They provide the structure and unity that group members need to work well together. But norms can also overshoot the mark in this collectivity and become too strict. The danger then is that they may actually hinder the group's functioning and that of its members.

Let's compare a soccer team. Normally, every player in the team has their own place in the lineup: the goalkeeper at the goalpost, the defense at the back, the strikers at the front, and so on. If that norm becomes very strict, for example, the backs are never allowed to go past the center line, and strikers must always be on the opponent's half of the field, then it not only literally robs those individual players of their playing space and creativity, but it also takes the spirit and creativity out of working together. A team like this has a much smaller chance of winning.

This is also how it works in our therapy groups. When norms become too strict, group members lose their individual space, to the detriment of productive cooperation. For example, the group norm that you should never interrupt each other can be very inhibiting because everyone very politely allows the other person to finish speaking. This creates a group with a norm of caution and inhibition.

The opposite is also true: if norms are too weak or too flexible, the group's outcome is also affected. Normlessness in a group produces chaotic cooperation and neglects the interests of individual group members. Because group members are given too much space, they feel unsafe in such a group; they are left to their own devices.

A helping norm

In an online therapy group for students with a fear of failure, there is a clear norm that you should cancel on time if you are unable to attend. The group and therapist are thus surprised to see that Denzel is absent without having canceled. Theresa: 'I am quite worried because Denzel was not feeling well last time.' Natalie: 'Yes, I have that same feeling. He seemed depressed.' 'Should I app him?' Wayne asks. The group therapist shares the members' concerns and perceptions: 'That's a good idea, Wayne. Shall I call him right away?' Wayne nods in agreement. The group therapist leaves his screen and returns a moment later. 'I have spoken with Denzel, and your instincts were right. Denzel was indeed depressed, but he'll log in and join us in a moment.' A short while later, when Denzel has also logged on, the group responds supportively. Marie: 'Good of you to join us, Denzel!' Natalie: 'We missed you, Denzel. Glad to see you.' Denzel: 'Sorry, I just wasn't up for it today. I think I might be in a dip again. Maybe I should go back on the medication.' Group therapist: 'I know you have used it before when you had a dip and that it helped you. Perhaps it would be a good idea to make an appointment with your doctor?' Denzel: 'I don't really feel like it, but I'll do that.' At the next meeting, everyone is present. Denzel is doing better; the previous meeting was a really important one for him. He saw his doctor, and together, they decided that antidepressant medication was not necessary yet. At the moment, group therapy is the best medicine for him.

Hence, in a therapy group, there must be a balance between the degree of uniformity of group norms on the one hand and individual space on the other. Exactly what that balance is varies from group to group. Some groups benefit more from a strict norm structure than others. Take, for example, a diet management group for people with eating addictions. If, in such a group, there were no strict rules and norms governing eating, the group would not produce results. The target group and the group task determine what structure optimum is functional. This optimum is especially important in our therapy groups. Unlike result-oriented teams, such as sports and work teams, a therapy group does not have a collective end goal (winning or a certain production quota, respectively), but the end product is measured individually: the individual end goals of the group members. In therapy groups, individual space is inherently indispensable.

Four factors interact to determine the balance between norm structure and individual space:

1. The strictness of the content of the norm
2. The number of group members who support the norm
3. The degree of group cohesion

4. The duration and embedding of the norm

1. The strictness of the content of the norm

As explained at the beginning of this chapter, a group norm always includes an opinion of what constitutes appropriate behavior in a given situation. That opinion can be intolerant to individual deviations, resulting in the norm having a strict effect, or tolerant, causing the norm to allow for greater individual space.

An intolerant opinion often contains words like 'never' and 'always,' whereas a tolerant opinion contains nuances. Therefore, it makes quite a difference whether the intolerant norm is used, 'expressing anger is never good, it only causes hurt,' or the tolerant norm, 'anger is a normal feeling that is not always easy to express, but you can talk about your anger.' Although a norm is primarily a collective phenomenon, it can still offer room for individual variation by virtue of its content (Postmes and Jetten, 2006).

2. The number of group members who support the norm

A group norm exists when the majority of group members support that norm. Power in numbers is an important factor in the strictness of a group norm. A group where almost everyone fully agrees on the main norms creates a compulsion to conform to the dominant opinion. Such a conformist group does not allow for deviation from the dominant norms. As a result, it is very difficult to change norms in such a group. For example, if all members of a therapy group for girls with anorexia do not consider it necessary to stop visiting internet sites that promote 'skinniness,' a group therapist will have a hard time convincing them from doing so.

Unanimity regarding norms by no means always occurs. There are often subgroups that adopt different norms among themselves, or there is a solid minority with a dissenting viewpoint. In that case, there are no *group* norms (yet) because people in the group have different views on a particular issue. A group therapist can use these differences when he wants to set norms in motion.

3. The degree of group cohesion

In Chapter 6, 'Group cohesion,' I showed that group cohesion and group norms are interrelated. They mutually reinforce each other. Cohesion always reinforces existing norms. Mutual acceptance plays an important role in cohesion. Group members want to fit in, not look out of place. Therefore, they tend to be loyal to each other and adapt to what is the norm. Cohesion in itself thus has a norm-conforming, assimilating influence. Here, we see the mechanism of normative social influence at work.

If the norms are content-tolerant, then their cohesive reinforcement is functional. Cohesion that reinforces norms that have strict content is less pleasant.

Such a combination can create stifling or coercive conformism, making any dissenting opinion taboo. It makes quite a difference whether cohesion reinforces the norm 'everyone is responsible for what they tell or don't tell here' or the norm 'here, everyone tells their biggest secret during the second meeting.'

4.   The duration of a norm: the group culture

The longer a group exists, the more obvious and implicit the group norms become. Group members are then often no longer aware of these norms: they are commonplace and have become a social fact (Hoijtink, 2001). Even if the composition of such a group changes, they will continue to exist. They are passed on to the new group members and become more and more embedded. In group dynamics, such a sustainable system of deeply embedded norms is called *group culture*. A group culture can take on a very tough life of its own and become virtually unchangeable. Consider an ongoing therapy group that continues to chat after the session, no matter how hard the therapists try to stop them from doing so. The group's composition has already been changed completely, but the habit has been passed on and persists.

The special nature and vulnerability of therapeutic norms

At the beginning of this chapter, I described how one of the most important functions of group norms is that they foster task performance. Each group therapist is happy when *therapeutic* norms arise, that specifically support that extraordinary method and task of a therapy group. Exactly what norms are needed depends on the particular task and method of that therapy group, but there are some therapeutic norms that are essential for any therapy group. In each therapy group, members are expected to present and talk about problems, fears and worries, respond sufficiently to one another, and reflect on each person's learning process. Therefore, each group therapist explains, as clearly as possible, what is expected from every member as tasks, in the 'pitch' at the start, or when a new member joins. And hopefully, those task expectations will become the group norm. But as we well know, that is not a given. Every group therapist, at one time or another, experiences a group where members contribute little or in which people hardly respond to each other. And that resistance is understandable. Therapy groups are a world apart when it comes to personal openness. In individual therapy, it is already quite a feat to bare your 'heart and soul,' but opening up and allowing yourself to be vulnerable in the company of seven or more people you sometimes do not know very well is extraordinary. However, in therapy, and therefore also group therapy, this is imperative. Sharing your problems, fears, and concerns openly is an indispensable task. And that is not only unusual but also very exciting. As children, we were used to showing our vulnerability, but as adults, we have unlearned this. Under the influence of upbringing and social conventions, we become accustomed to behaving socially and appropriately. This is logical because showing vulnerability, problems, or inability always produces negative feelings like fear, shame, or sadness. For those reasons, therapy groups are usually initially perceived as very exciting and unsafe.

But experience shows us that it can be done; we know enough safe and productive therapy groups where these extraordinary 'vulnerability' norms exist. These therapeutic norms only succeed when there is enough cohesion, accompanied by trust and safety, a clear and convincing explanation when organizing and starting the group, and, with a bit of luck, also with the composition. Then, a group can develop in which the sharing of personal thoughts and feelings has become the therapeutic norm.

Summary

- Norms can be strict or tolerant: they can allow more or less individual latitude.
- The balance between strictness and tolerance is determined by the strictness of the content of a norm, the dominant majority, the degree of cohesion, and the duration of a norm.
- Each group has its own (task) optimum in the balance between strictness and tolerance of the group norms.
- The therapeutic norms of openness, vulnerability, and interaction make a therapy group extraordinary.

9.6   Practical manual: utilizing norms in a therapy group

9.6.1   Introduction

Group norms arise naturally. The group therapist can steer this process in a natural way by making clever use of the two previously mentioned forms of social influence. Convincing (informational social influence) is applied by the group therapist when explicit norms are involved; sanctioning (normative social influence) works best when dealing with implicit norms. A third way for a group therapist to influence norms is to 'model' the desired behavior.

1.   Influencing explicit norms by convincing
In a situation where the group is openly concerned with the group norms, for example, at the start of a group or when the norms are being challenged, the group therapist steers the group in an open and direct way by engaging in the norms debate. In doing so, the group therapist can utilize his expertise by explaining his view to the members and convincing them thereof. As an expert,

he can explain why certain behavior is desirable or undesirable. Thus, he can influence the direction in which norms develop by applying authority. Here, the group therapist uses informational social influence. Take a skill-training group therapy in which none of the members complete the homework assignments. Not doing the homework has become the norm. A group therapist can reverse this norm if he succeeds in *convincing* the members of the importance of homework for themselves.

2.   Influencing implicit norms by sanctioning behavior
With implicit norms, when the group norms are settled, in other words, have turned into habitual behavior, the group therapist steers the norms indirectly. He does so by rewarding desirable behavior and ignoring, structuring, or putting a stop to undesirable behavior. In this case, the group therapist uses normative social influence.

For example, he may clearly reward a group member who had bravely practiced an assignment at home and briefly ignore the group member who complains and says negative things about the homework assignments.

3.   Influencing norms through 'modeling'
The third way a group therapist can influence norms is by employing himself as a role model. Because of the group therapist's position and authority, group members tend to regard his behavior highly. Therefore, group members naturally elevate that behavior into a norm. This 'modeling' happens continuously; it is never 'switched off.' It thus happens more or less automatically, and the group therapist does not have to do anything for it in particular except to be aware of it and take it into account whenever possible. Ideally, the group therapist himself naturally exhibits the desired behavior expected from the group. For example, in a therapy group whose members regularly arrive late, it would be wise for a group therapist to set a good example by always being on time.

In this process of influencing norm behavior, the group therapist again utilizes the following three techniques: organizational techniques to create conditions for appropriate norms, and the combination of verbal techniques and relationship techniques to guide norm development during the ongoing group. Verbal techniques are especially important as a tool for influencing norms. Because the essence of a norm is its content, namely, the opinion of group reality (social reality), steering a norm means that the group therapist must engage in substantive debate about that opinion. And that requires language. Given that group norms concern the entire group, the group therapist will need to regularly apply group interventions, the group-oriented form of verbal techniques.

As we saw in earlier chapters, the relationship technique is the preferred tool for creating the most influential cooperative relationship with the group. Because group members are party to the norms debate, the group therapist must primarily steer in a cooperative manner. Therefore, when it comes to norms, a negotiating and cooperative attitude, for example, (COOPERATING), will be help-ful. A directing attitude generally does not work as well here but is necessary when there is a risk of losing sight of the task, or the group norms take on a destructive character.

If a group therapist wants to foster certain norms, it is, of course, important that he know in which direction he wants to steer. In other words, he needs to know what norms are desired in our therapy groups. This varies from group to group and depends on the specific task and method. However, some group norms are desirable in all therapy groups:

- Norms that ensure the preservation of the group (attendance, arriving on time, privacy, working undisturbed, group as workplace)
- The functional norms that foster the method and task
- Norms about openness, sharing, safety, and respect

9.6.2   Fostering group norms in a beginning therapy group

Steering norms beforehand
As I said before a sound task organization ensures the correct holding and direc-tion of the processes that arise. This certainly applies to group norms as well. Some aspects of task organization are extra important when it comes to fostering desired group norms. A good selection of members aids the formation of desir-able norms. In doing so, it is important to ensure that the issues or needs of the selected group members correspond as much as possible.

Properly informing prospective members during the assessment interviews contributes to the creation of the right norms. Providing clear information about the expected tasks fosters the emergence of task-oriented norms.

Following this, the group therapist can explain the group rules (see Chapter 3) and their conditional importance for group formation (preservation) and safety. When a group member joins the group, he or she agrees to the group rules. With a mutual 'yes,' a contract has been concluded between the new member and the group leader. That 'contract' on group rules is the basis on which group norms can arise.

Steering norms at the beginning period of the therapy group
The beginning period of a new therapy group (or entry of new members into an existing group) is the best time for the group therapist to steer group norms. These are not yet fixed and can still be influenced. The natural uncertainty among group members necessitates clarity. Because the group therapist has substantial authority in the beginning, he can take advantage of this. This applies especially to the first session, during which group members are often extra tense. As an expert, the group therapist can use a 'pitch' (see Chapter 5) to explain and discuss

the group's goal, task, working method, and, by extension, the group rules clearly and encouragingly. Group members then already feel part owner of these rules and understand their necessity better. It works best if the group therapist does all this with an active and cooperative attitude (HELPING). The first norms that arise are then more likely to be an extension of the group rules, that is, focused on the task and the importance of group safety.

From the first session, the group therapist is also influential as a role model by exhibiting the desired behavior himself. During the beginning stage, group members will especially see the group therapist as a role model, imitate his behavior, and elevate it to a norm. For example, a group therapist who is not overly neutral during the beginning phase but also shares something about his own experience or feelings with the group from time to time to encourage transparency and openness.

What applies to the first session applies to the entire beginning period. It is advisable for the group therapist to regularly re-explain the group's task and working method so that the group fully understands them and becomes familiar with them. When the group starts to get the hang of the task-oriented work and safety increases, the group therapist has accomplished a great deal and can take a step back.

Table 9.1 Fostering task-oriented and safety norms at the start of a group.

Verbal technique	Relationship technique (attitude and tone)
During the first meeting (of a new member), the group therapist calmly *explains* and discusses the group task and group rules with the entire group, and thus help norms arise.	The group therapist uses an active and cooperative attitude (HELPING).

Example sentences:
'For a group to function productively, everyone is needed. Hence the always present ground rule.'
'If you only practice here, it will not be enough to change your behavior. That is why it is very important that you take your homework assignments very seriously.'
'What we expect from everyone here is that you are open about yourself and to others. That is sometimes difficult in the beginning, but I will help you. However, we do not force anyone to be open. You determine at your own pace when you want to be open about yourself.'
'Responding to each other is also very important for this group therapy. You learn mostly from each other, from the support and recognition that the other person offers you, or from feedback.'
'Everyone here can count on being respected as an individual and on safety. Naturally, we will sometimes disagree or confront each other, but that should not be at the expense of personal respect.'

Steering norms in the early days of a therapy group

In the second session of an educational group therapy, 'coping with ADHD' for adolescents, the two group therapists ask the members how they experienced the first session. Allen indicates that he does not yet fully understand the point of the group. Other group members concur. 'Let me explain the purpose again,' says the group therapist. 'We meet ten times to talk about how ADHD affects your home life. Now, it's not just about information from us; it's also important that you share the hurdles you face at home with us. We will discuss an informative topic on ADHD during every session, and we are curious about your experiences regarding those topics. In addition, you will be given assignments each time to practice at home.'

Carol: 'It's just like school!' Group therapist: 'That's a very valid comparison, Carol, because this group also works with information and assignments. We told you last time how important it is to attend all ten sessions and how important the home assignments are. These sessions aim to help you cope better with your ADHD at home.' 'And if you really can't on one occasion, what then?' Becky asks. Group therapist: 'That would be very unfortunate because you miss out on a topic. In our experience, the group yields the most results if everyone is present each time. After all, you also learn a lot from each other's experiences.'

'But my sister is getting married in two weeks, and I want to be there!' Becky exclaims. Group therapist: 'Of course, it sometimes happens that someone has to skip once, but I would like your commitment to keep that to a minimum. What do you think?' Bobby: 'Seems reasonable to me. Preferably not at all, and if unavoidable, then at most once.' Group therapist: 'Can you agree with Bobby's suggestion?'

Fostering the development of therapeutic group norms

At the beginning of a therapy group, the norm structure has yet to form. That means the group must develop a set of norms. Most groups require more than just two or three norms. The extent of that system of norms depends on the group task and the type of group. An educational therapy group that meets six times needs fewer group norms than an ongoing therapy group for people with unexplained pain symptoms.

In this beginning period, it is natural for group members to spend a great deal of time debating and negotiating all kinds of issues important to that group. Group members then compare themselves to each other in order to develop their own opinions and arrive at common norms. Because group tasks and cooperation are the main focal points of a group, we see that important themes often arise around them. Task-related themes include, for example, task distribution, working methods, or the purposefulness of the group. For example, a therapy group for people with obesities debates the issue of whether it is better to lose weight through restraint and exercise or through drugs and medical interventions. After some time, a common task-related group norm nevertheless emerges from such a debate. For example, 'exercise and restraint is our working method unless that completely fails; then, we may ask the doctor for help.' Cooperation then involves, for example, (developmental) topics related to safety or how confrontational, supportive, or personal one should be in the group. Consider a group therapy training group that believes interpersonal openness and feedback is appropriate for this training but that it should not turn into group therapy.

The group therapist can foster the emergence of valid group norms in this stage in two ways: first, by encouraging a substantive discussion, asking *questions*, *inviting* group members to respond, and stimulating debate and, second, by encouraging the active participation of as many group members as possible. He does this by *mirroring* all group members' responses and facilitating the meeting by *connecting* group members with each other.

If there seem to be few differences, it would be helpful for the group therapist to try to differentiate, meaning to look for distinctions in the norms by *questioning* and *exploring*. If group members have differing opinions, it will be helpful to reinforce those opinions using the *broadening* verbal technique. As this is done primarily in active cooperation with the group, a HELPING attitude is most appropriate here.

Table 9.2 Fostering the development of therapeutic group norms by engaging in debate and reinforcing a minority viewpoint.

Verbal technique The group therapist helps group members exchange opinions and test them against each other using *mirroring*, *connecting*, *broadening*, and *confronting*.	Relationship technique (attitude and tone) The group therapist uses an active and cooperative attitude (HELPING)

Initiating a debate on group norms

In a therapy group for managers suffering from burnout symptoms, the majority believe that burnout is solely the fault of a bad employer. In opposition, a small subgroup believes that burnout results from an excessive performance drive, a sense of duty, and a lack of assertiveness. Thus, they look for the cause within themselves.

The group therapist pays attention to the minority subgroup that is likely to be overshadowed by *mirroring* and *broadening* their views. 'William, do

I understand correctly that you think factors originating within yourself play a big role in burnout?' William: 'Yes, I do think so.' Group therapist: 'Is William the only one who thinks that way, or do more people recognize that?' Francis: 'I also think that because I know that's how it works for me. I'm way too dutiful.' Ronnell: 'But could it also be both? That you are partly responsible, but that your work also contributed toward it?'

9.6.3   Fostering therapeutic norms in an ongoing therapy group

Fostering desirable group norms in an ongoing therapy group
Later in group development, when the group functions as a *workgroup*, the norms become more natural and increasingly implicit. Group members then do not discuss the norms and their content as much but respond directly to each other's behavior. They react positively to desirable behavior and negatively to unwanted behavior. This often happens with subtle verbal and nonverbal signals that are not even that noticeable but are usually clear enough for the person involved. An interested question or a disapproving look is often enough to encourage or inhibit a group member.

Let's take a therapy group for women over 50 with physical and psychological age-related complaints as an example. They regularly discuss various age-related topics, such as menopause, depression, sexuality, and the 'empty nest' syndrome. The norm in the group is not to talk about delicate personal matters, such as for example sexual abuse in childhood, in detail. At her first meeting, a new member immediately starts talking extensively about the domestic and sexual violence that happened to her and her sister in her childhood. In doing so, she violated the group norm. She will notice from the others' behavior that talking about the domestic and sexual violence so intimately in this group is 'not done.' For example, a group member may continue to frown at her without saying anything, or another group member may thank her kindly for her input, after which the group moves on to another topic.

As mentioned earlier, a group therapist can base his influence on the same mechanism and apply clever normative social influence. He can implicitly co-steer norms by directly sanctioning the behavior of group members. A cooperative (COOPERATING) attitude is especially appropriate in this direct but subtle behavioral influence. The group therapist primarily uses the verbal technique in this process of *rewarding* (desired behavior) and *ignoring* (unwanted behavior). In the next section, I explain this important technique in more detail.

Rewarding and ignoring
By directly rewarding desired behavior and ignoring unwanted behavior, the group therapist promotes desired norms in an implicit, imperceptible way. He

can consciously use this technique to influence norms. A group therapist should preferably alternate rewarding and ignoring; when combined, they form one technique.

• Rewarding

Rewarding is praising desired behavior and responding to that behavior non-verbally in a positive way, such as by nodding in a friendly manner to a group member. As with most interventions, it is important to keep the rewarding intervention short and concrete and, where possible, link it to the task or the other group members. When it comes to a rewarding intervention, timing is crucial. This intervention has the most empowering effect if it immediately follows the desired behavior (Groot, 2004). Because rewarding must appear convincing and powerful, the group therapist often uses the stating form here.

There are several options when it comes to *who* does the rewarding. The group therapist himself can reward the desired behavior by positively naming it and praising the person. But it works even better if the group therapist has the other group members reward the group member. Sometimes, the behavior is so obviously successful or desired that asking the group for a response is a given. For example, when a group member dares to show new behavior, the therapist can ask, 'What do you think of the way that Rachel just gave feedback?' Group member: 'Very clever, Rachel!' The most powerful effect occurs when the group therapist lets the group member reward herself, such as when that group member expresses or shows satisfaction or pride in herself. See the following example sentences.

Example sentences of rewarding:
'How wonderfully clear you are, John!' (rewarding by group therapist)
'You seem to be very satisfied with this exercise, Laura. Are you?' (self-rewarding)
'What do you find positive about Raymond's presentation?' (rewarding by other group members)
'Anne, you are really good at dealing with criticism!' (rewarding by group therapist)
'I can see that you are proud of your performance, Aram. Am I right?' (self-rewarding)
'Cora, Am I correct in assuming you are a little jealous of James's assertiveness?' Cora: 'Yes, I am. I wish I could stand up for myself like you do, James!' (rewarding by other group members)

• Ignoring

The essence of ignoring is to pay *no attention at all* to unwanted behavior. Ignoring is a more difficult technique than rewarding. *Not* paying attention to noticeable behavior is usually more difficult than focusing on it, especially if it attracts strong attention. And unwanted behavior tends to do that. For example, nonfunctional complaining behavior can be annoying. In your capacity as a group therapist, you might say something about it, for instance, that complaining doesn't help. Group therapists often try to stop unwanted behavior by discouraging or criticizing it. But you are then still rewarding the unwanted behavior. Because it does not matter whether you give the behavior positive or negative attention, the attention itself is rewarding. In cases like this, a group therapist must often resist the temptation to give the negative behavior attention. It helps – just as with the verbal technique of *giving space with silence* – to see ignoring not as refraining from doing something but rather as doing something, to see it as an *active technique* for influencing a group situation.

The art of ignoring is to pretend that behavior is not happening. The group therapist does this by *not responding* verbally to the group member exhibiting the unwanted behavior and by *not looking* at this group member. Instead, he looks at and reacts to the group members he does want to give attention to. Ignoring may seem like a weakness, but in practice, it is an extremely powerful technique that often proves very effective.

One of the difficulties for a group therapist is that ignoring seems rude. In practice, however, this is not that bad. Ignoring is quite common; most group members are not surprised when there is no response to certain behaviors, as long as you do not ignore the same member too often.

Example sentences of ignoring:
'Please continue, Ann.' (ignoring the other)
'Is that what you just meant, Ahmed, that you think this topic is very important?' (ignoring two members whispering to each other)

Table 9.3 Fostering desired group norms by rewarding and ignoring.

Verbal technique The group therapist fosters desired norms by *rewarding* desired behavior and *ignoring* unwanted behavior.	Relationship technique (attitude and tone) For an advanced and independent group, a supportive attitude (COOPERATING) is appropriate when rewarding and in interaction with a group member who is being ignored, a WITHDRAWN attitude is appropriate (including nonverbal disregard).

Rewarding desired behavior

A forensic therapy group for perpetrators of domestic violence is meeting for the fifth time. The group is safe and running well. Group members input their home experiences according to prior agreement and take practicing behavioral restraint seriously. Whenever group members are successful or have performed an exercise well, the group therapist rewards this by giving them positive attention and praising the relevant group member (or having other members praise them). Group therapist: 'Sitting down at the table with your wife was very brave, Larry. Do you agree?' (turning to the other group members) 'Yeah, well done,' says Adam. 'Just last week, you couldn't keep your hands to yourself. Very good!'

Ignoring unwanted behavior

In a 'running therapy' group for people with a depressive disorder, Megan demands a lot of negative attention at the evaluation after the running session. Even though her depression is decreasing, she keeps interrupting the group discussion with her complaints. During the evaluation, the group therapist decides to ignore Megan's complaining behavior.

Megan: ' . . . and then I didn't succeed in getting out of bed, and that's why I'm so tired and would have been better off not joining today. And maybe that's why I won't come next week and . . . ' Group therapist: 'You jogged quite well today, Joyce. Do you agree?' Megan: 'Well, I didn't, because . . . ' Group therapist: 'And, Joyce, I thought you were also doing well. Am I right?' Joyce: 'Yes, absolutely! For the first time, it felt really nice!' Group therapist: 'Fantastic! And why do you think it went better today?'

Of course, ignoring is not the only possibility for a group therapist to influence unwanted behavior. Ignoring is a very strong influencer as long as the undesirable behavior is not too strong or too persistent. In that case, the group therapist has two more options: first, limiting the undesirable behavior and, if that does not help, discussing and exploring the disruptive behavior, possibly with a meta-conversation. See the following example.

Dealing with unwanted behavior in three ways or three steps

In a therapy group for mood and anxiety complaints, Donald attracts a lot of attention. He keeps talking constantly, also when the group or group therapist are giving attention to other group members. Roxane is talking about her sadness. Donald: 'I have those feelings too, Roxane, and . . .' Group therapist: 'Any idea, Roxane, where this feeling of sadness comes from?' (*ignoring* Donald). Roxane: 'No, that's why I . . .' Donald: 'I think I know what. . .' Group therapist:

'Wait, Donald, let's listen to Roxane' (*limiting* Donald). Roxane: 'I sometimes think it is my feeling of inferiority that weighs on me so much.' Donald: 'That is what I . . .' Group therapist: 'Donald, please stop for a moment . . . is it okay for you to let Roxane finish her questions and then we will reflect on you?' (*limiting* and *structuring*). Donald: 'Okay.' (Later in the session) Group therapist: 'I first have this question to you Donald, why do you think you have to talk so much?' *(exploring).* Donald: 'Ehh . . . I understand what you mean, but I really don't know . . .' Raymond: 'Could it be that talking is the way you keep your anxiety under control?' Donald: 'I really don't know . . . could be . . . maybe, I often feel quite miserable here.'

9.6.4   Changing and blocking undesirable norms in an ongoing therapy group

Changing norms in an ongoing group

Group norms can also evolve in the wrong direction. This means that group norms no longer support the task or the group safety. For example, a social skills training in which the group members share the view that there is no point in practicing exercises at home that the group therapist had given them. The group therapist can then re-explain the working method and try rewarding and ignoring in order to steer the group back in the desired direction. But if the negative norm is strong and has become a group culture, these subtle techniques will be insufficient. The group therapist must then pause the task and explicitly readdress the norms in a meta-conversation (see Chapter 5). His influence then derives from effective *convincing* (informational social influence). He can do this by engaging with the group in a substantive debate about the norms, 'prying them open,' so to speak. Such a debate is not always easy. It amounts to the group therapist having to *convince* the group members that a different view would be useful. In doing so, the group therapist must *confront* the group with the negative norm and its consequences (less results). Together with the group, he must explore the underlying causes. Subsequently, the group therapist can *challenge* the group to debate and negotiate a change from the negative norm to a better norm. The group therapist has additional influence due to his expertise, experience, position of authority, and helper role, but this influence should not be exaggerated. Ultimately, a group determines the group norm. In this example, the group therapist can use his expertise to try to convince the group that practicing at home is an indispensable part of the training and that the results will be significantly less if members do nothing at home. If a subgroup dictates the negative norm, the group therapist can mobilize the rest of the group and reinforce their alternative opinion to drive the norm debate. Similarly, he can use new group members as 'crowbars.' They can play a refreshing role in the norms debate by still being allowed to be curious (naive) about the backgrounds of norms or still deviate from the dominant norms.

When changing norms, the group therapist must steer with an active but not overly directive attitude (HELPING/COOPERATIING). Changing norms will not succeed without cooperation with group members. As the group members are the ones who set the norms, it will not work if the group therapist unilaterally imposes an alternative norm.

Table 9.4 Change the content of a group norm or try to create a new norm.

Verbal technique	Relationship technique (attitude and tone)
The group therapist pauses the task and *confronts* the group with the undesirable norm, *challenging* the group to discuss and negotiate a different norm.	With this firm intervention, the group therapist should adopt an active attitude (HELPING/COOPERATIING).

Example sentences:
'Many of you regularly look at such websites, even though they diametrically oppose what we want to achieve here together. What are your thoughts on this contradiction?'
'I have noticed that, for the third time, only a few of you have done the homework assignment, even though that is an important agreement in this group. Why is that? What is your reason for not doing it?'
'I really want to explore that together with you because what's going on here doesn't feel right.'

Change a norm

In a therapy group for people with unexplained physical complaints, members often cancel. The reasons vary: one has a cold, another has to work, or there is an important family gathering. Group therapist Mark is concerned because there hasn't been a full group of members for five consecutive times. He resolves to discuss and influence this harmful development at the next session.

At the start of that session, the therapist noticed that two people had canceled. After the group has started, Mark takes over. 'Samual, I have to interrupt you because I want to discuss something with all of you.' Everyone looks at Mark expectantly. 'It has been discussed before, but people keep canceling each time, and we haven't been a full group for five weeks in a row now.' Mark looks around and allows for questioning silence.

'Yes,' Rose says, embarrassed, 'I wasn't here last week either, but I did notice previously that everyone has been absent at least once. Except you, of course, Mark.' Kyle continues, looks at Mark, and asks, 'Are you asking us why this is happening, Mark?' Mark: 'Yes, I would like to figure this out with you and change it because this severely undermines your therapy. Do any of you know what the problem might be?' Rose says, 'It's very difficult for me with my work. I sometimes have to work overtime and can't say no.' Joan responds sharply, 'I think that's nonsense, Rose. I just tell my work that I have an obligation. It's not easy, even for me, but you can do it if you really want to.'

Blocking a destructive norm

The group therapist must intervene even more directly when there is a destructive norm that is harmful to the group or group members. He must then put a stop to the destructive behavior. If vital group norms are compromised, the group therapist must pause the group. Using a meta-conversation (see Chapter 5), he addresses the destructive norm and explains why the destructive behavior is unacceptable.

Next, the group therapist must help the group change the norms by using a very active and steering attitude (LEADING/COMPETING) and various verbal techniques, including *limiting, structuring, confronting, questioning, mirroring, connecting, broadening*, and *convincing*. If this intervention is unsuccessful, the group leader must end the group or change the composition of the group.

For instance, take a group of adult clients in an addiction clinic where a dominant male majority insults and discriminates against the female group members. A group therapist will then have to intervene very firmly by immediately stopping that harmful behavior and clarifying why it is unacceptable. It is then necessary to investigate why the men are exhibiting such behavior. In extreme cases, such as when this has become a persistent group culture, the group therapist must change the composition or dissolve the group within this composition.

Table 9.5 Blocking a destructive group norm.

Verbal technique	Relationship techniques (attitude and tone)
The group therapist pauses the task (*structuring*), limits the group's unwanted behavior, and *explains* and initiates a debate for a different norm.	This intervention requires a strong, tenacious, and directive attitude (LEADING/ COMPETING).

Blocking a destructive norm

In a therapy group for young adults with personality problems, the norm of constantly making jokes has predominated for some time. As a result, communication between members is hardly ever taken seriously. One joke provokes another, and the jokes become more grim each time. More and more members are being belittled. The group therapist decides to intervene by having a meta-conversation. 'Wait a minute, Rachid and Frank. What are you doing?' Rachid: 'What do you mean? What are you doing?' Group therapist: 'What do you think I mean?' Rachid: 'No idea.' Group therapist: 'Anyone else understand why I stopped the conversation?' No one says anything. Group therapist: 'Let me explain. All I see is you guys increasingly making fun of each other, and as a result, you are no longer serious about therapy, which worries me. That's not how I want to work with you.' Members are silent. Group therapist: 'Is it clearer to you why I have stopped the group?' Again silence. Group therapist: 'It is almost time; unless someone wants to say something, I suggest we stop and return to this next time.' At the next meeting, it is possible to have a conversation in which joking behavior may be gently explored.

Exercises

Tool training 'rewarding and ignoring' for students in a group therapy training

1. The students role play an 'assignment therapy group' in mental health care. In this group, each member comes up with a concrete self-selected, achievable, and meaningful assignment that he or she completes the following week. The next meeting begins by reporting how the assignment went, and this situation is role-played. Successful assignments are rewarded. Unsuccessful assignments are afforded limited reflection time (ignoring), only a brief examination of why it was unsuccessful.
2. Each time, one student (or, if time is short, a pair) plays the group therapist for five minutes.

   The practicing group therapist is instructed to practice only rewarding and ignoring interventions and not to worry about the larger process. It involves two or three interventions.

3. After five minutes, the trainer interrupts the role-play, and there is an opportunity for feedback from the role-playing group members to the practicing group therapist.
4. After about five minutes of feedback, the next student continues as the group therapist. The role-play continues as usual. The group member role-players are asked to play in such a way that the practicing group therapist is provided with sufficient material to try out the skills.

Chapter 10

Role behavior in a therapy group

10.1 Introduction

Over time, under normal circumstances, a stable group dynamic structure develops in a group. Like norms, *roles* are essential components of that group dynamic structure. The natural group system develops roles, which, like norms, are necessary for the group's efficiency and survival. Together, they provide the necessary structure and stability to the complex processes that take place within a group.

Both norms and roles deal with the predictability of behavior in the group. Norms involve expectations about collective behavior, about the behavioral codes to which everyone must adhere. Roles are about individual behavior, the typical behavior you expect to see from an individual group member. Norms are structures at the group level; they emphasize equality. Roles are structures at the individual level; they emphasize precisely the typical personal differences, in other words, the diversity in the group. Roles are extra important in a therapy group because they are related to the personalities of group members and are useful for the therapeutic change processes.

The following topics are addressed:

- What is a role
- The function of roles for the group and for the individual member
- The emergence and development of roles
- Negative role development: role fixation and role blurring in a therapy group
- The group therapist's role repertoire
- The function and value of role behavior in a therapy group
- Practical Manual: steering and utilizing role behavior in a therapy group

10.2 What is a role?

What is a role?

As an observer, suppose you follow the development of a group for some time. What do you observe? A beginning group usually makes an undifferentiated

DOI: 10.4324/9781003368786-13

impression on an observer. You watch the group at work; no details stand out. If you observe the same group again after some time, you will be surprised by how much you suddenly notice *individual group members*. Each group member can be identified by his or her repetitive behavior in group therapy. For example, one group member pays attention to the performance of the group task, while another member primarily ensures that everyone gets adequate attention.

As you continue to observe the group, you will not only notice the division of tasks even more clearly, but you will also start noticing *persons*. You then see, for example, that the task-oriented group member is a very precise person who sometimes seems a bit coercive. And the caring group member emerges as an exceptionally friendly person who evokes growing sympathy from you. Thus, in a (normal) group, individuals do not merge with the group completely. Over time, they become more manifest because they dare to show themselves more. The longer we observe the same group, the easier it becomes to recognize and predict this individual behavior within the group. That's because it repeats itself more and more clearly. What we see are roles within the group.

Roles bring a group to life

Roles make a group 'alive.' We see the people, the characters, and on the group 'stage' a whole theatre can sometimes develop between those characters. In one of my therapy groups for personality disorders, there was a middle-aged man called Frank (names are fictitious). When he first joined the group, everyone immediately found him congenial. He very quickly assumed a distinct role within the group, perhaps best referred to as 'the charmer.' He behaved very endearingly, especially toward the women in the group. He held the door for them and was always interested in everyone. Because Frank was so friendly and pleasing, everyone developed a fondness for him, and his role grew stronger and stronger. He began to dominate the group and took up a lot of space due to his 'showing interest' questions and responses.

However, Scott, a car mechanic with a no-nonsense character, was the complete opposite of Frank. Scott became increasingly annoyed with Frank. A confrontation was inevitable. At a certain point, Scott confronted Frank about his manneristic showmanship. He was extremely annoyed. Frank was completely taken aback; he was not expecting any adversity in this group. After he processed the confrontation, with the help of the group and myself, he was able to recognize his behavior more clearly. He remained charming but could now show and discuss the depressive mood hidden underneath it all. His exaggerated role behavior diminished over time, as he no longer needed that disguise.

Roles and role divisions arise wherever people meet. In society, we are familiar with countless examples of this, such as the roles of doctor and patient, teacher and student, and best friend and best friend or group therapist and group member. Our social interaction cannot exist without roles. Unconsciously, we make agreements, as it were, about standard behaviors that belong to the division of roles in such a relationship. This is needed to ensure smooth interaction with each other. This way, we do not have to rethink and agree on all of our behavior toward each other over and over again. In therapy groups, we encounter roles for the same reason. Therapy groups can be quite complex, and roles provide a natural division of tasks, making cooperation easier.

I define a role in a group as a *characteristic combination of personal behaviors* that group members expect from a particular group member over time and that the group member in question usually expects from himself. For example: 'Hey, typical Joe again, who is always serious and can put things into words so well,' or 'Look, there we see Marian, with her characteristic combination of humor and perspective, which can sometimes lighten the heaviness so nicely.' Thus, a role consists of several personal behavioral elements that the group member forges into a coherent whole. Nonverbal behavior, behavior through attitude and tone, is an important – if not the most important – part of this. Attitude and tone make a role quickly recognizable. I explained before how we perceive the nonverbal message of attitude and tone with our feelings. In fact, if someone always behaves submissively within their role, or authoritatively or in a very friendly way, we quickly sense that. Therefore, role behavior can largely be understood and mapped using the IPC model (see Chapter 2).

A typical characteristic of a role in a group is the *predictability* of its behavior. It is a group dynamic structure. After enough time, one expects certain behavior from a group member. The fact that group members' behavior thus becomes recognizable and repetitive is pleasant for all parties. In the role-formation process, typical titles for different roles often arise spontaneously, emphasizing recognizability; we use this playful way to outline the 'living theater' of the group. The number and type of role names are infinite; you will read many examples in this chapter. One example has already been mentioned previously, the 'charmer.' The need for predictability sometimes leads the group members to make a caricature of each other's roles. A group member behaving in a 'motherly' way, for example, is given the name 'Mom' over time, confirming or even stereotyping her role.

Various theories on roles

There are several theories on roles in group dynamics. In this chapter, I apply three theoretical perspectives: functional role theory, differentiation role theory, and interactional role theory. Each of these theories represents an important theme relevant to group therapy.

Functional role theory assumes that roles arise because groups always perform a function, both for the environment and for the members. Roles are one of the structures that ensure a group achieves its goals for both the organization and the members (Benne and Sheats, 1948; Parsons et al., 1953, in Forsyth, 2017, 167). Even in group therapy, it is nice if, in addition to the therapist, there are group members with functional task-monitoring roles. For instance, a group member who addresses a fellow group member's unacceptable behavior when the latter mercilessly insults and denigrates someone.

The second theoretical perspective concerns differentiation, an important research topic in group dynamics (Knippenberg et al., 2007). Roles help facilitate differentiation, different behaviors, views, and identities in a group. Group members generally behave differently due to their various personalities and other characteristics. Those different behaviors acquire structure in the form of roles. This behavioral repertoire of roles contributes to the flexibility, diversion, and purposefulness of any group (Benne and Sheats, 1948; Bettencourt and Sheldon, 2001, in Forsyth, 2017, 177). The importance of role differentiation for group therapy is easy to understand. The diverse roles of members in a therapy group are very valuable. They give room to different personalities and diversity in general. Consider roles such as a member who is very good at spontaneously expressing and verbalizing feelings, one who is great at listening and understanding, a member who is always good at putting his or her observations into words, or one who is good at dealing with anger, or someone who is very original and creative.

The third perspective is the interactional role theory. This assumes that a role arises in the interaction between an individual and the group, between individual dynamics and group dynamics (Goffman, 1959, in Forsyth, 2017, 177; Turner et al., 1994). This perspective is also very useful in group therapy, especially in situations of pathological role fixation and how to resolve it. I elaborate on this perspective in the next section.

A role arises from double dynamics

Roles arise from the *combination of and interaction between* group dynamics and individual dynamics. For example, a conflict between two members unexpectedly arises during a group therapy session. Apart from the group therapist, Jessica suddenly also becomes intensely involved. She proves to be very skilled at mediating and helping with conflicts, exactly the role needed at that moment. Because she is good at this, she also enjoys doing it. From then on, when disagreements occur during group therapy, Jessica again shines in her role of 'mediator.' Role behavior has a function for both the group and the individual group member at the same time. The behavioral needs of the group and those of the individual group member converge, leading to the creation of a role. I call this phenomenon *double dynamics*. Role behavior always reflects both the person and the group *simultaneously*. As a result, we can never immediately distinguish between what comes from the individual and what is related to the group. When we switch perspectives, we sometimes notice the personal side and sometimes the group side. This given of double dynamics in roles is the common thread in this chapter.

Types of roles

A well-known distinction is one between formal and informal roles. *Formal roles* are official roles. They are part of the job structure and stem from someone's official position in an organization. Formal roles have a job description that concretely describes behavior and authority (mandate). Examples in health care are socio-therapist, team leader, physical therapist, treatment coordinator, group therapist, client, resident, psychiatrist, and nurse. *Informal roles* are not predetermined but arise spontaneously, for example, the 'clown': the group member who makes the group relaxed by often making them laugh.

We also distinguish between *task-oriented* versus *process-oriented* roles. A group member in a task-oriented role explicitly supports focus on task and task performance. A group member in a *process-oriented* role is much more focused on the relationships among group members and the atmosphere and emotions within the group. Some group members have a personal affinity for roles that focus on the process side, while others have a strong affinity for task-oriented roles (Bales, 1950). The 'task keeper' is an example of a typical task-oriented role: this is the group member who notices that there are only 15 minutes left for the two group members who have yet to take their turn. The 'thermostat' is a typical process-oriented role: a group member who senses group tension and is good at putting it into words.

Another important distinction for group therapy is between *avoidant* and *constructive* roles. The informal role of 'clown' can become so overpowering that everything is laughed off, and the group no longer works on their therapy seriously. In group therapy, repetitive avoidant roles are valuable material for treatment because the underlying anxiety and avoidance of a member, as well as the group, becomes palpable and visible.

Summary

- A role is a characteristic combination of behaviors that group members expect from a particular group member (and themselves) over time.
- Roles have a function for the group and for the group members.
- Roles ensure differentiation.
- A role results from the interaction between individual dynamics and group dynamics – the *double dynamics*.
- We distinguish between formal and informal roles, task-oriented and process-oriented roles, and avoidant and constructive roles.

10.3   The function of roles for the group and for the individual member

The function of roles for the group

Role behavior always has a function for the group as well as for the individual group member. The main function for the group is *role differentiation*: regular group members in recognizable roles take on certain tasks. The group process creates a natural division of labor due to different roles. They provide the necessary predictability and stability in the interactions. While one group member is very good at overseeing group therapy and sees over time that some group members do not get much attention, another group member is very good at confronting and thus develops that role. Sufficient role differentiation is essential for a well-functioning group; it not only helps with the different group tasks but also facilitates important aspects of the therapeutic learning processes, such as diversity and spontaneity (Forsyth, 2017; Nijstad, 2009). The opposite, which I refer to as 'role blurring,' is detrimental to a group. In that case roles of individual members have not developed well and remain vague or weak.

Role differentiation is strongly associated with informal leadership. Bales (1950) found that members who talk a lot easily acquire a higher status and informal leadership role. Thus, role differentiation occurs not only horizontally but also vertically. The connection between roles and informal leadership can also be seen in the role typology of Brusa et al. (1994), which I discuss in the next section.

The role typology of Brusa; four essential roles

Much research has been done on group dynamics about the necessary roles, or the minimum role differentiation a group needs. Several role typologies have emerged, for example, those of Bales (2001), Belbin (Oomkes, 2002), Benne and Sheats (1948), and Brusa et al. (1994). For the purpose of this book, I favor the role typology by Brusa et al. (1994). Brusa and his colleagues developed a well-organized theory of role differentiation based on extensive factor-analytic research. They concluded that four roles are crucial for group functioning. Because these roles often coincide with informal leadership, the authors use the terms: Task Leader, Emotional Leader, Scapegoat, and Deviant.

The Task Leader

The Task Leader feels responsible for the task and task performance and will show his or her attention and commitment to it and foster a task-oriented culture, for example, by inviting group members to share their problems and feelings.

Having one or more Task Leaders in a group is useful because the group therapist has companions sharing his main responsibility, that is, task performance.

The Emotional Leader

The Emotional Leader takes care of the atmosphere in the group by paying attention to the level of tension and maintaining mutual involvement. He or she signals that the group is not coping with the tension or that there is not enough mutual support and solidarity. It is an essential role in every therapy group because tension regulation and emotions and conditional safety are crucial.

The Scapegoat

At first, it may surprise you that the Scapegoat is a functional role. But upon further consideration, this is understandable. This role is functional because the Scapegoat provides the tension reduction that every group sometimes needs. I also call this role the 'lightning rod.' By eliciting irritation, the Scapegoat sacrifices himself as the person on whom group members can take out their annoyance. For example, a group member known for his irritating and provocative jokes but who nevertheless remains a valued member. This role is functional as long as it remains within limits and does not necessarily belong to only one person. For example, a new group member could spontaneously take over this role.

The Deviant

The Deviant stands out because of the critical distance he or she maintains from the group. This allows the Deviant to observe and critically comment on the interactions within the group from a distance. The group member in the deviant role is good at looking at things from a different angle and putting forward a different view alongside the prevailing one. The deviant role is certainly useful for therapy groups where differences between individual members are important for learning and individual development. In addition, this role has an important function in the authority crisis and autonomy of the group in that the Deviant also dares to be critical of the group therapist.

What is notable here is that for a group to function well, it needs more than just task-oriented roles. It needs a mix of task- and process-oriented roles. Upon closer consideration, this is to be expected. After all, task and process are both essential to the functioning of a group. Hence, it is logical that both are represented in the repertoire of roles that a group develops.

This list of four necessities may give the impression that they are always fulfilled by the same persons, but that does not have to be the case. Members can switch roles, depending on their own development or that of the group. It is also possible that more people show the same role behavior during the therapy group sessions. This fact is especially important for group therapy where experimenting with different (role) behavior is part of the therapeutic method.

Learning from each other through different roles

A wary atmosphere prevails in an intensive interactional psychotherapy group. Group members are mostly nice to each other and hardly dare to confront one another until James joins the group. James has been referred to this psychotherapy group because of his depression and deeply rooted negative self-image. But his spiritedness also adds vibrancy. He is very good at confronting others in a subtle and humorous way. He soon takes on the role of 'feedback giver,' holding up a mirror to someone but also to himself, and this can be stressful but is appreciated by the group. After some time, others also dare to follow James's example, which raises the quality of the group therapy.

The function of roles for the individual member

Roles do not only serve a function for the therapy group and the therapeutic method but are also helpful for the individual member. Each individual more or less wants to show up and be useful to the group. Because role behavior is always fulfilled in a personal way, a role is one of the ways in which an individual can assert himself as a person.

However, a role never entirely coincides with the person. At first, we mainly see how a person performs the functional part of the role. Over time, we see that a role sometimes has very personal characteristics, especially if it meets the individual's needs. A role then gives the individual not only a foothold for interaction but also provides structure by which that person can manifest and make himself useful within the group. In this case, there is clearly a win–win situation: both the group and the individual in the role benefit from the mutually affirming combination (see the previous example).

Apart from a role being a vehicle through which a group member can manifest himself in the group, a role also provides the opportunity for masking, protection, and avoidance. The behavior of a role resembles a coat, like an outer layer that makes the person completely or partially invisible. For example, a group member in a 'reverend' role can indulge his talent for morality and 'how things should be' while hiding his fear of looseness and frivolity. A group member can play with this double-sidedness. Sometimes, he or she will conform scrupulously to the role expectation and display nothing of his or her own person, for instance if the group is not safe. Other times, if the group offers a lot of space for experimenting, a group member may interpret the role very freely and give it a clear personal character. The masking aspect of the role could also serve as a cover under which a group member can carefully try out new behavior (see the following example).

Group therapy as a spectacle

Human life is sometimes compared to dramaturgy (Helwig, 1958). Group situations lend themselves especially well to this, thanks in part to the phenomenon of roles. That is why theater terminology is the same as in this chapter. Roles bring a group to life. We see the people, the characters, and on the group 'stage,' a whole theater can sometimes develop between those characters. We can also extend this comparison with dramaturgy to where the action takes place. Roles require a stage and a play. In the theater, this is the stage; in our group, it is the room with a table or chairs in a circle where members get together for a session. Just like in a theater, the players who enter the group stage are watched by audience members: the other group members. This public situation always makes a group exciting. Just as audiences in the theater cheer or boo, the observing group members can be supportive or disapproving. However, observing others can be inhibiting, especially in groups dealing with sensitive issues. Shame then lurks. An important difference between our group and the theater is that the audience in the group is not only an audience but (alternately) also an actor. Unlike the audience in the theater, the audience in the group regularly participates as well. This, in turn, provides opportunities to make use of this observing third party. The observers are often invited in groups to respond with feedback, comments, support, or advice. Because they are familiar with the other position, group members can often give each other very good feedback, both in an accepting and confronting manner. The public function of group role-play is a valuable part of group therapy

A role as vehicle for experimenting

In an educational therapy group for people suffering from COPD, there is a need for someone who monitors the time because the sessions always run late. When it becomes apparent that no one wants to do that, everyone ends up looking at Harry, the least assertive group member. Again, he cannot say no and takes on the role of 'timekeeper.' After two meetings, everyone is surprised: instead of an introverted Harry, who always talks softly and mumbles, the group members see a very different Harry, who quietly but decisively cuts off group members and gives others the floor while pointing at the clock. And Harry develops in his role. As the number of meetings increases, he comes across more clearly and decisively. Harry visibly enjoys this role, which enables him more than ever to fulfill his deepest desire: to also show assertive behavior.

Summary

- Roles fulfill a function for the group: role differentiation helps the group in the division of labor and facilitates differences, spontaneity, and, thus, the interactional learning processes.
- There are four functional group roles: the Task Leader, the Emotional Leader, the Scapegoat, and the Deviant.
- Roles fulfill a function for the individual: a role is the vehicle for the individual to manifest (or hide), make himself useful, and interact.

10.4   The emergence and development of roles

The mechanism of role suction at the onset of a role

During the interaction, roles emerge from what I call double dynamics. The group needs these roles, and group members want to make themselves useful. Because attitude plays such a big part in role behavior, the principles of the IPC model apply in this interaction between the group and group members: Above behavior evokes Under behavior in the other and vice versa, just as Near behavior and Distant behavior evoke the same behavior in each other. Thus, a dependent group will quickly awaken a leadership role in an individual group member who possesses leadership qualities. An individual group member with strong cooperation qualities easily acquires the role of 'connector' in a group that needs help in cooperating.

A member does not merely assume a role; the other group members must assign it to the member. For example, if a group member would like to be 'the leader' but lacks the trust of the others to do so, this group member will not be allowed to assume that role. A role is a mutual structure.

How does this role assignment work? How do you explain why one person ends up with a particular role, and another doesn't? In group dynamics, one explains this phenomenon with the concept of *role suction* (Redl, 1963). Role suction is the power of the group to pull a group member into a role. Whether that group member takes on the role depends on the group member's own motivation for that role. If the group member feels that the role suits him or her, this process of role assignment will proceed smoothly and be hardly noticeable. If the group member does not wish to take on the role, it comes down to whether he or she is able to refuse the role. Then tension arises in the group around this role assignment. Usually, a group member is given enough space to be able to decline. But a group can also put a lot of pressure on someone in order to assign a role. Role conflict could then arise (Forsyth, 2017). An example: consider a group member who, under pressure, takes on a role while on the inside, he absolutely does not want to, for example, the 'patient,' the person whose problems are the worst and who needs help all the time. It works best, of course, if the role is mutually convenient. Then, the double dynamics create a pleasant win–win situation.

Role suction

An inpatient rehabilitation department for clients with psychotic vulnerability and addiction organizes regular outings as part of resocialization. Using a socio-therapeutic method, the clients do as much as possible themselves in the process, including the organization of a relaxation outing. The group therapist explains that there is money for a relaxation outing and that the organization is up to the group. Almost everyone is enthusiastic, and they spontaneously suggest various ideas. 'Let's go paintball shooting!' Peter shouts. 'What? No,' says Rose. 'Having dinner together somewhere sounds nice to me.' 'Whatever,' says Jeremy.

'Who is going to organize it?' the group therapist asks. After a while, during which most group members noticeably look out the window or look in the direction of Jeannette, Jeanette breaks the silence: 'I would like to give it a go.' 'Of course! Jeanette, our jack-of-all-trades!' Roger exclaims. Others agree: Jeanette must do it. Jeannette: 'Well, guys, you know me. That's just the way I am. . . . I like doing it, you know that. But not alone. Jeremy, are you in?' Jeremy nods. Spontaneously, Rose also offers to help. 'Okay,' Jeanette says to the group therapist. 'I will convene this little club to organize something nice.'

This process of establishing roles happens on a somewhat subconscious level. It is a subtle interactive negotiation process, sometimes consciously but often subconsciously. A role gains more 'body' in a further development process, which takes a while. There is no real role until the group has existed long enough for recognizable role behavior to emerge.

A group can exert a big influence on the role behavior of an individual group member, but the reverse also occurs: a group member can assume such an appealing or compelling role that he thereby determines the behavior of an entire group. The mechanism of role suction then applies the other way around: a group member in a strong role exerts strong suction on the group to meet the needs of an individual group member. The rest of the group may yield to this or not. For example, a person in a hefty victim role will strongly appeal to any rescuers and helpers in the group. Sometimes the sucking power of an individual group member is strong enough to pull an entire group into a counter role.

The development of roles

Roles – like norms – are influenced by the developmental stages in which they emerge. Because little interaction and development take place in the first phase, the parallel phase, the first roles that emerge are based on the familiar roles that group members were used to before the group began. Roles we often see in the parallel phase are those of the 'silent' one and the 'boss.' They represent the two solutions to the uncertainties and tension of the beginning group: withdrawing and creating certainty. The 'boss' thus regulates his tension and immediately meets the group's need for clarity. The notable silence of the 'silent' one legitimizes keeping quiet in the group. Two other complementary roles that we regularly see in the parallel phase are the 'helper' and 'patient.' In therapy groups, people who need help are naturally well represented, and in the 'dependent' initial phase of the group, some of them still expect the solution to their problem to come entirely from the group therapist. If the latter disappoints them in this, there are often group members who will fill that gap and take on the 'helper' role. The roles in the parallel phase are often somewhat rigid and adapted.

As the group continues to develop, these initial roles often disappear, and space is created in the inclusion phase to try out role behaviors. This 'fluid' phase is particularly well suited for this due to the experimenting space that characterizes it. Group members experiment with different roles and show more of themselves in their roles. The safety of this phase lies in the fact that they can try out roles 'on a trial basis' and let them go if they don't work out. For example, a group member who was quiet in the parallel phase can try out a more outspoken role in this phase. An ambitious group member can try out whether the 'task leader' role suits him. As a result of the space available for experimenting, role differentiation grows in the inclusion phase. This natural experimenting space in group development is important for group therapy, in which trying out new behaviors is an important goal.

In the mutuality phase, roles become less important as a 'foothold,' both for the group and for individual group members. This means that there is more freedom to fulfill the roles in a personal way. When a group reaches the *workgroup* phase, an appropriate role structure with sufficient role differentiation has been established.

Summary

- The process in which a group entices a group member to assume a group role is called *role suction*.
- A situation in which a group member sucks an entire group into a particular role can also occur.
- Roles develop analogously to group development.
- As the group develops, a varied role structure emerges that meets the needs of the group and in which the roles become more personalized.

10.5   Negative role development: role fixation and role blurring in group therapy

Role fixation

Ordinarily, roles in a group remain flexible. If necessary, a group member can let go or change a role, and the group can cope. However, it also happens that roles become rigid; they then become more noticeable because of their one-sidedness and immutability. Because of their rigidity, such roles lose their function and begin to hinder interaction. We call this *role fixation*. In some literature, it is referred to as 'role-lock' (Bogdanoff, 1978). Interaction throughout the group becomes fixated around a dominant role. An example of this is the 'jammer,' who keeps talking in a group that is becoming increasingly quiet. With role fixation, the behavior of the individual member is very strong and demands all the attention, making it seem as if the whole group revolves around him or her and the group task is sidelined. Role fixation almost always has an avoidance function.

Because the group member in a fixated role stands out so emphatically *individually*, it will appear as if that group member is the only determining factor. As I demonstrated previously, we have an individual bias in our observation of groups. This is a fallacy and a pitfall in assessing and addressing role fixation because individual dynamics are only half the story. Again, double *dynamics* is the cause. Role fixation occurs when both the individual group member and the group need a role *permanently*. The most severe role fixation occurs when group and individual dynamics complement each other. We call this role fixation, but essentially, group fixation always occurs simultaneously. Both parties interactively maintain a grip on each other, for example, a group that is prone to laughing a lot and has a group member with a particularly big need to be the group 'clown.' The two complement each other perfectly. And if they are strong enough, a balance is easily created with 'clown' role fixation at the center. As soon as someone in that group tries to upset that balance, for example, by being serious, the group will prompt the 'clown' to make jokes again. Another example is the combination of a rather inhibited and closed group and a group member who feels the need to talk a lot. As soon as there is even a moment of silence, this talkative member immediately starts babbling again, regulating this group member's own tension and that of the group.

If the group therapist wants to influence role fixation, she needs two leverage points: the dynamics of the individual group member and the group dynamics. If we zoom in on the individual side of role fixation, it always involves a person with a lot of rigidity. An example is someone who has spent his whole life accustomed to a dependent arrangement and ditto role in all previous groups. Such a person will most likely end up in a strongly expectant 'helpless' role again in the next group. If we focus on the group side, we see that role fixation always has an avoidant function of not facing certain themes or feelings because the group cannot handle them. For example, in a group where discussing sex is taboo, one will strongly reward the group member in the 'moral guardian' role, with the risk that this group member will become locked into that role.

Role fixation occurs regularly in therapy groups and is not always a bad thing. If the group and the group therapist can discuss and eliminate role fixation, it could turn out to be enlightening.

Utilizing role fixation therapeutically: the 'co-therapist'

In one of my intensive interactional psychotherapy groups, I had a persistent 'co-therapist.' This group member had had little support from her parents throughout her life and was used to always managing on her own – until she ended up incapacitated for work after a big conflict at her work. Then her 'I can do everything alone and don't need anyone' system fell apart. She opted for therapy in a group to develop more trust in other people and to lean on someone for once and not feel like she has to do everything herself.

But the first thing she did in the group was help everyone else. She was an excellent therapist buddy for me, but that was not in her best interest. She knew her pitfall well but found it incredibly difficult to let go of her helping behavior. She finally succeeded, thanks to the group's help. The group members cared for her and consistently confronted her when she played the 'co-therapist' role again. This delineating care was new, unknown, and good for her.

It took a long time before she could reflect on the parental care she lacked. After that, her behavior changed tremendously. She was able to let go of helping others and instead regularly seek attention for herself. After almost three years of therapy, she left the group with a positive result.

Role fixation can turn harmful if it becomes extreme, persists for too long, and becomes part of group culture. Several fixated roles and the typical avoidance thematic in which they thrive are mentioned in literature (de Haan and Pol, in NVGP, 2019; Yalom and Leszcz, 2020), for example, the 'helper' (avoidance of taking responsibility), the 'lightning rod' (avoidance of conflict), and the 'scapegoat' (avoidance of aggression). It is not always just a member who ends up in a fixated role. The object can also be, for example, a different group, the outside world, management, or the group therapist himself. The following section demonstrates in detail how role fixation works, using the scapegoat role as an example.

The fixated scapegoat role

The scapegoat is a distinct case of role fixation. Characteristically, this person does or says things that are 'wrong,' is disapproved of, and provokes aggression. We read at the beginning of this chapter that in a mild form, the scapegoat role is functional because it acts as a lightning rod and ensures that aggression in the group remains manageable. Like other roles, however, this role can become fixated. It always starts with stereotyping a member as 'the bad guy' by the group. In the mild variant, although the wrong is ridiculed, it is tolerated. In the case of a fixated scapegoat role, the aggression is more destructive: it can turn to hatred, and the fixation noticeably becomes more all-encompassing and extreme.

Where did the term 'scapegoat' originate?

The term 'scapegoat' is derived from a story in the Old Testament (Leviticus). It tells how the community is 'purged' of evil by sending (sacrificing) a goat who embodies evil into the desert. In a similar way, a group expels a group member after 'unacceptable characteristics' are projected onto that group member. The 'unacceptable characteristics' projected onto the scapegoat always involve feelings, experiences, or meanings that the group is unable to cope with (Scheidlinger, 1982).

Double dynamics and interaction between group and group member are also at play in scapegoat role fixation. The ratio of the individual dynamic share to the group dynamic share may vary. Sometimes, the group's share is bigger; other times, the individual's is bigger. When group dynamics dominate, the group accuses a group member of having done something 'wrong.' They project that 'wrong' onto that person. Their message to the scapegoat is that he or she, and what he or she represents, is *bad*, and it would be best to disappear. The wrong that this person represents must be 'eliminated,' destroyed. That 'wrong' can be anything: anger, sad feelings, vulnerability, red hair, wrong clothes, and so on. For example, in an adolescent mental health group, a shy boy may become fixated on the scapegoat role and constantly be told that his clothes are ugly – no matter what he wears. A scapegoat role fixation in which the group dynamics has the biggest share is the most damaging. It is the malignant, bullying, discriminating role fixation. In such a case, the group often chooses a vulnerable person who has difficulty defending himself to take their aggression out on, while the scapegoat himself hardly plays a part in it. If the role fixation lasts for too long, there is a big chance that the group member in question will be seriously damaged. But a fixated scapegoat role is also bad for the group. The offending group members may start to feel very guilty with an unlimited scapegoat role fixation.

If individual dynamics prevail, the group member in the scapegoat role will believe that he or she has unacceptable characteristics and, therefore, deserves the group's disapproval. It is usually someone with a strong inferiority complex or a tendency toward self-loathing. In the case of a very strong negative individual dynamic, the scapegoat role can be so powerful that the whole group is sucked in, even if the group members don't really want to. This is also harmful to both parties. Consider a new client with severe borderline issues whose severe negative self-image makes it impossible for even a healthy therapy group to overcome the pathology; over time, the entire group will start to hate and ostracize the new client.

Sometimes, the group focuses the negative attention on a 'scapegoat' because it dares not direct the focus toward the person for whom the aggression is really intended. We call this the shifting of interactions. We see this in a group where the therapist or group member shows very dominant behavior. For its own safety, the group then chooses a defenseless group member to whom they deflect their aggression.

Double dynamics in a fixated scapegoat role

Throughout his life, Roy has had an inferior view of himself. He is accustomed to expressing that view provocatively in groups. Cynical and defiant, he portrays himself as a loser. He does not act differently in a clinical therapy group for young offenders with psychiatric disorders. This group consists largely of group members with a criminal status. They have a choice: therapy or juvenile detention. Most group members don't like therapy at all, but they don't want to go to jail either. They take their frustration out on everything: the food, the coffee, and especially on Roy. He has to put up with an increasing load of 'shit.' For example, when the staff imposes sanctions for breaking house rules, or when the TV is broken, Roy is blamed for everything. And Roy doesn't defend himself but instead attracts criticism. The staff members are struggling to get a grip on the situation.

Role blurring

The opposite of role fixation is *role blurring*. In this case, the roles in the group are barely perceptible. The roles are 'weak' or very similar, so no role differentiation occurs.

Role blurring can have several causes. Inadequate selection opportunities for the group therapist are one of them. If a group therapist has few clients to assemble a group, it may result in a composition that lacks certain roles. Sometimes, the group task involves unilateral selection. For example, members of a therapy group for people with social phobia could saturate the group with personal anxiety that they all choose the 'coward' role, resulting in a failure to achieve the desired role differentiation.

Insecurity can also be the cause of role blurring. In the normal development of role differentiation, group members show increasing individuality in their roles. But in an insecure group, group members will keep a low profile so as not to expose themselves. Several issues may arise that cause group members to remain vague and invisible. For example, a conflict between two group members that is not properly resolved may result in continued insecurity and hiding oneself. In a different case, strict group norms can cause insecurity. A norm that disapproves of differences between group members ('everyone is complete equal here') or prohibits human feelings such as aggression and jealousy makes group members reticent. They are then unlikely to show themselves and certainly will not profile themselves in bold role behavior.

Inadequate role differentiation will lack the necessary different roles, which could significantly lower the quality of task performance. In this case, no one takes responsibility, or group members keep conflicting opinions to themselves. A group therapist should not allow such a situation to continue but rather address the underlying fear among group members. Often, that fear is excessive, and it helps to challenge it and put it into perspective. If that succeeds, group members will feel freer to show different behavior.

Summary

- With role fixation, the same double dynamics play out as with an ordinary role but then are more extreme.
- Even though role fixation seems to arise only from the individual group member, group dynamics always come into play.
- Role fixation occurs when the group avoids a particular theme or feeling.
- There are many types of role fixation; the scapegoat is one of the most prominent.
- A persistent role fixation is harmful to the group member in question and to the group as a whole.
- Role blurring lacks the desired role differentiation.
- Role blurring can occur due to inadequate task capabilities, such as inadequate preselection opportunities.
- When role blurring persists, the fear of exposure usually plays an important role among group members.

10.6   The function and value of role behavior in group therapy

Role behavior has various starting points for group therapy, as we have already seen before. I'll list them again.

Role differentiation promotes the quality of learning from each other in group therapy

Role differentiation is extra important for group therapeutic practice because it increases and deepens the learning capacity of the group. In group therapy, members learn primarily from each other and from each other's differences, and different roles increase the array of visions, insights, and solutions that can then be introduced.

Roles illustrate avoiding and pathological behavior in group therapy

A typical characteristic of a role in a group is the *predictability* of its behavior. In group therapy, this role predictability is very useful, because it makes the maladaptive side of a group member's behavior clear so quickly. For example, how avoidant someone behaves by constantly showing the role of 'helper' and never drawing attention to themselves. Because roles are so much a part of the person and role behavior is repeated in the therapy group, it is often quickly picked up by the other group members. Often that behavior is so familiar to the client himself that the other group members realize the inadequacy before the client himself, and that confrontation can be the beginning of an insightful change process. And this is where the big advantage of group therapy counts: complex avoidance behavior is more easily recognized in group therapy because group members are more likely to accept something from each other than from the professional group therapist.

Roles help to focus on the individuals in group therapy

In group therapy, the group is the therapeutic tool needed to help individual members improve. Thus, those individuals must always remain visible. Because roles are always performed in an individual manner, they help maintain that individual focus. Zooming in on role behavior means seeing the person behind that role. That is why role behavior, with its recurring behavior patterns, is rewarding material for group therapy, especially when treating personality problems (Trimbos Instituut, 2008).

Personality problems are often accompanied by role-fixated behavior. Take a client with a very scrupulous conscience and who sets the bar high for himself and his environment; he is stuck in the 'strict schoolmaster' role. The typical role (fixation) that this client displays will catch the attention of others and evoke reactions, for example, annoyance over his schoolmaster-like attitude. This feedback gives the client in question insight into his inappropriate role behavior, which then invites reflection on one's own behavior. The insight thus gained can encourage clients to let go of the role fixation and try new behaviors. Roles are an ideal vehicle for this.

Roles legitimize experimenting with behavior in group therapy

A therapy group is a flexible training ground, and ideally suited for experimenting with new behaviors. A role acts as a stepping-stone to try out new (role) behavior. Within a role a client can play with interactional and group behavior.

A therapy group with all kinds of roles and interactions is an instructive reflection of the real world, and experimenting with a role in the group is the preliminary stage of trying out new behavior in one's own world.

In intensive interactional group psychotherapy, this testing of new behaviors often takes place in the final phase of group therapy. And in some educational groups, such as a social skills therapy group, role-play is used as a method to systematically train new behaviors. A special form in this sense is group therapy that uses the psychodrama method (Gilhuis et al., 2014). By portraying and acting out important situations from a client's life and life history in roles, he or she experiences in-depth insight into the genesis and sometimes also the solution of his or her problems.

Summary

- Role behavior has an important function in group therapy.
- Role differentiation promotes the quality of learning from each other.
- Roles illustrate avoiding and pathological behavior in group therapy.
- Roles help to focus on the individuals in group therapy.
- Roles are helpful in group therapy on personality problems.
- Roles legitimize experimenting with new behaviors within and outside the group.

10.7   The role repertoire of the group therapist

Within her formal role as a group therapist, she has some important sub-roles that can come to the fore at appropriate moments. These roles arise in the same way as with group members, namely, when the dynamics of group and group therapist meet each other in a common need. The roles to be distinguished are to a large extent related to the functions of the group therapist, as I have described them in Chapter 4. These are the following sub-roles, the 'organizer,' the 'educator,' the 'therapist,' and the 'crisis manager.'

Before and in between, the group therapist is often the 'organizer,' especially when she designs the group therapy on paper and explains it in the pitch. This role naturally transitions into another important sub-role, namely, that of 'educator.' In every therapy group, even in the intensive long-term interactive psychotherapy groups, she regularly explains what the purpose of the therapy is and how it works. And when the therapy group marches, it is the 'therapist' who directs the task, guides processes and conversations, and stimulates the therapeutic interactions. In the complexity of group therapy, it helps the group therapist to be aware of the different roles that are needed at any given time, and also to really keep those roles apart at times. Take, for example, a crisis that arises suddenly. Then it is very wise to let go of the role of 'therapist' for a while and just be a 'crisis manager' for a while. And then discuss the experience again in the role of therapist. See the following example.

A crisis during group therapy

A newly started ongoing couples therapy group has been in existence for six months and is going well. The essential goal of the therapy group is for each couple to gain insight into the relationship problems, what causes them, what perpetuates them, and how they can be reduced. The core of the method is interpersonal and insightful feedback on each other as a person and as a couple. There are four couples, two of a man and woman, one lesbian couple, and one gay couple. All participants work very seriously by giving each other feedback but also by supporting each other, and sometimes also by giving suggestions for better interaction with each other as a couple. Unexpectedly, a crisis arises. Marjorie comes to the group without her partner Kelly, is very anxious and tense, and tells that she has been unexpectedly abandoned by Kelly. After the previous meeting, in which she was supported by the whole group, she had been angry at Kelly at home because she was often dominated and sometimes even humiliated by her.

After she told the group, she received a lot of support and compliments for her assertiveness, and members were vicariously angry with Kelly. When there had been enough response to Majorie, Jeff and Christine went further by bringing their sexual problems to the group. During that subject, the group therapist saw out of the corner of her eye how Marjorie seemed to pull away completely. She looked pale and had big frightened eyes. The group therapist interrupts the ongoing conversation by going to Marjorie: 'What's happening to you, Marjorie?' Marjorie: 'Ehh what? Ooh, I don't know, I feel myself becoming very strange, like everything is spinning, and like I'm losing myself. And I have very weird thoughts.' Group therapist: 'What about you? Sit back in your chair and take a deep breath.' Jeff: 'I'll get you a glass of water, Marjorie.' Group therapist: 'What do you mean by weird thoughts, Marjorie?' Marjorie: 'Yes . . . I don't know exactly, I'm confused and scared.' Group therapist: 'Also afraid to hurt yourself, Marjorie?' Marjorie: 'Yes, that comes up easily for me when I feel really bad, and when I was studying I made an attempt once, and that always comes up again.' Jeff: 'Here's some water, Marjorie.' Marjorie: 'Thanks, Jeff.' Marjorie gets a lot of support because other group members can feel her anger and also her fear after such a breakup. Group therapist: 'I suggest that we talk together after the group about what you need now, to be safe with yourself again, Marjorie, is that okay?' Marjorie: 'That's nice, please, but it does me good to talk about this now, this already helps. . . . Jeez.' Quisha: 'It's not nothing what you've been through Marjorie, I think you're brave, and for me that mindfulness exercise always helps so much, when I feel like a role.' Group therapist; 'Are you okay with us going back to Jeff and Christine, Marjorie?' Marjorie: 'Yes fine, of course. I'll sit quietly for a moment and take a deep breath.' Group therapist: 'Okay, Jeff, where did you go?' Jeff: 'Well when Christine yesterday evening did not want sex . . .'

The double dynamics of the group members and the group therapist do not always match the role of the group therapist. Group members, especially in a beginning group, expect the group therapist to take and hold the formal 'task leader' role. This is related to the hierarchical expectations of group members. They initially associate a group therapist with hierarchical roles such as teacher and doctor. Frustrating these role expectations creates confusion among group members, sometimes resistance but often a learning process. It would be unfortunate for the group therapist to be pinned down to this formal vertical task leader role. First and foremost, it is important that group members become co-responsible for task performance. For that reason alone, sharing the task leader role with group members is a good thing. In addition, it is important that the group therapist not be limited to one role, as she has more options in the therapy process. As the group therapy progresses, the more horizontal role becomes more prominent, such as the role of 'process facilitator' and 'connector.' The group therapist can steer the group through this by explaining the reason for the more 'horizontal' role behavior. For example, she can make it clear that these behaviors are designed to invite group members to participate, cooperate and share responsibility. It often works well if the group therapist then demonstrates the more horizontal, collaborative role behavior. For example, she may choose not to emphasize her leadership role, sitting among group members rather than at the head of a table or in a larger chair. A group therapist duo can also use their position and role strategically, for example, by not sitting next to each other, not forming a leadership front, but rather deliberately sitting opposite each other in the group therapy circle to emphasize the role of 'interactors.'

The natural development of the group's movement toward independence helps in this regard. A group therapist moves in tandem with that natural development by adapting her role to the phase the group is in. In the parallel phase, she has more of a leading role, which she exchanges – after the authority crisis in the inclusion and mutuality phase – for a more horizontal role.

The group therapist also needs freedom in role repertoire in order to respond to unexpected situations. It is very important in situations where group members exhibit extreme role behavior. For example, a group member in a fixated role strongly demands (role suction) affirmative role behavior. This applies to group members but equally to the group therapist. It is important that the group therapist be aware of this risk and know how to resist the suction.

Because attitude is such a big part of role behavior, the group therapist can benefit from her knowledge of the IPC model in this type of situation.

Summary

- A beginning group expects a formal task-oriented role from the group therapist.
- The group therapist benefits from not letting the group fixate (lock) her in this role.
- The group therapist moves in tandem with the development of the group by adapting her role to the phase.
- A group usually has to get used to a group therapist who is not directive.
- The group therapist must have freedom in role repertoire in order to handle unexpected situations.

10.8   Practical Manual: steering and utilizing role behavior in a therapy group

10.8.1   Introduction

As I explained in Chapter 5, you utilize group processes by giving them space and connecting them to the task. In doing so, the group therapist is free to stimulate process development. Even though role development often occurs naturally, this is also applicable to roles. The need for role behavior, both by the group and by the individual group member, is such that the desired role differentiation often occurs naturally. Affirmation and reward are often sufficient.

If the group is very inhibited and role blurring occurs, the group therapist can help eliminate the role blurring more proactively so that more role behavior can emerge. If role fixation occurs due to out-of-control roles, the group therapist must intervene firmly. When steering role behavior, the group therapist uses the following well-known techniques: the organization technique and the verbal and relationship technique combination.

10.8.2   Fostering role development and role differentiation in a therapy group

Fostering role development in advance
Opportunities for organizational techniques in advance are limited. Because roles arise during the spontaneous encounter between the individual and group, they allow only very limited influence in advance. In addition to using the standard conditions (such as a clear group task and working method), the group therapist

can try to facilitate appropriate role differentiation through the selection of group members. For example, the four necessary roles defined by Brusa: Task Leader, Emotional Leader, Scapegoat (lightning rod), and Deviant (see previously in this chapter). However, experience shows that a group therapist rarely has a sufficient number of potential group members from which to select all desired roles. Moreover, roles only really develop in the dynamic interactional field during group sessions. The role a group member exhibits during the intake interview could change due to group interactions.

Fostering role development in a beginning therapy group
In a beginning group, the roles of most group members have not yet been developed. However, usually, some roles emerge to eliminate the uncertainty of that initial period. These are often more straightforward and dominant roles, which disappear during the course of development because they are no longer needed. Therefore, it is important for the group therapist to provide sufficient safety during this initial period so that role development can continue. The group therapist does this by welcoming spontaneous (role) behavior with an inviting attitude (COOPERATING), *mirroring* and *rewarding* and, where possible, *connecting* it to the task or to the other group members.

Table 10.1 Fostering role development in a beginning therapy group.

Verbal technique	Relationship technique
The group therapist actively confirms role behavior through *mirroring*, *connecting* it to group members and the task, and *rewarding*.	**(attitude and tone)** This technique requires an affirmative attitude (COOPERATING).
Two example interventions: Group therapist: 'Gregory, am I correct in saying that you feel very responsible for the group task? And one thing I notice about you, Latoya, is how well you can observe.' Turning to the group: 'Have you guys noticed that, too?' Group therapist: 'It seems that everyone is happy with Jasmine's leading role. Am I right?'	

Fostering role development in an existing group
As long as the roles are open and varied enough and the group is working on its task, the group therapist does not have to do much except gently affirm the group and the individuals in their role behavior by displaying an inviting attitude (COOPERATING), supplemented by the verbal techniques of *mirroring* and *rewarding*. She can then use the role behavior as material for group therapy (see the end of this section).

Removing role blurring

Sometimes, too little role differentiation occurs. This can be detrimental to task performance. In that case, the group therapist must uncover the reason (often fear), discuss it with the group, and invite group members to broaden their repertoire. She does this actively and together with the group (HELPING). The group therapist uses the verbal techniques of *confrontation, questioning*, and *explaining* to discuss role blurring and the verbal techniques of *inviting* and *advising* to evoke new behavior.

When members leave, or new members join an ongoing group, it presents a perfect opportunity for a new role repertoire. Shifts in group roles almost always occur then. For example, when the 'senior' (often the longest-serving group member with a leadership role) leaves, a game of musical chairs always ensues, often followed by new positions and roles. The group therapist can also use that moment to promote role differentiation.

Table 10.2 Removing role blurring in a therapy group.

Verbal technique	Relationship technique
Step 1	(attitude and tone)
The group therapist *confronts* and *questions* group members to find out if they also see the lack of role repertoire and how they feel about it. She *explains* why more repertoire for the task is useful.	To help the group 'wake up,' she applies an active and activating attitude (HELPING).
Step 2	
The group therapist actively and playfully *invites* and *advises* group members to explore and experiment with new role behaviors.	

Three typical interventions:
Group therapist: 'Can I ask you something? Do you also feel like nobody in this group is allowed to just be silly for once?'
Group therapist: 'I sometimes see you almost becoming angry, Tyler. Am I right?' Tyler: 'Yes, you are, but I restrain myself.' Group therapist: 'What would happen if you didn't restrain yourself?'
Group therapist: 'You guys can handle a bit of constructive criticism, can't you?'

10.8.3   Changing negative role behavior in a therapy group

Influencing role fixation

Because role fixation draws too much attention to the group member stuck in the fixated role, it will seem like he or she is the sole source of the role fixation. This power of individual role behavior is sometimes so strong that even a group therapist must be on guard against inadvertently joining in the role fixation. A group therapist may have a strong tendency to push this individual group member to let go of the fixated role behavior. This one-sided way will not succeed because the group member's behavior in the fixated role is always partly caused by group dynamics. The one-sided attention role fixation attracts is a pitfall. The rule with role fixation is to assume double dynamics and take a two-sided approach. It is important that the group therapist try to clarify the role situation. Important questions are

- How strong is the role fixation (can the group member still step out of the role or resist the role suction)?
- What is the individual group member's share in this?
- What is the group's share in this?
- Are the group and individual group members reaffirming each other in their role positions?
- What theme or feeling does the role fixation resolve for the group member and for the group?

If role fixation becomes permanent, it will hinder the group task and become harmful to the group and individual members. The group therapist can allow this situation to continue for a while until everyone is aware of it. Then, she should firmly intervene with a meta-conversation, pausing the group task and discussing the role-fixation process. In doing so, it is recommended that the group therapist follow the succeeding intervention steps:

1. *Question* or *confront* the group and fixated members about the interaction pattern, and both parties' share in it.
2. If one of the parties does not recognize its own share, tactically *question* this 'blind' party about its own share (can also be done through the group).
3. If group members begin to recognize something, *analyze* the function of role fixation.
4. If the dynamics of the individual group member have a lot of influence, *advise* the group not to adopt the counter role and *explain* why they shouldn't.

The group therapist's attitude must be obviously directive (LEADING). She can safely repeat this intervention cycle (a toehold) if the group and the individual revert to the previous role fixation, which often happens in practice. Changing such fixated role patterns is difficult, especially if they have existed for some time. If the change does not succeed immediately or encounters difficulties, group members easily revert to the familiar role-fixation pattern. However, with persistence, the group therapist usually succeeds in eliminating the role fixation.

If the group therapist succeeds in controlling, investigating, and exploring the role fixation, it is sometimes possible to turn it into therapeutic experiences for the group and group members.

Table 10.3 Limit and change role fixation in a therapy group.

Verbal technique	Relationship technique (attitude and tone)
Step 1 In view of the (often denied) role fixation, the group therapist repeatedly *confronts* and *questions* first the fixated group member and then the group or vice versa. **Step 2** If the group or group member do not recognize their own share, the group therapist should *question* this. **Step 3** As the group and group member become aware of the role fixation, the group therapist can explore its function with *in-depth questions.* **Step 4** In cases where strong suction of individual dynamics of a group member occurs, the group therapist may *advise* the group not to adopt the counter role and *explain* why they shouldn't.	With this technique, the group therapist must adopt a strong, active, and persistent attitude (LEADING).

Two typical interventions:
Group therapist: 'I am again noticing the same pattern. Everything is directed at Peter, and it mainly involves criticism. I wonder if I'm the only one who sees this pattern.' Joyce: 'But Peter often acts very weird. It annoys me tremendously.' Group therapist: 'I'm sure it says something about Peter, Joyce. But apart from Peter, could it also say something about you or the others?' Gordon: 'I beg your pardon? What are you saying? Surely, you can see that Peter is not quite right in the head.' Group therapist: 'And yet the question remains applicable to all of you, Gordon. What does it say about the group?' Marja intervenes in the conversation: 'What is it that you want us to say? That we are using Peter as a scapegoat? He brings this on himself, you know.' Group therapist: 'Well, sometimes a group does take out their frustrations on a particular group member, and maybe that is what's happening here.' Aron: 'Maybe we are just as shitty as Peter sometimes, but we don't want to admit it.' Turns to the group therapist: 'I think this is the case because I can identify with what you are saying.'

Group therapist: 'You are correct in observing that Olivia is having a very difficult time. And I understand why you want to help her. But Olivia has a tendency to demand a lot of help from others and to make herself dependent on it, whereas Olivia would benefit more from first exploring what she is capable of on her own. Therefore, it would be better for Olivia if you stop helping her and giving her advice. Do you understand what I mean?'

10.8.4   Using role behavior to steer a therapy group

In this book, I emphasize the usefulness of group processes as a steering tool, which is certainly true regarding roles. Once the group is up and running, the appropriate role differentiation with informal leaders provides the group therapist with a convenient leverage point with which to influence and steer the therapy group. In Section 10.3, I explained how a group member in the deviant role can contribute to critical reflection on how the group is doing. Thus, that group member can be utilized if a group therapist wants to change something in the group, for example, by challenging an undesirable norm or introducing a different working method. As a group therapist, you can then seek out group members in a critical role (several group members can perform the deviant role) during the conversation and invite them to express their opinions. The group therapist can initiate change in the group with a COOPERATIVE attitude and inviting verbal techniques (*questioning, mirroring, connecting*). Table 10.4 summarizes this technique and is illustrated with an example.

Table 10.4 Utilizing group roles to steer a therapy group (initiate change).

Verbal technique	Relationship technique
During the conversation, the group therapist locates group members in different roles through *mirroring* and *connecting*.	**(attitude and tone)** An active but clear Under attitude is best suited to this technique (COOPERATING).

Utilizing group roles to confront a therapy group

Group therapist: 'So, the whole group is okay with mobile phones going off? That's not what we agreed on. Anyway, if everyone agrees, then we will try it for a while and see if that works.'

'What do you think, Leo? You look pensive.' Leo: 'I don't understand why you put up with this!' Group therapist: 'You don't understand why I put up with this? 'Well,' Leo interjects, 'I think this group is a lame mess. If it keeps going like this, I'll be leaving soon.' Caroline: 'Just because of a few mobile phones, Leo?' Leo: 'No, of course not, but that's sort of the cherry on top. I thought we would be working on our issues.' Group therapist: 'Leo feels that more serious work needs to be done, and that requires you to switch off your mobile phones. Do you agree?'

All roles can be utilized, for example, in situations where creativity is desired or where a particular aspect or feeling is being avoided. Consider, for example, the 'observer,' the group member who is often silent and records everything carefully. This role can also be utilized very often, for example, in situations where members do not want to self-examine and where concrete feedback would be appropriate. The moment the group avoids feelings, the group therapist can invite the 'emotional leader.' The 'task leader' role can be deployed precisely at times when the group is slacking on the task. These and other roles give the group therapist an important steering tool. Here is another example:

Steering a therapy group by utilizing different roles

Roger is a new member of a protocol therapy group for people with early childhood trauma. The group therapist begins to notice that Roger pays a lot of attention to others and hardly ever asks for attention. When Roger once again clearly exhibits that pattern of behavior, the group therapist decides to direct attention to it: 'I would like to take a moment and focus on you, Roger.' Roger: 'Why? We are busy with Josephine, and I have another question for her.' Josephine: 'Yes, I am considering what you said, Roger. I recognize that sad feeling.' Group therapist: 'Getting back to you, Roger. I think I see a pattern in you, and I want to ask you some questions about that.' Roger: 'I don't understand what you mean.' Group therapist: 'Do you understand what I mean, Rose? It looks like you do.' Rose: 'Sure, I think you mean that Roger keeps talking about others and never about himself. And you never show your own feelings either, Roger. I think that's a real shame.'

10.8.5   Utilizing role behavior for the working method in a therapy group

Role behavior is rewarding material for most types of group therapy. This is because of the typical behavioral patterns that clients repeat in their role behaviors in the group. The most useful situation is when a participant demonstrates clearly maladaptive role behavior within the group. Very often, a client is only partially aware of this. At an appropriate moment, the group therapist *confronts* the client with his not-very-productive role behavior, always with a questioning and accepting attitude (HELPING/COOPERATING), and compares that observation with the client's goal and the group goals. And of course, it is always helpful to involve the group members in this therapeutic process. In addition to being an aid in the diagnosis of maladaptive behavioral patterns, roles also lend themselves as therapeutic tools. In Section 10.6 I described the various forms of group therapy in which roles are explicitly used as therapeutic tools, such as in social skills, group therapy, or psychodrama. See the following example and previous examples in this chapter.

Utilizing maladaptive role behavior

Joseph is participating in a social skills therapy group to gain more social contacts. What is striking about him is that he always talks about himself and rarely shows interest in others. He then glories in the role of 'orator,' camouflaging his social insecurity. Even now, as he practices with the role-play 'Making contact by having a chat,' he does not ask the other person anything about themselves but only talks about his hobby of restoring vintage cars.

After the exercise, the group therapist decides to confront Joseph with this behavior. Group therapist: 'Joseph, may I point out something I have been noticing for some time now?' Joseph: 'Go ahead, Willem.' Group therapist: 'During this role-play, I noticed that you are good at talking about yourself.' Joseph: 'That's good, right?' Group therapist: 'Indeed, it's good that you're not afraid to show yourself, but perhaps you do that too well. You did not ask the other person much, and the purpose of this exercise is to 'Make contact.' Joseph: 'I don't understand. I never used to talk, and now I'm glad that I'm finally able to talk about myself.' Group therapist: 'That is wonderful, of course, but if you want to make contact, and that is your goal with this group therapy, then it will be even better if you combine telling with asking questions and showing interest in the other.' Joseph: 'Okay, I get it. Can I then practice that again?' Group therapist: 'Absolutely, Joseph, go ahead.'

Chapter 11

Termination and saying goodbye in a therapy group

11.1 Introduction

This chapter deals with the termination of a therapy group or a group member's treatment. It is an extension of Chapter 8, 'Group development,' and also based on Levine's theory (1979).

Termination is an important phase in the life of a therapy group. This final phase is important because of the evaluation of outcomes and the specific termination processes evoked in it. Termination is a therapeutic process in itself because it can help group members become disengaged and independent and learn how to cope with goodbyes and loss (Daemen and Van Paassen, in NVGP, 2019).

The following topics are covered:

- Termination of the group task in a therapy group
- The process of termination: separation crisis and termination phase
- The therapeutic value of termination processes
- Practical Manual: steering and utilizing termination in a therapy group

11.2 Termination of the group task in a therapy group

Termination is an essential part of the task of a therapy group. It is the final piece of the group enterprise. At that final moment, the client takes stock and sees what he or she has achieved in terms of results. The clients who have realized their intended goals will feel empowered and satisfied. For example, they no longer have symptoms, have learned new skills, have gained more self-confidence or have gained new insights. These group members will confidently complete the task and detach themselves from the group. The group is no longer needed. Group members who have not yet or incompletely realized their goals will use the evaluation to see where they stand in the treatment process. They still need the group for longer or – in the case of a time-limited group – an alternative, appropriate continuation of their treatment.

DOI: 10.4324/9781003368786-14

The more concrete both individual and group goals are defined in concrete end terms at the beginning, the easier they are to test at the end. In Chapter 3, I explained the importance of always envisioning the end at the beginning and making concrete predictions about where the group and group members will end up. The beginning and end of a group are connected like a loop.

Summary

- The therapy group follows a cycle: everything about the beginning and end of a group is connected.
- At the end, the beginning returns, namely, the goals agreed upon at the time.
- The more concrete the goals are at the beginning, the easier they are to evaluate at the end.

11.3 The process of termination: separation crisis and termination phase

Termination is part of group development

For group members, termination does not end with the conclusion and evaluation of the group task. The peculiarity of group therapy is that group members have entered into a relationship with each other to accomplish a group task. When terminating a group, group members must not only conclude the task but also terminate the relationships between them. Termination also impacts the nature of the group process, namely, the attachment between members. As with the termination of the task, the termination process revisits the beginning. When group members let go of each other and say goodbye, the bond they formed with each other at the beginning of the group is always reawakened. The amount of attention paid to this depends on the type of therapy group. In a group with strong attachments, this personal parting is often given a lot of space. In a group in which attachment between group members has remained minimal, for example because the group had only four meetings, the personal parting will be less intensive.

In Chapter 8, I outlined how a group undergoes natural *regression* in addition to natural *progression* during development (Levine, 1979). Completion and departure are parts of the natural developmental arc. Progressional development was the focus of Chapter 8. This chapter focuses on the regression, the development of the group in its final phase. If we assume a new group, the sequence of developmental steps will look like those shown in Table 11.1.

Table 11.1 Developmental phases and crises according to Levine.

Phase 1		Phase 2		Phase 3		Phase 4
	Transitional crisis 1		Transitional crisis 2		Transitional crisis 3	
Parallel phase	Authority crisis	Inclusion phase	Intimacy crisis	Mutuality phase	Separation crisis	Termination phase

The last two steps, the separation crisis and the termination phase, involve the termination of the group. Within these, completion and separation take place.

When separation or loss occurs in a group, a two-step process emerges. The process begins with the awareness of *feelings and thoughts* regarding an upcoming separation and the group's efforts to deal with them. Step two in the process is the *actual* parting (saying goodbye) *itself*, in which the group must find a way of wrapping up and saying goodbye. According to Levine's theory we call the first step the *separation crisis;* the second step is the *termination phase.*

11.3.1 The separation crisis

The separation crisis belongs to the list of developmental crises in groups, including the authority and intimacy crises (Levine, 1979). Each developmental crisis deals with an essential human theme that comes into play at some point. Such a theme always evokes an emotional conflict of contradicting desires and fears. Separation is also such an essential human theme. The separation crisis involves the *fear* abandonment or loss, of not being able to cope with the separation, and remaining dependent. At the same time, there is a *desire* for autonomy, to be strong enough to deal with separation and loss and to be able to leave the group. Although separation always evokes painful feelings, we can view the separation crisis as a positive developmental crisis. Separation also always marks a transition and new beginnings. For example, forensic clients in the end phase of their detention following a group therapy aimed at resocialization. Their separation and completion are a big transition. They will sense some anxiety to do it alone again and at the same time feel the desire to be free.

A separation crisis occurs when themes such as termination, parting, abandonment, and loss become the key issues in the therapy group. This crisis can be triggered by an imminent parting but also by the mere thought of a possible parting. For example, a separation crisis may result from a touching story about a serious loss a group member recently suffered. Such a moment can make group members realize that they have to deal with loss in their own lives. The impending end of the group is another trigger of a separation crisis. Characteristically, group members are either surprised or frightened the moment they become aware of it. A separation crisis can best be seen as a 'preparation moment': it is the prelude, a kind of virtual goodbye, in which the group members emotionally adjust and prepare for the actual parting.

The fear of separation stems from our basic human need for attachment, which I described in Chapters 1 and 6. We need others to make us feel secure and supported. Once we have established a secure attachment with someone, we would rather not part with that person. If someone we are attached to unexpected leaves, we can feel left alone. For example, if a good friend suddenly announces that she has another job and is going to live abroad, or a sympathetic neighbor announces that he will be moving, we are very unhappy about it; we are startled. It is not uncommon that underneath we even feel a little angry about such a sudden departure.

The same thing happens within our therapy groups. For example, a group may be heavily engaged in the group task and not realize that they are well over halfway through the total number of meetings. If an observant group member suddenly realizes this and brings it to the group's attention, anxiety may set in: 'Are we that far along already?' or 'Gee, I don't want the group to stop, it's going so well,' and 'That scares me because I'm not ready to be without the group!' Group members are startled to realize that they will soon have to deal with everything on their own again and that they will miss the support the group provided them.

A separation crisis in a therapy group

In an intensive interactional psychotherapy group for people with neuroticism Joyce is one of the longest-serving group members. She is well liked for her engaging personality and open manner. Thus, group members are startled when Joyce announces her departure during one of the sessions.

As usual, the group therapist begins with the announcements, 'Are there any announcements?' Joyce: 'I do . . . um . . . how shall I put it . . . I want to announce that I am going to quit the group. Or rather, I want to discuss my plan with you guys. I really think . . . no, I'm pretty sure I'm done here. I've learned so much, gained so much from the group, and . . . um . . . well, I'm doing really well.'

'Nooo!' Chantal exclaims. 'Are you leaving us?' Roger: 'Joyce, you can't abandon us like that!' 'Oh, Joyce, I don't believe you,' Kelly says. 'When are you stopping?' Joyce: 'Well, you guys will have enough time to get used to the idea of not having me around. I'm still here for another whole month.'

The group therapist notices that the group has difficulty letting go and realizes he feels the same way about Joyce leaving. She is such a great group member. But he knows this does not suffice as a good reason to keep her in the group; she is more than ready to stop. After a long discussion, the group members and therapist support her departure. In the four-week termination phase, Joyce's departure is often a prominent topic entailing grief about her departure, as well as old wounds about broken relationships and goodbyes, which result in teachable moments for several group members. At the final meeting, the members eat cake, cry, and give Joyce cards and a heartfelt goodbye.

The loss is palpable and discussed within the group even after Joyce is gone. The group mourns the loss of a beloved group member.

A separation crisis in a therapy group for the elderly

Group therapy for elderly people with depressive symptoms is going well. Most group members learn a lot about how to manage their depression. Some notice how actively making contact helps, others how important it is to have enough activities, especially when you are alone at home. The theme of loneliness comes up a lot. Some group members do have a partner, some are alone. A shock occurs when the partner of one of the participants dies unexpectedly. When Rosalie is present again, everyone is very supportive and understanding toward her. Two days after the group is the funeral, where not only the therapist but also all the group members are present, except George. In the next meeting George starts saying: 'Sorry, Rosalie, I wanted to be at Marian's funeral so badly, but I couldn't. I fell completely back into my depression in the past few days. And the whole event also scared me a lot. I don't have a partner at the moment so that wasn't it, I think I felt fear for my own vulnerability, my own mortality. I got so scared that I didn't dare to go. I'm ashamed of that and feel guilty, Rosalie.' Rosalie: 'That's okay, George, we missed you, but I get it . . . and it's great that you guys were there' (looks around the group with tears in his eyes). Group therapist: 'How good of you to tell this, George. When loss or separation suddenly comes very close, it is not surprising that we are shocked and think of ourselves, right?' When the group therapist looks around, he sees several group members nodding affirmatively.

The group always seeks a solution to this contradiction between fear and desire in a separation crisis. Such a solution is always a compromise between fear and desire. The solution acts as a practical tool to make the upcoming separation manageable.

The compromise may lean more toward the fear side or, conversely, the desire side. If the desire was most prominent, we speak of an enabling solution. Such a solution sufficiently takes into account fear and allows plenty of room for the desire side of the conflict. In this case, group members will be able to face the impending separation openly, discuss the associated fear and desire openly, and prepare well for the parting, allowing for the desire for independence. For example, a group may come to the conclusion that separation, while painful, is not insurmountable, that experience shows that talking about it helps and that others are confident that they can stand on their own two feet.

When the solution is primarily motivated by fear, we speak of a restrictive solution. Such a solution has the effect that thinking about, feeling and discussing separation becomes fraught with anxiety for abandonment and loss. We then see that the group members begin to avoid these anxious thoughts and feelings that the impending separation raises. They try to avoid these emotions associated with abandonment and loss in two different ways (Levine, 1979). The first way is to deny them. For example, a group member may downplay the upcoming separation day or pretend that the separation does not affect him or her at all. This avoidance is a flight into *counter-dependence.* The second way is the opposite, which is a flight into *over-dependence.* In such a case, group members react with regressive helplessness and disappointment; they feel that the group has accomplished nothing or is 'far from finished.'

Both such situations could appeal to the group therapist to actively help (by confronting the group with the reality of the separation) or even to rescue (by making the disappointed group members realize that the group did help them). Because this avoidance is a defense mechanism, such an active response usually backfires. It is better if the group therapist recognizes that this is an *emotional* reaction and tries to *mirror* the feelings (e.g., disappointment).

What we frequently see in a separation crisis is group members complaining that the initial symptoms or problems are returning. This can cause the group member and group therapist to worry that the group member has regressed to square one. However, if this group member showed good results up until the separation crisis, the group therapist can reassure him or her. After all, the relapse is then a side effect of the separation crisis, masking the actual successful end result of the treatment.

The group therapist can be of great help to group members in a separation crisis, as it is often a tense battle between desire and fear. He can steer the solution to the separation crisis in the desired direction. Usually, this is in the direction of an enabling solution, which will make separation a meaningful and discussable topic. Because the fear of separation is such a defining factor in the separation crisis, it is the best pointer for influence (Levine, 1979). The group therapist is most effective when he discusses and helps put the anxious feelings and thoughts regarding separation into perspective. Then separation becomes a normal reality that group members do not have to avoid but can face and handle. For example, suppose a group member harbors the unrealistic thought that parting means his whole world will collapse and he will be left helpless. If the other group members do not challenge this overly dramatic idea, the group therapist should do so and subsequently engage the other group members. If discussing and putting the fear into perspective is successful, the group members will be better able to handle the actual parting and may feel the desire to stand on their own two feet more.

The solution to the separation crisis that the group and group therapist eventually reach together has implications for the actual parting that takes place in the subsequent termination phase. The more enabling the separation crisis is resolved, the more openly and concretely the termination phase is used for closure and parting between group members. If the separation crisis has been solved restrictively, group members will not dare to be as open in the termination phase because the parting has remained fraught with anxiety. The group then needs additional help with parting during the termination phase.

A restrictive solution to a separation crisis
A therapy group for 'revitalizing after cardiac arrest' has ten meetings. There are two more meetings to go. The group therapist notices that the group is acting as if the therapy program will simply continue, as if there is no impending end. When the group therapist reminds the group that he wants to evaluate the group termination at the next meeting, he is confronted by sulking group members. Although the evaluation is on the agenda, the group does not take it seriously. When the group therapist gently inquires whether the group might be reluctant to stop, the sulking and resistance increase rather than decrease.

An enabling solution to a separation crisis
In a psychotherapy group for students with identity problems, David told the others during a previous meeting that he was thinking about quitting group psychotherapy. He said he felt much stronger and no longer felt as dependent on his parents, especially now that living independently in his room is going so well. And also, very importantly, he has energetically resumed his studies in economics, and that is going well. In this meeting, however, he again expresses doubts about his intention. Isn't it too early? Has he improved sufficiently that it will stick, he wonders.

Several group members give David feedback on his personal goals. Most feel that David is ready to stop. However, two other members believe he is not ready at all yet. David listens to the feedback and, after a brief pause, says he will think about what he wants to do: quit or continue for a bit longer. The group therapist suspects underlying motives in the pair and asks why they feel David is not ready. During the conversation that follows, both group members discover that they are very attached to David and do not want to let him go. After clarifying their motives, the two members can look at David's intention more objectively and now agree that he is ready.

11.3.2 Termination phase

This phase is the second step in the termination process. As the separation crisis resolves, the group moves into the termination phase, where the real completion and real parting take place. As in the separation crisis, the termination phase is about separation, detachment, and autonomy – only now, it is for real.

A serious and thoroughly organized evaluation of the goals is the most important issue in this final phase. Sometimes, this involves the whole group (in a closed group) and sometimes only the members who have agreed to quit (in an open group). In the Practical Manual, I explain how the group therapist can organize the evaluation to be as reliable a measuring point as possible.

As I described previously, during the termination phase, not only is the task (the goals of the members) evaluated, but also the process side, the relationships. And this happens spontaneously, as it is part of the natural process of parting, of detachment. When group members have worked together for a while, there is always bonding between them, so it is normal for them to feel extra what they have meant to each other now that they have to part. When parting, the natural need then always arises to say something to each other about this, to evaluate and appreciate the relationship, as it were. An example from our daily life. If two members of a group trip to Bolivia establish a friendly interaction, they will not only reminisce about how beautiful the Andes were when they part but will also express how much they enjoyed each other's company. They will smile at each other, say something positive about their interaction, and give each other a heartfelt handshake, hug, or kiss.

The duration and intensity of the group therapy determine how deep the contact has become and how intense the parting will be. Sometimes, a group has meant very much to a group member, sometimes less. Other times, group members are relieved to be able to let go of each other, and the end of the group comes as a release. In more structured and short-term therapy groups, parting is usually not a major topic, whereas, in more long-term group therapies, it receives more attention because the bonding has been more intense. In a long-term intensive interactional psychotherapy group, the members can become so attached to each other that saying goodbye is accompanied by grief and mourning.

Even if the separation crisis is resolved enabling, that does not mean that the actual parting between group members in the termination phase will be a breeze. Termination is primarily an emotional event involving a few difficult emotional aspects.

Termination is emotion under high pressure
Actual parting becomes a boundary; it is an all-embracing happening. We do or do not part; there is no such thing as partial separation. Termination makes feelings more intense than usual. Consider the official farewell of a loved colleague who is retiring. What else could you say when you shake hands with him or her at the end of the reception, knowing that you might never see each other again? Now, you still have interaction and can still say something; after that, no more. That compelling ultimate, that now-or-never quality, puts great pressure on parting and creates an extra emotional charge.

Termination from a group is very public

Saying goodbye requires group members to be open with one another. This is always a delicate moment. The parting members allow themselves to be vulnerable to each other and must dare take the risk of hearing something disappointing. Will the group member allow and be able to understand the farewell message? This tension is complicated in a group because an audience is always watching. The group members present will often be helpful and empathetic, but it only becomes apparent once you have dared to be open. When a group member is at the point of saying something personal to another group member, a group that is watching can be inhibiting. A group member may have anxious thoughts, such as 'Will they think I'm crazy?' and 'Is this appropriate?'

Termination feelings are double feelings

Next to intense feelings termination always evokes double feelings. Double feelings are the rule rather than the exception when breaking up. For example, a group member feels anxious about missing the group but is happy about stopping. In addition to sadness, a group member feels relief. He or she is proud of the results achieved and, at the same time, uncertain about whether they could achieve more. Or the group member notices that he or she has gained positive feelings for another group member whom he or she previously disliked for some time. This ambiguity creates confusion and makes expressing feelings back and forth difficult. Even more confusing for many group members is the feeling of anger that often accompanies saying goodbye. Noticing that you are disappointed or angry with the group, even when you yourself choose to quit, is often difficult to understand. Feeling abandoned by a departing group member you really like is confusing. Yet it is precisely the anger at goodbye and loss that is very important to be able to feel because it helps with processing and facing reality. It helps to cope with the 'illusions' that always go along with treatment, that symptoms never disappear completely, that life after group therapy is not the dream you imagined, that reality is sometimes disappointing.

Organizational procedures and education as a termination aid

Structure and regularity are some of the most important tools for making evaluation and goodbyes easier to handle. When parting, we always see three main forms of structure emerging: *procedures*, *rituals*, and *education*.

Organizational procedures

It is wise for the group therapist or the mental health institution, especially in the case of long-term or clinical group therapy, to record the organization of the evaluation and farewell. In the Practice Manual I elaborate on that.

Rituals as a tool for parting

When it comes to parting, we almost always see the group using *rituals* (Michaels, 2006). Rituals are a common phenomenon in social situations in which an important existential transition occurs with accompanying, often intense feelings and are intended to make it easier to accommodate or express those feelings. Such transitional situations in our daily lives include the birth of a child, passing an exam, or getting married. As we know, all these situations are accompanied by appropriate ritual customs. For example, when a child is born, the Dutch send a birth card and serve rusks with colored aniseed-flavored sprinkles, and we complete our education with a solemn graduation ceremony. Parting is also such an existential transition situation that is accompanied by rituals.

Rituals that we see when saying goodbye are often symbolically meant to hold on to something of the one who is leaving. For example, we bury a loved one by collectively shoveling a bit of sand onto the coffin, and at silent marches commemorating tragic violence, we leave candles and flowers at the scene of the crime. Rituals are *meaningful customs* that offer comfort and make it easier for a group to give something a place to express feelings and cope with reality. The *symbolic acts* that form rituals are very important and useful in shaping farewell moments (Michaels, 2006).

What do these parting rituals look like in our therapy groups? They vary from group to group and depend on the group task, duration, and intensity of the interaction. For example, in a group that has only run for a short time and in which there has not been very intensive collaboration, a shared cup of coffee at the end may already act as a ritual. In a long-term therapy group or therapy groups in a clinical setting, the rituals are usually more elaborate and connected to the therapeutic method. Then, the evaluation is accompanied by subsequent rituals, such as special ways of giving feedback or characteristic graduation. Sometimes, group members give each other a memento or a card with a therapeutic message. If a group exists longer, the rituals become part of the fixed habits at recurring farewell moments. Like norms (meaningful customs), they become incorporated into group culture.

Education as facilitating action

Saying goodbye and the contradictory and sometimes intense feelings that come with it can feel so confusing that group members withdraw. Education is always important in group therapy, but especially when saying goodbye. It helps if a group therapist explains at such times that these conflicting feelings are normal and that they are part of saying goodbye.

Summary

- People are built to become attached, not separate.
- The process of termination is like a two-stage rocket: first comes the separation crisis and then the termination phase.
- Separation crisis and termination phase share the same emotional conflict: the fear of abandonment and loss, not being able to cope with the separation, versus the desire for autonomy.
- In the separation crisis, that conflict takes place prior to the separation, in the termination phase during the actual parting.
- When parting, feelings are often stronger than during group sessions due to its ultimate and public nature; thus, delicate attachment feelings and dual feelings come into play.
- To handle these feelings, a group therapist helps with structures, including procedures, rituals, and explanation.
- The group dynamic structure loosens during the termination phase.

11.4   The therapeutic value of termination processes in group therapy

The themes of termination are inseparable from health care, and we thus often deal with them in our therapy groups. Loss, parting, and death are never far away when it comes to geriatric and somatic care. In addiction care, saying goodbye to life as an addict is the goal and in mental health care, it is about letting go of unfruitful patterns of thought, feelings, and behavior. In rehabilitation, dealing with limitations is part of daily life. Of course, the effort of group therapists is aimed at improving and curing, but that is not always possible. Hence, learning to cope with limitation, loss, and parting is part of it and is an equally legitimate goal, just like improving skills or curing symptoms are.

Generally, it is useful to pay attention to termination in therapy groups. Besides the usefulness of evaluating outcomes, the theme of separation in more intensive therapy groups, in particular, has broader therapeutic value. In these therapy groups, members learn not only how to attach but also how to detach in order to learn how to part in a healthy way. Many clients in mental health and addiction care have negative or sometimes even traumatic experiences with both attachment and separation. Therapy groups are an ideal tool to help correct those negative associations and facilitate saying goodbye in a new and healthy way. We see this regularly in practice as well. For example, during the farewell, someone may articulate, 'It feels like this is the first time in my life I'm actually saying goodbye; it's quite difficult and heavy, but still better than running from it, as I've always done until now.' Through positive experiences with termination, clients learn to cope better with life situations in which they face loss, limitations, or parting (Daemen and van Paassen, in NVGP, 2019).

A good separation also facilitates a very important general therapeutic goal for our clients, namely autonomy, daring to stand on one's own two feet. An enabling resolved separation crisis and an open and realistic termination phase promote a healthy 'letting go' and ditto autonomy. A restrictively resolved separation crisis and termination phase in which the parting and the feelings associated with it cannot be openly discussed keep the client more dependent than necessary; unrealistic fears remain, which is a missed opportunity to promote autonomy.

Another important therapeutic value of termination is the fact that in the termination phase, when detachment occurs, the original attachment from the beginning and the associated feelings can be experienced again. Often also the attachment of a long time ago. In some groups where past and old learned patterns are important to group therapy, living through the parting and old attachment has therapeutic value.

Old attachments and separation

During termination, it is normal to touch on positive and negative experiences of attachment and separation from the past and for it to surface spontaneously. This happens during a separation crisis and during the termination phase. Both can stir up anxious memories of loss and abandonment but also memories of good attachment and warm relationships. Whether the group therapist uses that material or only listens to it depends on the type of therapy group and group task. In many types of group therapy methods, previous experiences of attachment and separation are used to better re-create the current parting happening in the group, to make it a corrective experience. However, in the last session of, for example, a social skills therapy group, there is no need to explicitly address past attachments. The past is used only in situations where it is functional.

11.5   Practical manual: steering and utilizing termination in therapy group

11.5.1   Introduction

As with the other group processes, the group therapist can influence the termination process and use it in a positive way. To do so, he must again use his three techniques: *organizational techniques* (to create the conditions for termination prior to and during the group) and the combination of *verbal techniques* and *relationship techniques* (to direct the evaluation and termination process during the ongoing group). Organizational technique plays a distinct role here. Because termination benefits so much from structure, the group therapist makes additional use of organizational techniques in this phase.

The group therapist facilitates the termination process using a combination of verbal and relationship techniques. Separation involves increased emotional intensity; thus, listening carefully to feelings is an important skill to promote the process of termination.

11.5.2   Organizing termination in a therapy group

Organizational techniques allow the group therapist to provide structure prior to or during group therapy to make termination and separation easier and more productive for group members. Previously, I showed you how structure can be provided with organizational procedures, rituals, and education. Next, I discuss how to handle these aspects of structure in practice.

Organizing termination in open or closed therapy groups

A closed therapy group involves a collective termination, while an open group involves a termination phase in which one member says goodbye to one or a few group members. The processes described in this chapter are similar in both types of working methods. However, the open or closed way of working each requires its own organization of the termination.

With a closed working method, the composition of the therapy group, the group duration, and the end date are all fixed from the beginning. The group stops collectively. The termination, as it were, is ingrained in this working method. Group members either automatically encounter it or collectively avoid it. The group therapist makes it easy for the group and himself by integrating the organization of the termination. He can best do this by clearly marking the final period as a separation phase and regularly bringing it to the group members' attention right from the start.

Collective termination in a therapy group with a closed working method has the advantage that termination is a joint undertaking and subsequently pleasantly clear to the whole group. Even if the therapy group collectively avoids termination, it is often very clear in a closed working method and, therefore, easy to deal with. A separation crisis is often clearly recognized and experienced by everyone in a closed group. Because everyone says goodbye to everyone else, a proper termination phase can take place collectively.

In a therapy group with an open working method, the group member stops individually while the rest of the group continues. Everyone says goodbye to the group member leaving the group and vice versa. An open group lacks the concentrated collective termination but has its own characteristics. One advantage is that group members in an open group have already dealt with termination before. So, before it becomes time for a group member in an open group to quit, he or she has encountered several separation crises when other group members have departed. Termination is, therefore, more continuous and natural in open groups. It is easier to convince a group with an open process of the reality of the group's finitude and of finitude in general.

Another advantage is that the group member can decide when to stop. This does, however, mean a heavy responsibility for individual group members. The decision of a group member in an open therapy group to stop treatment is therefore often made in consultation with the group and the group therapist. Termination in an open group needs additional organizing because the end is not as ingrained in the group organization as in a closed group. It is not uncommon for a group member to overwhelm the group with an impulsive decision to quit, which is rarely to the benefit of both the group member and the group. The decision is often ill considered, and the group becomes unstable when members unexpectedly quit. What helps is for the group therapist to explain some ground rules at the beginning of treatment on how an individual group member can responsibly terminate in an open group, ensuring that the termination is a well-considered and shared decision rather than an impulsive act. Next, I outline what such a termination protocol looks like.

The key steps follow:

1. Termination must exist as a reality for group members right from the start. The group therapist is well advised to refer to the end (and hoped-for outcome) of group therapy as early as the first meeting. Concretely, this means that he, in addition to the other group rules, also explains these ground rules for quitting.
2. If a group member wants to quit, he or she should discuss it before the decision becomes definite – thus, at the time of *consideration*.
3. The group member considering quitting discusses his or her consideration by asking the group and group therapist for feedback. Is it a wise decision? Is he or she ready, or is it too soon?
4. The group member then weighs all the facts at home and makes an autonomous decision independent of the group: quit or continue.
5. Once the decision to quit has been made, the end date must be determined and agreed upon, leaving sufficient time for the group and the departing group member to complete the process of stopping and saying goodbye. Depending on the intensity of group therapy, between one and four weeks.

Organizing the task evaluation in a therapy group

As I have indicated several times in this book, good organization of the task evaluation is indispensable for the success of any group. Next, I discuss two useful tools for such task evaluation: *evaluation questions* and *concrete feedback*.

• Evaluation questions

Any evaluation of group therapy treatment should always address three questions (Daemen and van Paassen, in NVGP, 2019):

1. What were my individual goals, and which ones did and did I not achieve?
2. What about group therapy helped me?
3. What do I want to continue working on, and what do I need to be able to do so?

The first and last questions are about the individual group member; the second question is about the group therapy applied. Knowing what aspects of group work helped is important information for both the group therapist and the departing group member. The group member can determine from this what works for him or her as a learning tool. With this information, the group member can benefit in his or her life after the group or in a follow-up treatment. From the collected answers to the question of what has and has not worked in the group, the group therapist can determine which elements of the working method can be maintained and which should be modified or omitted.

The results of these evaluation questions can be supplemented by the results of an appropriate measurement instrument. Some therapeutic methods have associated measurement instruments. In mental health care, treatments are routinely evaluated using routine outcome monitoring (ROM). There are several well-validated questionnaires that can be used to conveniently and quickly track (monitor) treatment outcomes and client satisfaction. The data from those ROM questionnaires are good to use as individual outcome measures (De Jong and Spinhoven, 2008; Koementas-de Vos et al., 2018). I do not discuss this further as it is beyond the scope of this book.

• Concrete feedback

The key tool for evaluation is the feedback group members and group therapists give each other. Feedback is the concrete and objective information one gives back to a group member during an evaluation. Here, I refer again to the Johari table (Chapter 7), which clearly demonstrates how interpersonal feedback can bring about useful information. By using objective feedback from fellow group members and the group therapist, group members can test their results. The originally formulated goals are the measure.

A well-functioning group is very capable of providing reliable feedback. Collectivity allows a group to very powerfully convince a group member of certain feedback. For example, such a group member could easily override unpleasant feedback from one person but will not be able to do so in the case of similar feedback from four or five serious fellow group members. Such feedback usually sinks in and makes the receiver think. The reliability of a group's feedback can also come from its variety. If a group member receives diverse feedback from a number of serious fellow group members, it can also be thought-provoking. It may cause the group member to take a more nuanced view of himself or herself or to recognize that the problem is multifaceted. In all of this, it is essential that feedback from group members be concrete and reliable. The ground rules in Table 11.2 help guard that reliability.

Table 11.2 Rules for concrete and reliable feedback. Based on Remmerswaal (2015). Translation by author.

Rules for reliable feedback	Example (with continuous text)
Give feedback in a descriptive way, in a nonnormative and objective I-message form.	'I noticed how, during the last two meetings, you . . .'
Use concrete and clearly indicated behaviors.	'When criticized by Roy and Rachel, you didn't say 'yes, but' once, as you used to at the beginning of this group when criticized.'
Use a concrete experience.	'I find that pleasant because it makes you more approachable.'
Make sure the timing is precise and ensures accurate context information.	'I wouldn't have dared say what I'm saying to you now before that.'
Show that the feedback is meant to be positive and useful.	'It is clear to me that you have learned a tremendous amount from this group therapy.'

In most therapy groups, it is appropriate to have one group member evaluate himself first. Then, the other group members take their turn. Finally, the group therapist gives his feedback, possibly supplemented by the results of a completed questionnaire. Because of our defensive tendency, it helps to start with the positive remarks followed by the critical ones. The group therapist's task is to summarize the evaluation in the form of a conclusion and again present it to the group member in question. If the latter agrees with the conclusion, resulting agreements between the group member and therapist will automatically follow.

There are numerous variations that the group therapist can use to shape the evaluation of a group. The standard way is that one or two sessions before the final session, the group therapist asks departing group members to review their personal goals and 'pre-evaluate' the group therapy at home. During the final session (or sometimes the last two sessions), he ensures that each departing group member is given adequate time to evaluate. It is best to use a format that fits the way the group is used to working.

Appropriate rituals

As I explained earlier in this chapter, saying goodbye in a group usually involves rituals. Rituals are a nice vehicle for the expression of emotions while regulating concomitant anxiety. However, not all rituals are equally appropriate and functional. An ongoing therapy group for adolescents that has developed the habit of giving expensive gifts at farewells is overdoing it – so rituals can be exaggerated and then often have an avoidant function. A group therapist is well advised to allow the group a great deal of individual input when designing rituals but to guard the boundary of functionality. The best guide for rituals is to ask whether they are a reflection of the group task and whether they are proportionate.

Take, for example, a group of severely overweight people. An appropriate farewell ritual could be the preparation of a healthy farewell meal together. An appropriate farewell ritual in a grief support group is for members to give each other a symbolic gift in the final meeting from which they can draw comfort. For example, one group member might give another group member a stuffed animal as a gift to draw comfort from in sad moments. Another group member can gift someone 'the beach' so they can regularly take a breath of fresh air and clear their mind.

An overdone farewell ritual

In one of my therapy groups, intended for students with an anxiety disorder, a habit developed of celebrating a group member's departure with cakes and lots of pastries. With each farewell, the cakes got bigger, and the group members ate more and exchanged fewer and fewer feelings about the goodbye. When I questioned this custom, the group at first reacted angrily and indignantly. It became clear to me that cakes and pastries expressed a great need to give something to each other at farewells. Later, they understood my concern, and the group could see that the cake and pie did indeed serve the function of avoiding difficult farewell feelings.

But the need for a ritual remained strong. I then used the subsequent farewell situations to experiment with different rituals with the group. On one occasion, it resulted in a collective poem by the group for the departing group member. Another time, each group member gave the departing group member a symbolic gift, similar to the example of the grief support group. In turn, the departing group member gave each of the remaining members a symbolic gift in return. The group soon came to appreciate these creative rituals; they no longer talked about cake.

11.5.3   Fostering the termination process in a therapy group

Fostering termination at the start of a therapy group
If the group is running, the group therapist can positively foster termination. This can be done from the very beginning of the group. It is advisable that he clearly points out the end of the group or treatment already in the first session in order to remind group members of the finality of the group. By connecting the 'developmental arc' with the usefulness of the end result, the group therapist immediately promotes the task orientation of the group members. He does so in a persuasive and encouraging manner (LEADING) and uses the verbal technique of *explaining*.

Table 11.3 Foster termination in the first session of a therapy group.

Verbal technique	Relationship technique (attitude and tone)
In the first session, the group therapist *explains* to the group that they are working toward an end and final outcome.	An encouraging style and attitude are appropriate here (LEADING).
Typical intervention: Group therapist: 'As we get started, I want to express the hope that later, at the end of the group, we will have achieved a good result together.'	

Foster termination at the beginning of a separation crisis
The beginning of a separation crisis is an important but delicate moment in the entire termination cycle. This is the 'startle moment' when it dawns on group members that the group is really going to end, that a group member really intends to leave the group, and that loss is a reality that can affect anyone. This is an important moment because it is precisely this moment that can be used to put feelings about the finality of the group on the agenda. The moment is delicate because the unexpected shock can send the group into flight mode. If there is too much fright and fear, the whole group drowns in avoidance and termination then becomes a 'scary' topic.

The group therapist must support and understand group members with separation anxiety. In doing so, he lays the foundation for an open attitude toward termination and all that it evokes. Therefore, he primarily uses verbal techniques of *mirroring* (feelings) and *connecting*, combined with an actively supportive attitude (HELPING).

Table 11.4 Helping the group at the beginning of a separation crisis.

Verbal technique	Relationship technique (attitude and tone)
The group therapist *mirrors* the group's feelings of fear about the upcoming separation and *connects* group members with each other.	At this event, the group needs an understanding and supportive attitude from the group therapist (HELPING).
Some examples of typical interventions: Group therapist: 'Do I understand correctly that you are startled that the group only has four more sessions left and will then stop?' Group therapist: 'Do I understand correctly, Ricardo, that you suddenly realize that your buddy Bob is going to leave? Aren't you actually telling Bob that you're very sorry he's leaving and that you feel sad about it?' Ricardo: 'Yes, that's right. That's exactly how I feel, Bob!'	

Foster termination by helping to resolve a separation crisis I: countering separation denial

As the separation crisis unfolds, a conflict arises between the tendency to avoid the reality of the impending separation and the desire to cope with it. Avoidance can manifest itself in two ways. In both cases, group and group members evade responsibility for the separation. The first way becomes apparent by the denial of the impending separation. Group members downplay it or do not want to acknowledge that it is going to happen. To make the avoidance visible, the group therapist primarily uses the verbal technique of *confronting* and an active and sometimes steering attitude (LEADING or HELPING).

Table 11.5 Help resolve the separation crisis I: countering denial.

Verbal technique	Relationship technique (attitude and tone)
The group therapist *confronts* group members about denying the separation, *asks* about it, and *explains* again the benefit of discussing the end of the group	This requires an active and incisive attitude on the part of the group therapist (LEADING or HELPING).

(Continued)

Table 11.5 (Continued)

Typical example:
Group therapist: 'I have a question for you. Isn't it better to face the end of group therapy throughout the next three weeks and learn to deal with it instead of pretending it's not going to happen?' Roxane: 'Three weeks is still so far away. What's the use of thinking about it now?' Group therapist (turning to the other group members): 'Do you guys think three weeks is far away, too?' Jimmy: 'No. Three weeks will be over in no time, I think. But (turning to the group therapist) what should we do now? What do you suggest?' Group therapist: 'I get the impression that you are avoiding the issue of the group ending, and I want to help you figure out why you are doing that.' Jimmy: 'So, in your opinion, are we supposed to be broken up about it already?' Group therapist: 'No, but I notice that it's not being discussed, nor what you all plan on doing once the group has stopped. You act as if the group will go on forever, as if there will be no goodbyes when it in fact ends in three weeks.' Judith: 'All this whining about the group stopping is annoying me. Can't we just get on with today's session?'
The group therapist sees Judith's comment as indicative of her trying to sweep the goodbye under the rug. He decides to ask further questions. Group therapist: 'I get a strong impression that you don't want to face the ending and saying goodbye, Judith?' Judith: 'Yes, well, I'm not sure that's quite the case. But it is true that I would rather not think about the end of the group yet.' The group therapist replies that there may be benefits to facing termination and presents these benefits to the group. Judith: 'Well, maybe you have a point. I hadn't looked at it that way before.' Group therapist: 'Do you have any idea, Judith, why you find it annoying that the group is shutting down?' Judith: 'Well, no, I don't know, I just don't like it, it almost makes me a little angry.' Group therapist: 'Do I understand correctly Judith that it irritates you that the group can't just go on, but has an end?' Judith: 'Yes, maybe so, I don't know exactly, it's confusing.'

Fostering termination by helping to resolve a separation crisis II:
helplessness in response to separation

The second way of avoiding, the group also evades responsibility for the separation. In this case, the group members respond helplessly and 'down'; also because their initial symptoms have resurfaced. Table 11.6 demonstrates how the group therapist can handle this avoidance. He resists the temptation to rescue group members by realizing that this is an emotional response to termination. Instead, he consistently *mirrors* the direct or indirect feelings of the group members. To avoid affirming the helpless attitude, the group therapist uses a COOPERATING attitude as a relationship technique.

If the group is open to information, the group therapist *confronts* group members about their tendency to not take responsibility for the fact that the group is going to stop. He then *explains* the importance of termination, *connecting* group members to each other. Education about what termination can do emotionally, such as feeling disappointed, worried, and sometimes even angry, because initial symptoms return again, is an important part of this approach. A HELPING attitude is best suited for this active approach.

Table 11.6 Help resolve the separation crisis II: countering helplessness.

Verbal technique	Relationship technique (attitude and tone)
The group therapist *mirrors* the feelings of disappointment and sometimes angers the group members with their helplessness. In the second instance, he *confronts* the group members with the impending stopping and parting they are avoiding. He *explains* the purpose of parting and *connects* the group members with/to each other. In doing so, the group therapist also *explains the aspects of* termination, for example, that original symptoms may resurface.	Since the group members are behaving helplessly, a strategic Under (IPC) attitude is best suited (COOPERATING). Because the group therapist is tempted to save the helpless group members (which, of course, is not possible), it is wise not to act too actively and instead tolerate the helplessness and try to discuss it.

Two typical examples:
Rick: 'I don't know what's going on with me. I've been feeling so down lately.' Catherine: 'Same here. And I notice that my enthusiasm for this burnout group therapy is completely gone.' Group therapist: 'What exactly do you mean, Catherine?' Catherine: 'Well, at first, I thought I would fight these feelings; I want to be able to handle my work again. But now that therapy is almost over, I think: what have I learned now? I'm still as tense as I was at the beginning when my boss kept looking over my shoulder. And that is very disappointing.' Group therapist: 'Do I understand correctly that you are disappointed with your accomplishments so far?' Catherine: 'Yes, indeed. I expected more from this therapy.' Group therapist: 'We are going to have a comprehensive evaluation next week, but I am curious, could that also have something to do with group therapy ending?' Melissa: 'Yes, I think so. In any case, I feel like it is almost over, and my feelings are conflicted. On the one hand, I am happy about having Monday afternoons to myself again, but on the other hand, I would have liked to learn a bit more.' Group therapist: 'I understand, Catherine (turning to the group), when it comes to the end of a group, we often see that disappointment or those double feelings that Melissa described. Original symptoms often resurface briefly near the end of therapy, and that is usually triggered by the realization that the group will stop. By no means does that say anything about what you've really accomplished.' Rick: 'Oh, I didn't know that.' Group therapist: 'Are you also sad that the group is stopping, that you will no longer see each other?' Catherine: 'Well, as I said earlier, I would have liked to continue. I find this a very pleasant group where I feel safe and can tell my story. I'm going to miss that a lot, and it may sound weird, but it almost feels like I'm being let down.'
Group therapist: 'Okay, Catherine, that's certainly not my intention, but that's how it sometimes feels for group members when the therapy stops.'

(Continued)

Table 11.6 (Continued)

> Group therapist: 'I am sorry, Denzel, it is not possible to extend the group therapy.' Denzel: 'Shit man, I don't like that.' Group therapist: 'That makes you mad at me, doesn't it?' Denzel: 'Yes, do you think it's crazy, I'm just doing so well and I'm very scared of relapsing. Stupid group therapy!' Group therapist: 'I can understand your feelings, Denzel. Fortunately, we still have a few sessions to go before the end, and we can see together how we can help you and if you need anything after the group, okay?'

11.5.4   Utilizing termination in the termination phase of a therapy group

In the termination phase, the main topics of group therapy are the evaluation of results and saying goodbye to each other. It is a period in which concrete measures regarding evaluation, farewells, and what's next are taken. In this period, feedback on results, cooperation, and relationships are the main activities for group members. Much is learned throughout group therapy, but this final phase is often of additional value, a harvesting period, when the finishing touches, or the cherries, are put on the cake. In a mature adult group, the group therapist can productively use the termination to complete the treatment. In intensive group therapies, the parting of group members is given lots of space, along with all of the associated emotions. In structured therapy groups, the parting is usually simple. Also, the personal attachment possibilities and limitations (how much a group member has really bonded) are especially noticeable during the farewell. And that final phase is often confrontational to those group members who are not used to consciously saying goodbye.

The group usually does a great deal itself, but the group therapist must always be on standby to help. It is especially the interactive moments that the group therapist can take advantage of with the *connecting* verbal technique. Since the group does a lot itself, a COOPERATING/HELPING attitude is best suited.

Table 11.7 Utilizing termination during the termination phase of a therapy group.

Verbal technique	Relationship technique (attitude and tone)
The group therapist *mirrors* the group members' separation feelings and thoughts. He *connects* these to the group task while simultaneously *connecting* the group members to each other.	With such a farewell, an interaction-facilitating attitude is appropriate (COOPERATING/HELPING).

(Continued)

Table 11.7 (Continued)

Some typical interventions:
Group therapist in the final session of a therapy group for assertiveness:
'Ethan, are you in fact saying to Olivia, "I would advise you to do this
therapy again; you can get a lot more out of it"?' Ethan: 'Yes, that's how
I see it, Olivia. You got a lot out of it, but certainly not all you can. Your
goal of being more direct, for example, you could be much better at that.'
Olivia (turning to the group therapist with a questioning look): 'Is it possible
to follow another group therapy?' Group therapist: 'If someone can still
benefit from many learning opportunities, it is certainly possible. But what
do you think about Ethan's opinion about your goal of becoming a little
more direct?'

A group therapist in the final meeting of an educational therapy group for
rheumatoid arthritis patients: 'What is it that you are trying to say to Joan,
Evelyn?' Evelyn: 'I want to thank you, Joan. I benefited very much from your
compassion, and we often had the same opinion about rheumatoid arthritis.
That was also pleasant. Maybe we can keep in touch once the group is over?'

Group therapist: 'What is going on with you right now, Patrick?' Patrick: 'I
don't know exactly . . . um . . . this last meeting with the group feels very
weird. I feel sad but also relieved. I'm very grateful for your supportive feedback. This is all very unusual, even scary.' Claire: 'Is it perhaps that you have
never properly . . . or . . . um . . . ever really said goodbye, Patrick?' Patrick:
'Yes, that's it, I think, Claire. I've always run away from it, also with relationships. I would usually end it very abruptly; now, I'm not doing that here, and
that's so crazy but also kind of good.'

Separation is different in every situation. In a therapy group, two group
members left shortly after each other. The first was Brian, who had only
briefly participated in group therapy and had not really bonded. Despite
advice from the group and group therapist to continue, he decided to leave
anyway. His farewell during his last meeting was modest and formal. It was
painful to notice that the group members didn't really mind Brian leaving.
John's farewell was very different. The fact that John was leaving was difficult
for everyone, not only because he had participated longer but also because
of his character – he was kind, showed interest in others, was straightforward, had humor, and had really connected with the group.
People loved John. Many group members were in tears at the farewell.

Chapter 12

Depth processes in a therapy group

12.1 Introduction

Sometimes, the members of a therapy group exhibit puzzling behavior that we cannot fully understand. In such cases, this could insinuate *depth processes*. These are characterized by regressive behavior with complex and sometimes intense emotions such as anxiety, distrust, and anger but also infatuation or admiration. These depth processes often exist under the surface but become visible when triggered by an incident. Consider a group therapy session in which a group member suddenly and unexpectedly lashes out violently at another member. When this outburst is discussed, it becomes apparent that the angry group member for some time has been annoyed with the other member, whom he perceives as haughty and elitist. Some group members recognize this annoyance very clearly, others not at all. The group becomes divided, resulting in a tense and unsafe atmosphere.

Depth processes cannot be explained through the group dynamics concepts discussed so far. Although they have an effect on the group level, an individual perspective is needed to understand them. They take place primarily within the layered inner world of individuals. They come with inherent concepts, many of which originated in theories other than those of group dynamics, particularly psychoanalysis (De Wolf, 2002). In the 1940s, when group dynamics popped up, there was more of a connection between group dynamics and psychoanalysis than what there is today (Lewin, 1951/1997; Whitman, 1963). Over time, these two currents became disconnected, which is unfortunate (Schruijer and Curseu, 2014; Shaffer and Galinsky, 1976). Both assume layered behavior with sublevel motives: group dynamics at the collective level and psychoanalysis at the individual level. Together, they form a good combination to better understand the underlying depth processes and their complex effect on group members' interactional behavior.

This chapter discusses the following:
- Different types of anxiety in a therapy group
- Typical forms of avoidance that occur in therapy groups

DOI: 10.4324/9781003368786-15

- Regression and transference in a therapy group
- Countertransference and transparency of the group therapist

12.2   Anxiety is part of it

Depth processes are always accompanied by emphatic feelings. The affect anxiety plays a key role in depth processes and, therefore, is a common thread throughout this chapter. Groups in general always evoke some tension in human beings, and this is especially true for members in a therapy group (Shay, 2021). Anxiety is part of the therapeutic challenge that a therapy group presents to group members. Entering a new group is always exciting, and change or learning something new rarely succeeds without fear of the unknown. For example, spontaneous feedback from a fellow group member, however well intentioned, could be perceived as confrontational and provoke anxiety (De Dreu and Weingart, 2003; De Haan and Pol, in NVGP, 2019). Some degree of anxiety is functional in any group.

So, in principle, anxiety is not unhealthy, but too much anxiety is not beneficial. Group members may suffer too much or even be harmed by it. Often participants do not directly tell that the anxiety is too high, but the group therapist sees increasing regression in the behavior. Clients behave in a more withdrawn and passive way and show relapses in their symptoms. And this causes the therapeutic learning process to stagnate. Therefore, regulating the anxiety level in any therapy group is an important task for the group therapist. Continuously ensuring that the level of anxiety does not become too high but also not too low is an art in itself.

Table 12.1 shows how the group therapist can do this through her technical tools. An important tool is variation in structure in the group task (see Section 5.3 and Figure 5.1 in Chapter 5). The group therapist can experiment with the structure by tailoring it. More structure reduces anxiety; less structure increases anxiety. The group therapist can add more structure to the process using organizational techniques. For example, she can make the working method and member tasks more concrete, add new rules, or create a schedule for taking turns. The group therapist can apply the verbal technique to reduce anxiety by providing information, *explaining* something or emphasizing the group rules. It often requires the group therapist to discuss the anxiety (using the verbal technique and relationship technique) with the group, try to understand it, and if possible reduce it.

The desired structure and clarity also extend to the group therapist herself. By understanding the group members' anxiety but also being transparent about her own feelings, thoughts, and intentions, she invalidates the anxiety related to herself. An active, helpful, and open attitude by the group therapist (HELPING) is best suited for this structure and transparency.

Table 12.1 Reducing a too-high anxiety level in a therapy group.

Organizational technique	Verbal technique	Relationship technique (attitude and tone)
The group therapist provides more structure to the group task and working method.	The group therapist provides information by *explaining*, structuring, and being transparent about her intentions. Discuss group members' anxious feelings and thoughts using the verbal techniques of *mirroring* and *broadening*.	This requires an active and supportive attitude from the group therapist (HELPING).

Example sentences:
'I understand that there is a lot of unease among you because the purpose of the working method is unclear. Let me explain it again.'
'Camaron, you feel like you are being forced to be open here. I want to reassure you that it is up to you to decide when you want to talk about yourself.'
'Does anyone else recognize this anxiety that Chuck has explained so clearly?'

Anxiety in beginning group members deserves special consideration (Shay, 2021). Many beginning group members suffer from fears relating to groups and group therapy. These are fears that often occur, but because those fears are often magnified, the members suffer unnecessarily. They especially deserve a lot of attention and care from the group therapist, who explains and knows how to reduce the anxiety to a realistic and manageable level. This is not only necessary and good for the new or just starting members but also prevents early client dropout. It often involves one or more of the following fear-filled examples.

Fear of not fitting in or being rejected or humiliated

Part of being human is that we like to feel safe and accepted. We do this by attaching ourselves to each other and forming a cohesive therapy group. As described in Chapter 1, every human being is familiar with the fear of being excluded, of not fitting in. A person who is about to join a therapy group is easily overcome with such anxiety. 'Do I fit in here?' and 'Suppose they don't like me' are fearful thoughts many beginning group members suffer from. In a stronger form, such anxiety becomes malignant. Group members have then imagined that the group will solely focus on them and ridicule them or force them to tell shameful things about themselves.

Fear of intensity

The fact that you are up close and personal with each other in a therapy group, and on top of that, with unfamiliar people often quite different from you, tends to evoke feelings of anxiety in a beginning group member. He or she fears that reactions toward each other will be overwhelming and that the therapy group will become emotionally out of control or trigger uncontrollable feelings (Jongerius, 1993).

Fear of having to adapt or blending in with the group

The idea of connecting with a 'mass' of group members evokes fear of coercion or losing individuality. The fear then is that joining the therapy group means not being allowed to have your own opinion and having to conform to the majority. On a deeper level, the fear of disappearing as an individual (Jongerius, 1993).

These fears are not irrational, but they can become too powerful in the individual's imagination. In this case, they say more about the beginning group member than about the group. In the group member's mind, the fears are greatly exaggerated. Nevertheless, it is advisable for the group therapist to take the group member and his or her anxiety perceptions very seriously and respond to them appropriately. This can be done by reassuring the group member when his or her perception is unrealistic and explaining again how the group works, including the group rules for safety (see also Chapter 3).

The anxiety mentioned in this section is not reserved for group members only. A group therapist may also suffer from the aforementioned fears, although she will be better able to guard against them thanks to her professional training. I agree with Van Paassen (2023), who believes that anxiety is a normal phenomenon in the group therapist that can help with the insight into oneself as a person–professional but can also help in understanding countertransference to clients. Every group therapist must be able to withstand a certain amount of anxiety and dare to feel and explore it.

12.3   Different forms of avoidance in a therapy group

Avoidance of the group as a whole

Avoidance is a normal phenomenon in groups and certainly in therapy groups. The complaints for which members seek treatment are often related to the avoidance of important personal feelings and thoughts, and practically all therapeutic methods include ways to explore avoidance and reduce the underlying anxiety. Avoidance at the individual level often stands out the most, and working on it is part of group therapy. But sometimes, the whole group shows avoidance, which is difficult for the group therapist because these collective group dynamics are so strong. When the entire group avoids engaging in the group task or avoids difficult issues, the group and group therapist will experience this due to its massiveness. Even if only a few group members are vocal, we can still sense the entire group resisting or fleeing. In Chapter 9, I explained that a norm is a collective view with an underlying reason. Such a reason is a vision or belief about how you view the group or the outside world. This collective underlying belief can also have an avoidance function. British psychiatrist and group therapist Wilfred Bion first described this phenomenon in 1961. He called a group in such an collective avoidance mode a *basic assumption group* (Bion, 1961). What he means is that, in such a situation, the whole therapy group has an avoidant assumption concerning itself and reality and behaves accordingly. This is an often persistent belief, which, although not grounded in reality, is no less real to the group. A therapy group in the mode of a basic assumption group is an avoidance group because it proposes a different solution to the problems than simply addressing the problems with the task as the *workgroup* is supposed to do (Bion, 1961).

Bion distinguishes three types of basic assumption groups: the dependent group, the fight–flight group, and the pairing group.

1. Dependent group

A group with a dependent assumption assumes that the leader of the group – the group therapist or a dominant group member – will help the group and solve the problems for the group. A therapy group with such a basic assumption believes that it is unable to handle the problems. In practice, we see a group in which the group members take a wait-and-see attitude, take no initiative, display their helplessness, and strongly appeal to the group therapist or a 'rescuing' group member to solve their problems.

2. Fight–flight group

This basic assumption group collectively has the distrustful belief that danger is imminent and that the group must protect itself by fleeing or going into battle. The group can see danger in anything, for example, in the group therapist, the organization of which the therapy group is a part, the task of the therapy group or in some group members. The tense and distrustful atmosphere in such a group can be clearly felt. Attempts to come closer cause group members to react defensively and distance themselves. They often verbally attack the group therapist or other group members.

3. Pairing or paradise group

Because we don't observe such a basic assumption group as often, it is less easily recognized. In this group, avoidance is related to a subgroup or duo where the members have a visible exclusive relationship with each other. This duo gets a lot of attention, and, in the process, they are idealized as a kind of Adam and Eve in paradise. This is accompanied by all sorts of hopeful expectations, such as that the complaints will pass automatically or that life should be completely harmonious and blissful. This idealization allows the group to avoid the reality of group therapy, especially its confrontational aspects, such as feeling disappointed or angry. Here, too, the actual group task is shifted to the background.

Avoidance by way of subgroups

Subgroups are a normal occurrence in therapy groups. In Chapter 8, I described that one of the developmental phases, the inclusion phase, is characterized by subgroup formation (Levine, 1979). In group development, subgroups have a transitional function – cohesive unity is not yet possible in the whole group, but it is already possible in subgroups. These subgroups have different views of the therapy group. The discussion of the conflicting views of the subgroups and the resulting synthesis then often advances the group's development.

But subgroups can also take on an avoidance function when they become fixated on their conflicting views, thereby halting development. The representatives of both sides then remain in endless debate with each other without reaching a solution.

In another case, subgroups can become 'bonds,' closed off and keeping secrets from the rest of the group. The previous pairing group is a good example. This always creates an atmosphere of secrecy, ambiguity, and suspicion that is disastrous for open task performance. Some members of the therapy group know about the secret 'pairings'; others don't know anything about them but sometimes feel that something is going on or is not right. An extreme example is the development of a romantic relationship between members or even between the group therapist and a member. In the Troubleshooting guide at the back of this book, I discuss in detail how a group therapist can deal with subgroups, destructive 'bonds,' and exclusive relationships.

Avoidance is a normal part of the therapeutic learning process in a therapy group. The group therapist cannot ignore it and should always investigate the avoidance together with the group members. This always results in learning experiences for the group members. This becomes more difficult as avoidance becomes more collective and severe. Then the task of the therapy group can really come under pressure. In extreme cases, a collective avoidant therapy group develops into an 'anti-group.' In the next section, I explain this phenomenon.

The 'anti-group'

Nitsun (1992, 2004) describes an extreme form of collective avoidance. As an extension to Bion's assumption groups, Nitsun speaks of the 'anti-group.' With this term, Nitsun emphasizes the destructive potential of groups to counterbalance what he perceived as too positive an image of them in the 1970s and 1980s (Foulkes, 1964; Nitsun, 1992). He normalizes, as it were, the negative side of groups. This ties in with the realistic intent of this book: how every group therapist can use and utilize the processes in therapy groups but also how negative processes can be prevented, stopped, or turned into learning material.

According to Nitsun, every group harbors potentially aggressive and destructive powers that can significantly influence the group. These are the aggressive and destructive emotions and processes *within* the therapy group, as well as those *toward* the group. They may come from within the group itself, from the organization of which the group is a part, or may come from the group therapist. We have encountered them throughout this book: groups with a negative culture, scapegoating and rejection, disturbed interaction, destructive subgroups, rivalry and conflict, group members anxious about being perceived negatively in the group, a group therapist who is acting out her countertransference, and, finally, the organization that underestimates and inadequately supports groups. Destructive processes can paralyze therapy groups, divide them, or dissolve them entirely.

Depth processes also underlie the anti-group. According to Nitsun, there are two causes. First, our early childhood expectations, which are always activated when we ask for help, are at odds with what group therapy offers. When problems or tensions arise, we long for the safe, redeeming relationship with a trusted caregiver, especially if the relationship with the original caregiver fell short. This, of course, is an idealized desire that will be frustrated in any treatment, including individual therapy. However, a therapy group contrasts sharply with that expectation. We desire a warm, accepting individual therapist and not a group of other people with problems. On top of that, compared to an individual therapist, a beginning therapy group is often extra unsafe and frustrating. This explains why it is common for clients to reject group therapy offers and why they prefer an individual approach.

The second cause for the emergence of an anti-group stems from the expectations of the group members. Members in a therapy group typically have their own individual expectations, which they project onto the group. If those projections are very negative, a collective belief of negativity and disappointment about the group will quickly develop. This belief can remain persistent and become the reality of that group (Janzing, 1992). It does occur that group members' expectations and projections differ, which then enables the group therapist to evoke a discussion on the opinions. See the following examples.

When negative beliefs about therapy groups dominate

Shortly after the start of a new therapy group, questions such as 'What do you think about this group therapy?' or 'What did you guys think of our session today?' often arise. Sometimes, there will either be a positive or a neutral response, but in other cases, there might not be any response or, when questioned further, only a critical one. For example, 'I am not keen on group therapy, and today was another confirmation of that; for me, it was all very slow and gloopy,' or 'I didn't actually learn anything new today, so I wonder how useful this group will be.' This should alarm any group therapist. If there is a dissenting voice from the remaining participants, for example, 'I thought it went all right,' then ambivalence prevails. It is important that the group therapist takes the various feelings and thoughts very seriously and tries to further explore whether hesitations can be removed. If most of the members concur very negatively as well, the group therapist has a problem. The negative belief about the therapy group then dominates so strongly that it will not be easy to reverse it. Regardless of the group therapist's strong conviction about the potential of a therapy group, if the members themselves do not believe in it, an anti-group will quickly arise.

So, a therapist who recommends group therapy will have to be very convincing in her explanation of the results of therapy as a treatment for the client's complaints. And once a client has agreed to group therapy, promoting the processes I described in Chapter 6 are vital. If there is anything that helps make group therapy successful, it is cohesion, acceptance, and inclusion. Both an individual person and a group can serve as a secure attachment object, as I explained in Chapter 6.

In addition, clear task organization and good leadership are usually effective antidotes to the anti-group (Van de Loo, 1995; Van Vught and Wildschut, 2012). Concrete group goals clarify what is and is not intended but also what is to be gained. A typical characteristic by which we can recognize the anti-group is the violation of group rules. Nitsun calls it 'boundary violation' and cites 'boundary management' as the remedy. Good leadership in this context means daring to intervene firmly, confront group members or the group with transgressive behavior, and motivate them to discontinue that behavior. Reminding group members of the primary task is an essential part of this. Containing, discussing, and analyzing the intense negative feelings is also a challenge, which, if successful, can keep the group afloat and sometimes even provide deepening (Moeskops, 2006; Nitsun, 2004). In addition to this firm structuring, it is of great importance that the group therapist know how to understand, tolerate, and contain those intense feelings (see also 'Intense feelings' in the group in the troubleshooting guide).

12.4   Regression and transference in a therapy group

Regression

People carry their history in their brains and bodies (Pesso, 1973). They store memories and past behavior patterns that were useful when they were much younger but that are no longer needed now. These faded with development to make way for other, more mature behaviors. But they are not really gone. They are still hidden somewhere in a remote corner of our brain and body.

A therapy group can reactivate those old emotions and behavior patterns in group members. Such a situation is called *regression*, which literally means *going backward* (De Wolf, 2002). Often, without being aware of it, group members then start behaving in the present as they did when they were much younger. There are two group situations that can trigger regression. One situation occurs when there is *much* anxiety in the group, and the other when there is *very little* anxiety in the group. I briefly discuss these two situations next.

Under threatening circumstances, when there is a lot of anxiety, people usually revert to old, familiar 'survival mechanisms.' We also see this happening in our therapy groups. We often recognize these regressive survival reactions by extreme forms of behavior. For example, in a very threatening group situation, people become so dependent that they can't do anything anymore, or they suddenly become very determined and boss everyone around. This form of regression can be seen as an impulsive protective reaction against anxiety.

Take, for example, a therapy group for the elderly with depressive symptoms sitting in the therapy room, ready and waiting for the group therapist to arrive. When this group suddenly learns that today's meeting will not take place, it can trigger a regressive reaction. Some group members react anxiously and helplessly and have feelings of doubt; others say nothing and promptly leave.

The second group situation, one in which very little anxiety is present, also provokes regression. For example, when people do not have to do anything for a while, that is, because they are on vacation, regression always occurs – we don't have to do anything, we can leave things as they are and let it all go. We lower the bar, give in more to pleasures, such as good food and drink, and do more entertaining, relaxing, and sometimes even childish things, such as sliding down a slide. This regression allows us to rest while on vacation and, once back home, to again cope with the responsibilities of adult life.

We also encounter this type of regression in therapy groups. The atmosphere in the group is then often giggly and passive; the group is no longer genuinely engaged in the task at hand. This regression is functional insofar as it relaxes the atmosphere. However, if the regression continues, it becomes dysfunctional because it does so at the expense of the group task. The group is then 'on vacation' instead of being at work.

The group therapist must take regulatory action when there is too much regression. In case of regression due to anxiety, she must reduce the anxiety level in the way described in Section 12.2. And in the case of 'vacation regression,' she must confront the group with avoidance and remind members of the agreements concerning the group task, somewhat increasing the tension, so to speak.

Eliminating excessive 'vacation regression'

A dietitian at a neighborhood health center runs a therapy group for overweight people. This is the fourth group session. A distinct culture of joking around, not taking each other or the group therapist seriously, constantly giggling and not getting down to business is developing. The group therapist gradually becomes annoyed with the group's loafing and worries that the group task will fail. Halfway through the session, when the biggest joker in the group is just about to tell a joke, she intervenes: 'Excuse me, Lee, but I'm going to interrupt you for a moment. I'm wondering how you all feel about this group. Whether you are satisfied with the outcome and the way the meetings are going.'Lee: 'Well, you certainly know how to catch a person off guard. Uh, I think I'll finish my joke first if you don't mind. . . . And then the manager said . . .' Group therapist: 'No, Lee. I really want you to not speak for a minute. I'm interrupting you for a reason. I'm worried about this group.' Lee: 'Worried about the group? Aren't you exaggerating a little? I actually think this is a fun group,' Heather responds while some group members giggle. Joan interjects: 'Well, I'm also worried. This so-called jolly atmosphere annoys the hell out of me. Maybe I'm too serious, but I come here for therapy about my weight, not to listen to jokes all the time' (looks at Lee). 'There, I've said my peace!'

There is a third situation in which regressive behavior occurs in therapy groups: a situation where the group feels safe enough for group members to engage in regressive behavior. Regression can then become part of the treatment. Therapy groups that strongly connect present-day problems with past causes particularly use recalled old behavior patterns as essential material for treatment. Regression in such a therapy group serves the group task: investigating the causes from the past. This is called *therapeutic regression*. The old, awakened patterns are valuable historical material for these therapy groups. The process involves *partial regression*. The client can experience old feelings and memories clearly, while his observing and investigating 'ego' remains alert in the present moment (Berk, 2005; De Wolf, 2002).

Transference

Regression has a special effect on interactions in therapy groups. The interactions that group members in a regressive situation engage in with each other and with the group therapist are then based on recalled old feelings and thoughts. The group members and therapist notice this by the 'distorted perception' of how a group member (or even an entire group) sees and experiences them. This is called *transference* (De Wolf, 2002). Expectations, behaviors, and attitudes from the past are *transferred*, or projected, onto others in the present moment without stroking with current reality.

The group member himself experiences this transference situation as realistic; the person receiving the transference experiences it as non-accurate. For example, the recipient may not recognize himself at all in the characteristics, feelings, or opinions attributed to him, or he experiences the uncanny feeling of being placed in the wrong box. Transference can confuse the interaction because the projecting group member is unaware of the distorted reality and acts as if it is real.

Three transference objects

Transference is a relational phenomenon. As there are always three relationships at play in a group, there are also three objects of transference. A group member can experience transference to a group member, the therapist, or to the whole group.

In addition, transference feelings are not only distortions; they generally also contain an element of truth. We usually link the reality bias to the realistic characteristics of the group member receiving the transference. For example, if a group member used to fight a lot with a strong rival sister, a firm and decisive group member will evoke transference feelings more easily than a gentle, withdrawn type.

What if there is a lot of transference directed toward the group therapist? Should she do something with that transference? No, not at first. In fact, some degree of transference always occurs within a therapy group. If this transference is mild and positive, the group therapist must simply allow and tolerate the transference. If the transference becomes very strong and simultaneously very negative or overly positive, an intervention is required. Intense transference undermines the cooperative relationship with the group therapist, which is undesirable because that relationship is fundamentally important. The group therapist can then help by contrasting her own reality with the transference, thus helping to correct it. It is very useful to utilize the group for this by asking other participants how they perceive the group therapist. Other group members often recognize strong transference bias, and this mutual reality correction often works even better than that of the group therapist herself. Through transparency and visibility, the group therapist helps the group member or the whole group face the 'distortion' and, if possible, correct it.

12.5   Countertransference and transparency of the group therapist

The depth phenomena described here evoke emotional responses not only in the group members but also often in the group therapist. No one is insensitive when it comes to issues such as anxiety, group avoidance, regression, transference, or intense feelings following interactions in the therapy group. It is normal for a group therapist to respond to these through her own feelings.

Sometimes, the group therapist experiences a very emphatic feeling that imposes itself on her, without its origin being readily apparent. Such an emphatic but somewhat puzzling emotional reaction by the group therapist is called *counter-transference* (De Wolf, 2002; Hafkenscheid, 2014). There are two types of counter-transference, aptly referred to by Hafkenscheid (2014) as 'subjective' and 'objective' countertransference. Subjective countertransference is therapist-specific; this occurs during group therapy when a sensitive issue personally affects the group therapist herself. A good example is a therapist who finds it difficult to receive compliments and feels unpleasantly embarrassed by a well-meant compliment from a group member or a group therapist who is especially sensitive to a group member with authority and charisma within the group because that group member evokes the same feelings in her as her own dominant father used to evoke.

Objective countertransference is the client-bound countertransference. Even then, the group therapist has an emphatic and not immediately understandable feeling, but now it appears to be mainly related to the client's behavior and feelings. Consider a group therapist who begins to feel increasingly powerless with a client who strongly presents himself as a victim of his life. Suppose the co-therapist also experiences this strong powerlessness with this client, then this could well be a case of objective countertransference; that is, the group thera-pist's powerless feeling says more about the client than about her.

Countertransference feelings are an important source of information for the group therapist. Sometimes, that information says something about the group therapist herself; sometimes it says something about a group member.

Can the group therapist use that information? Should she do something with it? Sometimes yes, sometimes no. A first important rule of the game is not to react impulsively to one's own countertransference feelings. Countertransfer-ence can sometimes be so irritating that a group therapist blurts out a reac-tion before she realizes it, often resulting in regret. This 'acting-out' behavior is often an impulsive defense reaction that is not helpful in the contact with the group member in question. It is always important to control your initial impul-sive reaction and first explore and understand the countertransference feelings (Moeskops, 2006). The group therapist can then choose whether or not to pay attention to them. If the feelings of countertransference are so strong that they get in the way, the group therapist should always address them. In this respect, it matters whether the emotional reaction concerns a sensitive issue of the group therapist or whether it is the registration of a severe emotion of a group or group member.

1. How should a group therapist react when something affects her personally?

If the group therapist notices that she is being affected by an issue personally, it is important to recognize this personal reaction. Therefore, it is helpful if a group therapist is sufficiently familiar with her own sensitivities or pitfalls. If a situation arises in which she feels personally affected, it is important that she does not react immediately but takes the time to first carefully examine her instant reaction.

If her own pitfall becomes clear, it is usually not functional to burden the group with it. The group therapist should see to it that she has her own *support system* where she can tell her story and, if necessary, ask for support and advice. In many health care organizations that work with therapy groups, such systems exist in the form of peer intervision or supervision by an expert in the field of the target group or group therapy.

Sometimes, it becomes necessary for the group therapist to tell the group something about her triggered reaction. This is certainly necessary when, due to personal sensitivity, she has exhibited behavior the group finds difficult to understand. It will then be functional if she provides a limited explanation of her own part in and background to this reaction. Group members usually appreciate that, not only because of the clarification but also because of her personal openness: it shows that the group therapist is not only a professional but also a human being made of flesh and blood (Arendsen Hein, 1998).

2. How a group therapist responds to behavior or an emotion of a group or group member

In this case, the amount of attention the group therapist pays to her countertransference feelings depends on the type of therapy group. In all cases, recognizing one's own emotional reaction to a client's or group's behavior can help better understand the client and his pathology. In some psychotherapy groups, the group therapist may share her own countertransference, giving the client an example of how others may experience her. In this instance, the client and the group must be strong enough to weather such a confrontation.

Chapter 13

Troubleshooting guide

Groups, and especially therapy groups, are complicated. Therefore, it is normal for a group therapist to run into issues he does not know how to deal with. This troubleshooting guide is designed to provide group therapists with concrete solutions to unexpected questions and problems.

DOI: 10.4324/9781003368786-16

Prior to the group

The department or the colleagues do not believe in group therapy

It often happens in health care that a professional becomes enthused (for example, because he heard a colleague at a conference talking enthusiastically about an effective group therapy) and decides to treat a certain group of clients as *a group* instead of on an individual basis. In the process, it is common for such a therapist to encounter considerable skepticism from colleagues or department heads – they doubt whether group therapy works.

Causes

The cause of skepticism toward groups as a form of treatment stems from two interrelated issues. First, our judgment of group therapy always involves our bias toward the individual. In our culture, the focus has shifted to the individual person (see Chapter 6). As a result, even in health care, the idea of *individual treatment* being the norm often still prevails. It is difficult for many professionals to understand that, in some cases, individuals can be treated just as well in a group setting. Yes, the individual is central, but group treatment as a method is often as effective as individual treatment and sometimes even the preferred choice (Spijker, 2010). The efficacy of group therapy has been demonstrated for a multitude of diagnoses (Burlingame and Strauss, 2021; Factsheet Groepstherapie, 2019)

Second, there are persistent misconceptions about groups and group therapy. For example, the notion that group therapy is a second-rate, 'diluted' form of treatment. After all, the client must share the therapist with several other group members. But that is certainly a misconception because group therapy has its own efficacy that is due precisely to the presence of those other group members. More misconceptions and how to dispel them can be found in Chapter 3.

Solutions

So, how does one convince colleagues or management that group therapy can be effective? The best way is to give them the facts. The advice: set aside some time to inform your colleagues or management in detail about the usefulness and power of group therapy. Make that conversation interactive so the organization's needs are also discussed. If you feel you cannot do this convincingly by yourself, invite an experienced group therapist. He can support the efficacy of group therapy with facts such as guidelines and scientific research and explain under which circumstances and for which problems group therapy is recommended. This way, colleagues and management will get a realistic and differentiated picture to replace the black-and-white image of group therapy versus individual therapy.

The client has no confidence in group therapy and prefers individual treatment

Sometimes, besides mistrusting professionals, you will also encounter potential clients who are doubtful about the effectiveness of group therapy. They find groups scary and believe they will not be able to achieve the desired result. The advice to participate in a therapy group is by most clients experienced as a counterintuitive choice. These clients will opt for individual treatment (De Haas and Van Hest, in NVGP, 2019). See also Chapter 12, 'Depth processes.'

Causes

The biases and misconceptions I described previously also play a role in this case. And – not to forget – fear of the group. Groups and therapy groups in particular always evoke fear in the client, who is advised to do group therapy (Scott Rutan, 2021; Shay, 2021). It is normal for beginning clients to have anxious fantasies about 'not fitting in' or 'being criticized by the whole group' (see also Chapters 1 and 3).

Solutions

The best way to approach a doubting client is to interactively give objective information and factual explanations about what group therapy entails and what it can do for him or her. Most importantly, explain clearly – referring to guidelines – why group therapy is an appropriate treatment form for the client's problem.

In doing so, it is just as important to positively welcome the 'critical consumer' in the client. The outcome of group therapy is always better if the choice for it has come from two sides. The client must ultimately convince himself or herself whether or not to opt for the proposed group therapy. The following step-by-step plan will help you in such an interactive conversation:

- Take the time to explain to a client why you think a particular group suits them.
- Clearly explain to the client the task of the therapy group.
- Discuss and put into perspective the overly anxious fantasies about group therapy.
- Show what results the proposed group usually achieves.
- Explain which guidelines and research describe effectiveness.
- Invite the client to ask critical and informative questions and try to answer them as specifically as possible.
- Refer the client to more sources of information: provide a flyer about the group. Encourage him or her to search for relevant information on the Internet.
- Make a follow-up appointment in which the client can then communicate his choice for group therapy or why not.

It is important to respect the client's choice, of course. But if, in doing so, he or she sells himself or herself short because he or she rejects a very appropriate group therapy offer, it is in the client's interest that you convince him or her of the benefits of participating in the therapy group. Two more 'reality facts' come into play here. First, some clients have had a negative group experience. Sometimes, their resulting suspicion is well founded. Ask them about it and be mindful and understanding. Second, group therapy is not suitable for everyone. There is much overlap in the indications for individual or group therapy. Still, some clients are better off with individual therapy. For example, individual treatment is preferred for complex, multiple problems, as this makes it more possible to give separate attention to the various components of a complex issue. Learning from each other is also not always necessary for simple problems. A single depression, for example, is sometimes already sufficiently treated with medication. Then a group therapy is not useful (Berk, 2005; De Haas and Van Hest, in NVGP, 2019).

Insufficient group members

Therapy groups regularly suffer from a shortage of members. This is annoying for all parties: management is concerned about a shortage of clients and declining productivity, and the group therapist worries about the survival of his group while clients have 'too small a group' to learn from.

Causes

A group therapist is more vulnerable to hiccups in the supply of clients than an individual practitioner. Whereas an individual therapist treats about six clients in a working day, a group therapist needs at least triple that (assuming three group treatments of one and a half to two hours per day). No wonder group therapists sometimes complain, 'My group has had five members for three months' or 'The enrollments keep dropping.'

Solutions

What many group therapists do in such cases is announce during an indication meeting or referral meeting that there is still space in the group for several clients. It is also useful to check with your most loyal referrers. Talk with them and casually mention that you still have space in your group.

If the supply of clients remains meager, this informational strategy is not working adequately. Repeated requests then appear as if you are begging for group members, which is unpleasant for all parties. Your group then gets a bad image among your referrers (a group with few applications is probably not a very good one), which will incline them to refer less rather than more (De Haas and Van Hest, in NVGP, 2019).

Then, to begin with, ask yourself the following questions:
- Is my group offering and what it can bring to a client sufficiently known to referrers and clients?
- Is my group still viable? Is there enough need, or has it run its course?

It is all about public relations and market research. And that makes sense because offering group therapy only makes sense if there is a demand for it. For the group therapist, in such a case, there is not much else left but to also become a bit of a market researcher and spot the need in the field. Your most important customers are your clients and referrers. For example, you can reach your clients as follows:
- *Referrers.* Get invited to a team, indications board or referral meeting to inform them about your group therapy program. Make that conversation interactive. Ask the referrers if the information is clear and whether the referrals have been handled well so far – have you given them enough information about the treatment of previous clients – and if there is a need for this group or perhaps a different program. Also, ask if the name of the group is clear and whether it is recruiting enough. In Chapter 3, I explained how important the name of a therapy group is as an information source, calling card, and signboard.
- *Clients.* Create a clear, attractive information flyer (in print and digital) for referrers and clients. In it, inform them about your group, what it is called, what kind of problems it is intended for, how it works, what the participation costs are, where more information can be obtained, how to refer clients, and how to reach you for questions, among other things. The group organization design from Chapter 3 helps to create such a flyer.
- *The organization.* In large mental health organizations in the Netherlands, good experience has been gained using a 'group therapy coordinator.' It is not realistic to expect referrers to be able to oversee the full range of therapy groups, let alone to know where there is space. With the combination of a group therapy coordinator, and a digital information system, it is easier to coordinate referrals and group therapies (De Haas and Van Hest, in NVGP, 2019; Wermers, 2006). Such a digital information system shows an overview of the supply of group therapy, the starting date of each group, how many open spots there are, whom to contact for a referral, and so on.

If you have done this, I am sure your questions will be answered. Should it become clear that there is no longer a need for your group, it will be unfortunate, especially if you believe in that group and have put a great deal of effort into it. However, such circumstances offer opportunities and challenges to set up something new for a change. Finding out if there is a need for a different group offering is often fun and inspiring. Setting up and promoting something new keeps you as a professional alert and up to date.

When the group is running

A new therapy group struggles to get going

Sometimes, as a group therapist, you set to work with a new group in good spirits, but it is like a dead horse: no sign of life. The group members vacantly stare at you in bewilderment or with expectations. Before you know it, you put all your energy into trying to revive that dead horse. Without results, of course. A group cannot exist without energy and dynamics from within.

Causes

What could be going on? As this is a new group, the first thing you should consider is the group task. Is it clear to the group members? Do group members understand what to do? Is the task perhaps too difficult? By asking group members these kinds of questions, you will find out soon enough whether or not the task is the flaw.

If the task does not seem to be the problem, then look at the composition of the group. If group members do not sufficiently recognize in each other the vital reason (the main problem and the help request) for participating in the therapy group, then the basis not only for the task but also for group cohesion is missing. For example, suppose one group member's reason for coming is completely different from another. In that case, the group never becomes the collaborative task-oriented enterprise it should be.

Solutions

Often, a renewed, clear explanation is enough for group members to be able to pick up the task and get started. Sometimes, the task needs some adjustment to make it easier for members to handle it afterward. This strategy also helps when an unhappy composition is the reason a therapy group cannot get going. After you clarify the task again, it will become apparent if some group members feel they do not fit in that group. If that is the case, you should help them obtain more appropriate treatment (and apologize if you have selected them incorrectly).

The group therapist does all the work

This is a common problem among novice group therapists. The group therapist works hard and does a lot, while the group members sit back passively and watch it happen. They do not seem to feel co-responsible for their group therapy.

Causes

One of the main causes is that the group therapist steers too much and spoils the therapy group too much by overly taking care of them. This is often due to the therapist being hesitant to sit back, be quiet, and watch and learn for a while, thereby giving the group space to do it themselves.

Solutions

I refer to Section 6.7.3.2 for this, where I detail what techniques and attitudes the group therapist can use to actively participate without becoming the workhorse.

Members focus only on the group therapist and not on each other

This is another common problem among novice group therapists. The group therapist would like group members to start talking to each other, but they fail to do so. During the group therapy, everyone keeps quiet and looks expectantly at the group therapist. They continuously address him. It then becomes very difficult not to respond to their appeal (role suction; see Section 10.4).

Causes

In the beginning, every new group always focuses on the group therapist. The first interaction is thus mainly between group members and the therapist. This is normal. After all, the group therapist is the formal leader; group members expect hierarchical leadership from him, just like at the doctor's or with a schoolteacher in the classroom. The group therapist's job and trick is to change the direction of the interaction and get group members to talk to each other. Group members sometimes find that change difficult, so they stay focused on the group therapist longer than necessary.

Solutions

A client often has difficulty imagining what group therapy would be like. Therefore, the first thing to do is clearly *explain* the group therapy method again and why the mutual interaction between members is an essential part of the method. Like any treatment, you have to 'learn to do' group therapy, and the cognitive rationale of the interactive task helps with this. In addition, the group therapist has various techniques at his disposal to encourage interaction between members (see Section 7.5).

The therapy group does not perform the group task

The group members are not doing what they are supposed to: cooperating on the task. Instead, they act negatively by resisting, ridiculing your methods, or making fun of group therapy. It is the avoidant 'flight or fight' group I discussed in Chapter 12, 'Depth processes.' For example, a therapy group that routinely fails to complete requested homework assignments or a group in which jokes are constantly being made, and no one takes group therapy seriously. A therapy group that systematically neglects its task soon becomes a very frustrating enterprise for the group therapist. The powerlessness evokes feelings along the lines of 'don't be so silly' and, if the group continues to be difficult, even feelings of anger. Then, the group therapist must be careful not to give in to these dismissive impulses. After all, Distant behavior easily evokes Distant behavior (IPC).

Causes

The reasons for this can be very diverse. For example, the task may be unclear or not suitable. However, various process phenomena, such as insecurity, insufficient cohesion, strict norms, and difficult people in difficult roles, can also play a role. In terms of solving these problems, the exact cause is not that important. As a group therapist, you can use those dynamics, the energy of group rebellion and avoidance, as a point of leverage. After all, under the surface, a group's rebelliousness is always an attempt to make something clear to the group therapist.

Solutions

The group's critical and avoidant attitude conveys a message. That message can be uncovered by luring out the rebellious group and engaging in dialogue. To do this, the group therapist must silence the group and confront it with its avoidant behavior in a meta-conversation (see Chapter 5). Then, together with the group members, he tries to find the reason for their negative work attitude. This is not always an easy conversation, but it could illuminate what lies beneath the flight or fight attitude. Once the cause is clearer, the group therapist can work with group members to figure out what they need in order to start doing the work.

The therapy group does not adhere to group rules

Group rules are vital for the group to function properly. The most important rules are the *continuity rule*, the *privacy rule*, and the *group-as-workplace rule* (also see Section 3.3). Both regular absence of group members and violation of the privacy rule are fatal to a group. Discontinuity of group members creates a disruptive information backlog and impedes the cohesion and cohesiveness of a group. Sooner or later, this leads to a dysfunctional group. Violation of the privacy rule makes the group very unsafe. After such an incident, group members are not likely to talk about confidential matters with the group again. Unfortunately, violation of these basic rules occurs more often than we care to admit.

The group-as-workplace rule is important for many types of therapy groups. That rule is designed to encourage group members to meet only in the group setting and to actually do the group work together with the whole group. When group members make a habit of seeing each other outside the group, it leads to the leaking of important information and always results in an unsafe group.

Causes

Privacy-rule violations are usually not intentional. It often involves a combination of coincidences and inadvertence. For example, it sometimes happens that group members live close to each other or appear to have a common acquaintance. This can lead to privacy-sensitive encounters ('How do you know Josh? Is he in your therapy group?'). It also happens that group members take privacy-sensitive information (e.g., a report of a meeting) home with them and do not store it properly, giving third parties insight into group participation.

Failure to keep the continuity agreement is usually the result of an established culture of noncommitment. In such a therapy group, the belief that coming late or regularly skipping a meeting 'should be possible' has then become the group norm.

Noncompliance with the group-as-workplace rule has two causes. First, any group is challenging, which makes it tempting to 'socialize' with another group member at a separate time. Second, members do not always understand, especially in the beginning, why meeting in the group is so essential and why it is counterproductive to have conversations outside the group.

Solutions

If group members violate any of these three fundamental group rules, the therapist must see it as a signal and take it very seriously. In fact, neglected group rules rarely re-establish automatically. The group therapist should address the violations immediately and reexplain them in a directive manner. The renewed joint reinforcement of the violated rules is crucial because repeated violations of these fundamental group rules are disastrous for the group. The group therapist must always prevent the noncompliance with group rules from becoming part of the group culture. It is very important that the group therapist design the renewed agreements together with the group so that the group will support them. This provides the best guarantee that the group rules will become the group norm and that the group will comply with them.

Sudden stagnation of the therapy group

It sometimes happens that a group gets off to a good start and runs smoothly, only to suddenly collapse for seemingly inexplicable reasons.

Causes

If a therapy group runs well but then suddenly collapses, the cause is most likely related to the developing group process. The group is running well, so looking for the cause in the group task is less obvious. Apparently, something happened during a meeting that caused so much confusion or insecurity that the therapy group could not move forward and has become stagnant. It could be anything, but the following some common causes:

- An event that caused a feeling of insecurity, for example, an unexpected conflict between two group members, an untimely personal outburst, strange and frightening behavior by a group member or a group member remaining closed off and silent for a long time.
- A change in the composition of the therapy group. Some regression of the group is normal when new group members join. If the therapy group does not pick up after that, some members may feel unsafe because of the newcomers.

Solutions

When unexpected stagnation occurs, the group therapist should stop the task and discuss the process in a meta-conversation (see Chapter 5). At this point, he does not need to know the cause of the stagnation. Often, this is not even possible because nobody knows. His concern serves as a cue and is sufficient to discuss the stagnation with the group members and find the cause together.

If group members dare to talk about what is making them anxious or holding them back, a great deal will already have been gained. The cause then often becomes clear. If it is in the relational sphere (i.e., a group member is shocked by a new group member's foul language), the group therapist can make the group safe again (remove the stagnation) by helping the group members to speak to each other and possibly come to agreements on effective social (conduct) rules.

Dropout: a group member leaves the therapy group prematurely

This problem arises when a group member indicates that he or she will stop group treatment, even before any therapy results are possible, or, more annoyingly, unexpectedly does not return without notice. Ending treatment prematurely is not good for the person in question or the therapy group. Said group member often acts impulsively, without having considered and deliberated sufficiently about the decision, and may regret it later. A dropout is also a negative experience for the therapy group. Such an incident essentially constitutes a rupture in the relationship that damages the established trust in the therapy group and cooperation. The group is often left with a 'hangover' and feelings of inadequacy. The group therapist and the group failed to retain that group member, making them feel like they had personally failed.

Causes

There are roughly three causes for dropping out prematurely:

- *The group member does not fit the group task.* In this case, the group member is right because he or she was wrongly selected for this therapy group. He may differ from the target group in terms of important characteristics. For example, a working person with a mild alcohol addiction may feel out of place in a ward for addicts with a criminal past.
- *A group member is a loner in terms of important social characteristics.* Such a group member fits the group task perfectly but is the only one with a particular social characteristic. For example, he is the only one without a job, the only male in the group, the only transgender, or the only one with an immigrant background.
- *Fear of the group.* Sometimes, fear is a motive for dropping out. For example, a group member may be anxious about what to expect in group therapy or feel intimidated by another group member.

Solutions

Such an 'I quit' announcement often overwhelms the therapy group and group therapist. It is then important to persuade the group member not to act on the intention immediately but to discuss it in the group first. The therapist asks the other group members to express their feelings about the intended departure. If group members see that their fellow group member is selling himself short by suddenly dropping out, they will use their feelings to express how sorry they would be if he left. Fellow group members can sometimes provide very strong and convincing arguments. This is where cohesion also plays a big part; a cohesive therapy group would not be keen on losing someone prematurely.

If the group member is not sensitive to this and sticks to his point of view, this will often provoke aggression, with the possibility that the departing group member will still become ostracized (Daemen and Van Paassen, in NVGP, 2019). The group therapist needs to prevent that from happening. At such a moment, the group therapist is well advised to direct the aggression toward himself by wondering aloud if that member's anger is perhaps meant for him because he has not done his job properly (Daemen and Van Paassen, in NVGP, 2019). Sometimes, a sudden 'quitter' is the interpreter of general dissatisfaction with group therapy, which now becomes negotiable. This way, the departing group member is again embraced and included as a messenger of the critical views felt by the others but that have not yet been shared (Daemen and van Paassen, in NVGP, 2019).

Occasionally, this will help keep the person in question in the group, but sometimes there is no stopping him; he leaves immediately. In the latter case, it often turns out that the group member had already made the decision independently and is not receptive to reflection and consultation with the group.

If the group member does want to examine his intention, the group therapist and therapy group must do so as openly and objectively as possible. After all, the group member's reason for quitting could also be valid. (See also Chapter 11, 'Termination in a therapy group.')

If this requires more time than expected, or if the intention is based on complicated considerations, the group therapist can propose to explore the matter further with the group member in an individual meeting and discuss it with the group afterward.

Complex group members in difficult roles

As I explained in Chapter 10, there are always 'double dynamics' at play in conspicuous individual (role) behavior. The individual member and the group both always play a part. I also made it clear that the ratio between the two can vary. Sometimes, group dynamics play a large part; other times, individual dynamics do. If it involves complex group members, individual dynamics play a large part, even though it is always important to keep group dynamics in mind. They are usually group members with a one-sided and sometimes rigid personality. The group therapist can manage their influence by addressing those predominant individual dynamics in a specific way.

Causes

These difficult members occur regularly, of course, because clients with personality disorders are an important target group for group therapy. They are often anxious individuals who use rigid behaviors to control their anxiety. They inherently convey a fixed behavior pattern and lack a variable behavioral repertoire. Complex group members often take center stage to the point that they begin to interfere with normal interaction among group members. Their rigidity is easily confirmed by the group, reinforcing the role behavior. As a result, it usually does not take long for the role behavior to become fixed and thus dominate the group even more emphatically.

Solutions

Because complex group members are at such high risk of assuming a fixated role in the group, the group therapist must intervene in time. He can best address them according to the ground rules of double dynamics (see Section 10.8.3). In short, the group therapist tries to get both the group member in the fixated role and the role-affirming group to critically look at themselves. He can explain ways in which they can minimize role affirmation of the complex group member. In addition, he can help the complex group member face their own fears, let go of their own rigid behavior somewhat, and introduce the possibility of a different role repertoire.

With their rigid behavior, complex group members not only risk becoming fixated but may also find themselves isolated. They keep – each in their own way – the other at a distance. That is why it is important for the group therapist to free the complex group member from his isolation (de-isolate) by helping him or her to let go of the rigid behavior and talk about the underlying anxiety.

Next is a description of the most commonly occurring complex individuals in a therapy group.

The silent group member

Some group members are extremely quiet for long periods of time. Their withdrawn behavior corresponds to the withdrawn attitude as defined by the IPC model. This behavior often reflects their enormous shyness and shame; no one is allowed to get close. Sooner or later, the therapy group becomes troubled by these silent individuals. 'What is Woody really thinking?' 'Why is Kelly always staring at the floor?' 'Why does Tyler never join the conversation?' These types of questions then increasingly burden the other group members.

After a while, the group will start tugging at a silent group member by inviting him or her to open up. If that is successful, the problem will be solved. However, in some cases, the group member is too anxious and shy, and the invitation will only reinforce withdrawal and silence. A therapy group typically then gives up after a while. That is when the silent group member becomes fixated in that role. To avoid this, the group therapist must try to get the silent group member to participate sooner.

How can the group therapist do that? Not by continuously inviting the silent group member and thus putting them on the spot. The group did not succeed in doing that, so neither will the group therapist. It increases the silent group member's anxiety to such an extent that he or she might drop out. Likewise, the group therapist cannot allow the silent group member to remain silent, as this only affirms that person's silence. Ideally, the group therapist should use one or more of the following strategies (Berk, 2005):

- Just after the end of a meeting, when group members leave the group space, the group therapist establishes contact with the silent group member to show him or her that they are being noticed by the therapist. For example, 'Get home safely, Hunter.'[1]
- Observe whether the silent group member is participating nonverbally. The group therapist can connect with a friendly attitude by *mirroring* the nonverbal cues and *asking* if the silent group member would like to say something about it. For example, 'I see you nodding, Hunter. Would you mind telling me which part you recognize?'
- Connect with the group's attempts to invite the silent group member. The group therapist can use *mirroring, connecting,* and a friendly attitude

(COOPERATING) to indirectly (through the group) try to free the group member from her isolation. For example: 'Evelyn, do I understand correctly that you are saying to Hunter, 'I respect your being quiet, but you also deserve some attention time in this group?' 'How do you feel about that, Hunter?'

- Voice your own observation of the silent attitude and ask the silent group whether it bothers her and if she would like some help. If the silent group member responds to the invitation and joins the conversation, it is helpful to take a moment and ask her why she is so quiet.
- If a silent group member says nothing for a very long time, the risk of fixation increases. The group therapist is well advised to ask the silent group member at the end of a session for permission to approach her and ask how she is doing. For example, 'Hunter, can I ask you something?' 'Yes.' 'What do you think of the group so far?'
- If the silent group member dares to speak about her anxiety, it is important that the group therapist immediately 'de-isolate' this group member using the *broadening* verbal technique. For example: 'Are there others who recognize the kind of shyness that Hunter has described so clearly?'

The 'jammer'

A jammer is an inflexible talker who always reacts to everything or immediately 'switches on' when silence occurs. He or she is afraid of connecting with his or her own painful feelings and of appearing vulnerable to other group members. The preferred remedy is to use talking to keep everyone at a distance. The jammer's reactions usually lack a degree of 'fine-tuning.' The jammer talks for the sake of talking and way too much. This starts to irritate everyone after a while; this is when the role becomes fixated. Therefore, the group therapist should not let the jammer go on for too long and discuss the disruptive behavior before the annoyance becomes overwhelming. It is best if the group therapist limits the jammer politely and confronts him about his talking habits directly or indirectly through the group members. It is good to ask whether the jammer recognizes his or her behavior and knows why he or she is exhibiting such behavior. If the jammer reveals something related to the underlying anxiety, the group therapist should 'de-isolate' this group member using a *broadening* verbal technique. For example, 'Are there others who also find the silent moments unpleasant, like Becky?'

The dominant group member

This group member is afraid of being belittled or dependent. He or she resolves his fear by being bossy and, if it becomes more extreme, by behaving in a threatening manner. The dominant group member controls everyone through a bossy, controlling attitude (LEADING). Other group members are usually afraid of this group member and try to avoid him or her. To prevent this group member from becoming too fixated, someone must confront him or her at some point about the threatening behavior and put it forward for discussion. If the group members fail to do this, the group therapist must assume that task. He does this in exactly the same way as with the disruptor.

The scapegoat

This difficult group member does not consider himself worthy and seeks confirmation of these feelings of inferiority by invoking the disapproval and hatred of the group. This behavior hides the fear of being liked.

With a persistent scapegoat, the group therapist must be alert to the group's part. Group dynamics can sometimes play a large part in the creation and persistence of a scapegoat. I refer to the detailed description in section 10.8.3 on how a group therapist can address this problem.

The complainer

The complainer's weakness makes him strong. It is the group member who, with victim behavior and through his strong Under attitude (IPC), evokes rescuer behavior – read: lots of help and advice – from group and group therapist. However, when given advice or offered any help, this group member will respond with something like: 'Yes, but I already tried that, and it failed as well.' This complex member has been aptly described by Yalom and Leszcz (2020) under the name 'Help-rejecting-complainer.'

If the person in the complainer role ignores the many triggered help offers from the group, the group will become fed up and reject this group member. The group therapist must then intervene to prevent overly severe fixation. He can best do this by explaining to the group that advice and tips are not helpful for this group member and then confronting the complainer with a friendly but decisive attitude (LEADING/HELPING) about his destructive complaining. If the underlying anxiety is open for discussion, broadening it will be appropriate. The group therapist helps by asking the therapy group whether more members recognize this kind of fear.

Strong emotions in the therapy group

Sometimes, considerable commotion arises in the group. For example, when the entire therapy group can no longer recover from laughing at the clumsiness of another group member or when a group member becomes very furious because he feels he has not been treated fairly by the group therapist. Or if someone has suffered a severe loss, where the entire therapy group starts to sympathize and resonate and everyone becomes very sad. And sometimes individual clients can experience strong and complex emotions like jealousy, hatred, humiliation, or deep shame.

Causes

By definition, therapy always deals with emotional things. Group members are not there for fun, but because of problems they are facing in their lives. Think of intense social anxiety, PTSS, I'm-not-good-enough feelings, solitude, a persistent physical illness, great shyness, a depressive episode, personality problems, or mourning. These kinds of problems always arouse strong feelings. The intention in many therapy groups is to feel those emotions and express them in words because that expression helps a member reduce and cope with the symptoms (Helderman, 2021; Scott Rutan et al., 2014, 255–260).

But when those emotional expressions become very intense, it causes problems. Group members then fear that the emotions will get out of control or become unmanageable, that they will overwhelm them. In cases of intense anger, a person will fear impulsivity – being unable to control himself or herself – and the anger will become destructive. When there is a lot of sadness, group members fear the emotions will overwhelm them. It is the group therapist's task to not let the degree of emotions rise too high (to regulate) and especially help make these emotions manageable.

Solutions

It helps if the group develops a group culture where expressing feelings is considered normal. Such a norm must be accompanied by a second norm, namely the norm that it is customary to explore feelings. Together, these two norms make a group skillful in dealing with emotional situations and the feelings released in the process.

The following are guidelines for the group therapist in the case of intense expressions of emotion:

- Tolerate their feelings by allowing them to exist, consciously feel and recognize them, and remain calm ('containing').
- Acknowledge the feelings (and their intensity) by *mirroring* them.
- Show support and understanding.
- Keep enough distance; don't get carried away.
- Help group members deal with it ('coping'), but don't be too quick in wanting to solve the issue.
- Limit feelings when they become too intense or when enough is enough ('holding').
- Look at and reflect on the feelings on a meta-level: ask group members who are not among the 'feeling expressers' for a response, or, if the whole group is emotional, ask the whole group to view the feelings from a distance for a while.
- Discuss the emotional situation and connect it to the task in order to learn from it.

- When a lot of anger is floating around the group, pull the anger toward your-self as group therapist, showing there is an object it can be expressed to, and demonstrating that the group therapist will not fold under the pressure.[2]

A conflict between two group members

Interaction can become too intense, making it very stressful and unsafe for group members. Such a situation arises, for example, when a conflict between group members gets out of control.

Causes

We identify two types of conflicts: *value conflict* and *conflict of interest* (Gal-tung, 1969, in Van Riet, 1988, 160). In a value conflict, two group members have disagreements because of differing personal viewpoints on an important issue. For example, two group members may clash because they differ on the cause of their depression. One firmly believes that depression is congenital and that this group should primarily educate members about suitable medi-cation and learn how to cope with the illness. In contrast, the other member believes that depression occurs when a person suppresses his or her feelings and that the group should teach group members to allow and express feel-ings. Because our values and vision of reality are so closely related to our personal identity, it can be frightening when they are compromised. This is why a value conflict between two group members could quickly escalate. There is no easy solution. Very often, the more diplomatic group members will suggest a compromise and find solutions to the conflict. Resolving a value conflict is only possible after a substantive debate about the different beliefs. A solution is only possible when the members concerned dare to take a critical look at their own beliefs.

A *conflict of interest* can also escalate. An example is when two group mem-bers clash because they both feel like they are not getting enough attention in a group therapy session because the other demands too much attention. The group therapist and other members can also be useful helpers in a conflict of interest. As a conflict of interest is less tangential to deeply held beliefs, it is somewhat easier to reach a compromise, making it easier to resolve (Van Riet, 1988).

Conflict is very distressing for most members of a therapy group and by no means always productive (De Dreu and Weingart, 2003). If a conflict can be expressed and resolved together and with the group, it can obviously be instruc-tive for the whole group and even strengthen cohesion (de Haan and Pol, NVGP, 2019). If a conflict escalates, it is often difficult to resolve and carries the risk of negative repetition and damage.

Because conflicts are so unpleasant and distressing, group members would prefer to resolve them immediately, preferably eliminate them. This is often not possible because the deeper causes cannot be resolved immediately. The best solution for the group therapist is to help by providing plenty of structure, understanding and support to make the conflict negotiable.

Solutions

An intense conflict must be 'managed' by the group therapist. In doing so, he can best stick to the following step-by-step plan (after Van Riet, 1988):

* Let the conflict run its course for a while, possibly letting it build up a bit so it is clearly visible as a conflict. Then, acknowledge the conflict by confirming its existence out loud.
* If the arguments, accusations, criticisms, or destructive escalation (i.e., insults or condemning) are repeated, halt the conflict with a resolute, steering attitude (LEADING) and with the verbal technique of *limiting/structuring*.
* Show understanding for one party and then the other by *mirroring* the various viewpoints and feelings.
* Take turns asking one party to express their viewpoint or position and ask the other to listen only. Let them talk to you as group therapist.[3]
* If the arguing parties fall back into their pattern of polarization or stereotypical accusations (which happens easily), immediately intervene again by *limiting* and *structuring*.
* Ask other group members about their feelings or thoughts regarding the conflict (dilute).
* When the conflict has sufficiently fizzled out and been expressed, space sometimes arises in both group members for the opposing party. The group therapist can then ask the 'arguers' to switch perspectives so they can empathize with the opposing party's viewpoint.
* Later during the session, or at the next session, debrief the conflict with the whole group and explore together the compromises or solutions that emerged from it.

With his leading attitude, the group therapist shows that he is in control. The trick is not to nip the conflict in the bud. By acknowledging the conflict and allowing it to happen in moderation, the group therapist can show that he can handle a conflict and can take a beating when things get rough. This allows group members to feel safe. It does not necessarily mean the situation is a breeze for the group therapist. On the contrary, it is normal for him to experience tension when a conflict occurs in the group.

Table 13.1 summarizes the combined techniques the group therapist can use to limit and structure interaction in an escalating conflict.

Table 13.1 Managing a conflict between two group members.

Verbal technique	Relationship technique (attitude and tone)
The group therapist *limits* and *structures* the escalating conflict and then *mirrors* the feelings and opinions of the conflicting group members. Using the step-by-step plan, he discusses the conflict and de-escalates the interaction back to a normal level.	The group therapist maintains control with a leading attitude (LEADING)

Handling a conflict between two group members

In a group of parents of children with ADHD, two mothers heavily clash with each other. They share the experience that their children occasionally become so hyper that they sometimes don't know how to handle that behavior, but they differ in their approach. One mother often gives her son an 'educational spanking,' which she believes helps curb the hyperactive behavior. She was subjected to that when she was a child: her father regularly spanked her. According to her, it made her stronger. The other mother, however, is adamantly against a physical approach and vehemently condemns the first mother for her physical behavior toward her son. The latter feels rejected by this and, in turn, accuses the other mother of disrespect.

The conflict escalates considerably, and soon, accusations start flying back and forth. The group therapist intervenes and limits the accusatory interaction. He then mirrors first one mother and then the other. He shows understanding for the 'hands-off' mother and for the helplessness when her son drives her crazy. He then mirrors the other mother's indignation about hitting a child.

He continues by asking the other group members about their experiences handling their children when they become unmanageable, hyperactive, and out of control. Hesitantly, some parents confess that they have also spanked their children when they didn't know what else to do or at least felt the urge to do so. Other parents say they have learned to use other means because they never wanted to hit their child. The group therapist shows an understanding of the different experiences and viewpoints and then explains as objectively and expertly as possible that spanking is not the most effective way to calm a child with ADHD. He reminds the parents that the purpose of this group is to learn more effective ways from each other on how to calm and limit their children.

In the course of the discussion that then unfolds, the group therapist turns his attention back to the two mothers who were arguing with each other. He asks them about their feelings. Both appear satisfied, having felt heard and understood. By discussing the conflict in the group, the severity has been reduced, and space has been created to look at it constructively.

Subgroups

Problems and causes

Almost every group is familiar with the phenomenon of 'subgroups': two (or more) groups within the group have different opinions on a particular topic and are at odds with each other about it. We consider these subgroups a normal part of group development (during the inclusion phase). All sorts of things can underlie the distinction between subgroups. For example, talkers versus the silent on the theme of openness, doers versus the timid on the theme of responsibility, 'positivists' versus 'negativists' on the theme of hope for improvement. Normally, this contradiction resolves itself over time as the subgroups interact and seek out the nuances. The subgroups then disappear because they are no longer needed. But things do not always run smoothly. We saw in Chapter 12, 'Depth processes,' that persistent subgroups are often a sign of avoidance. Opposing views between subgroups can become fixated and cause stagnation. Typically, this escalation process will assume one of the following three forms:

1. Splitting
2. Isolation
3. In-crowd

1. Splitting

This is subgroup formation, plain and simple. Subgroups split the group into veritable camps, which increasingly dislike and argue with each other. It is a conflict, not between two people, but between two groups. The causes often involve differing values or beliefs, stereotyping, scapegoating, and power struggles. During the struggle, the subgroups stereotype each other, eliminating all nuance from the group, which only exacerbates the antagonism. If a group therapist does not manage to halt this process, the struggle between divisive subgroups will escalate into a very unpleasant conflict rife with hatred and envy. Divisive subgroups can sometimes arise among a few group members and could eventually split the entire group in two and sometimes even dissolve the whole group. It is a disruptive group process that demands all the attention and makes working on the group task impossible (De Wolf, 2002).

Solutions

Interaction is the best solution to a subgroup problem. Subgroups always have something to say, which makes for interesting dynamics. They represent opinions that are, or, perhaps more accurately, appear, in opposition to each other. When a group therapist succeeds in connecting the subgroups, it usually turns out that the antagonism is based on stereotyping. When that distorted image is corrected, the subgroups often find that they have many similarities. Because the group therapist has to 'fish' and find out a lot to achieve this, he mainly uses the verbal technique of questioning and – to avoid letting the group escape – a decisive attitude (HELPING/LEADING). The step-by-step plan in Table 13.2 could be of help.

Table 13.2 Eliminating subgroups.

Steps	Example intervention
1. Try to identify as early as possible when subgroups become stagnant, fixated and dysfunctional; voice this and try to analyze this with the group.	'I don't know if you have the same impression, but it sometimes seems like this group is made up of a group of silent members and a group of talkers.' 'Who are the talkers, and who are the silent members? Can anyone tell me?'
2. First invite the one and then the other subgroup to explain their viewpoints.	'What do you think is so important about first quietly waiting and see-ing?' (turns to the silent)
3. Ask them to respond to each other's viewpoints.	'I am curious about your reactions to what Richard just said.'
4. Reflect with the group on the meaning of the subgroups; in doing so, find possible neutral group members; usually, there will be a few group members who are not committed to any of the subgroups.	'Why these two groups? What do you guys think?' 'What's your opinion, Don? You've been watching silently for a while. You probably have your own opinion about it.'

2. Isolation

It often happens that one group member does not fit in and assumes the role of a loner. This could result from coincidental random characteristics that influenced the selection: the only male in a mixed group of women, the only one without children in a group where all other group members have kids at home.

Isolation can also occur during the process. For example, someone may be unable to see what connects the others or vice versa; a group member may talk about something that no one identifies with and that they consider very strange. As time progresses, there is a big risk the group will confirm the 'different' loner more and more in his isolated position and eventually exclude him permanently.

Solutions
The group therapist must use interactive verbal techniques (especially *con-necting* and *broadening*), combined with a helping attitude (HELPING), to try to *de-isolate* the loner and *connect him* with the rest of the group.

Table 13.3 De-isolating the loner.

Verbal technique	Relationship technique (attitude and tone)
The group therapist connects the loner with the other group members through *mirroring, connecting*, and *broadening*.	The group therapist uses a friendly, active approach (HELPING).

De-isolate

In the second session of a therapy group for people with burnout complaints, Scott, who already does not make an overly confident impression, tells the group for the first time how afraid he is of attending the therapy group meetings. He explains that he is often nauseated with fear beforehand and then doesn't really want to come at all. The rest of the group hears Scott's outpouring, but no one responds verbally. Most group members look at Scott disdainfully; others raise their eyebrows. Scott has been isolated in the group.

The group therapist compliments Scott for being there and being open about how he feels. He then turns to the group, 'Is Scott the only one who finds it stressful to be here?' Bryan immediately responds: 'I don't mind being here, you know, I don't feel stressed.' Christine jumps in: 'Neither do I. I don't have a problem with this group.' The group therapist repeats his intervention: 'Okay, I'm curious if there are people who recognize the anxiety that Scott has mentioned.' 'A little,' says Debra. Helen: 'I do, too. Perhaps not as bad as Scott, but like Debra, I feel a bit anxious.' Group therapist: 'So, Debra and Helen, can you tell me what causes you to be anxious about being here?'

3. In-crowd

Sometimes, subgroups emerge with a tight-knit, closed character, the 'in-crowd.' The 'privilege' of belonging to this subgroup is reserved for only a few. A select club of group members has made the covenant to seek support only from each other and not from the larger group. Such an exclusive union is known in practice as an alliance. Members of an in-crowd distrust the group and keep their internal information to themselves; in-crowds are often directed against the group. In-crowds almost always have an avoidance function. Group members take refuge in their safe alliance and avoid the real work that needs to be done. An in-crowd hinders the cooperation of the group as a whole; thus, everyone suffers.

Perhaps the most extreme form of such an exclusive alliance is a romantic relationship between two group members. Friendly feelings are a normal side effect in any group. As in many groups, some people discover that they like each other: interpersonal cohesion. As long as the task remains paramount, there is nothing wrong with that. Things tend to go wrong when friendship or love becomes the main objective. A romantic relationship is exciting and therefore attracts even more attention than a regular alliance.

Solutions

If the group therapist learns of such a romantic relationship (which is by no means always easy, as the surrounding group is often complicit in the secret relationship), he must discuss and challenge the relationship in a steering manner. Sometimes, he will succeed in convincing the couple that their relationship is getting in the way of their treatment and find a way for both of them to participate constructively again in the broader group process. However, it often happens that the romantic relationship and group therapy prove incompatible, and the group therapist is forced to take organizational measures. Sometimes, one of the partners has to quit, but often, both. In that case, the group therapist must arrange other treatment settings for them.

The secret in the therapy group

Problem and cause

In-crowds already have a secretive quality, but sometimes, they are related to an actual secret within that group. If a secret keeps important information hidden from the group, it eventually causes interference. When secrecy has been going on for some time, group members and the group therapist will notice. In particular, nonverbal signals between certain group members, such as mumbling together, always leaving together, frequent furtive glances of understanding toward each other, as well as many silences and inhibitions in the group, become noticeable. Because the other group members do not understand what is going on but sense the secrecy, a strange atmosphere in which distrust and suspicion prevail develops within the group. Something is going on, but no one knows what or is saying anything about it. Naturally, a secret does not contribute to the open atmosphere that a group needs for cooperation on the group task.

Solution

At times, it is necessary for a group therapist to actively try to uncover the secret. When he detects the suspicious and inhibited atmosphere that accompanies a secret, he should actively investigate. If the secretive atmosphere remains, he can share his suspicions with the group and ask if group members also noticed the strange atmosphere. If they recognize his hunch, it is important to continue asking for their thoughts on what might be going on. Because a secret is not easily unraveled, the group therapist must often sustain this detective role for a while.

Mandatory therapy groups

Problem and cause

Motivation is an important factor in the success of group therapy (Berk, 2005; Jongerius, 1993). One's own need for help, suffering, or self-perceived need is an important motivation for members to work together toward the goals of the therapy group. Nevertheless, groups with non-motivated members occur regularly. We especially encounter them in forensic care and addiction treatment domains. Think of resocialization group therapy for forensic patients who are ready for their first step out of prison just before the end of their sentence or a group of adolescents with recurrent addiction problems and delinquent behavior participating in a 'motivation group' as an alternative to detention. The desire to participate does not stem from within these members; they are more or less forced to participate. These are 'mandatory groups.'

The lack of motivation among these members leads to a typical 'mandatory group therapy' dynamic. Resistance is evident in all therapy groups, but these groups are characterized by resistance in optima forma. Overt opposition, unwillingness and sabotage of the entire participation are prevalent, making these groups especially difficult. Next, I explain the tools a group therapist can use to optimize the efficacy of a 'mandatory group.'

Solutions

There is no simple solution for these difficult groups. What helps is to be especially mindful throughout the initial process of organizing the group and to emphatically involve the members. A second important point is to use a 'guiding' attitude in the process. This term from the motivational verbal technique means that the group therapist keeps an eye on and understands the lack of motivation of the members but, in addition, helps the members find motivation and purpose (Miller, 2004). Such an approach involves the following steps:

1. Make a good analysis of the target group

   - What is the core or main problem (e.g., addiction)?
   - What are important secondary problems (e.g., psychiatric problems, intellectual disability)?
   - What are typical behavioral characteristics (e.g., distrust, major lack of motivation)?
   - Does it involve a mandatory situation or not (e.g., a judicial order)?

2. Help participants *explicitly* and *actively* discover and make a modest request for help, or in other words, look for some kind of motivation

   - What could be a request for help (e.g., more calmness with ADHD)?

- What could be or become motivators (e.g., not ending up in jail, some pleasure in visiting this group, loneliness)?
- Make it clear to the participants that it is their choice whether or not to participate and that you as a group therapist do not force them to be here

3. Make a clear pitch about the task, goals, and methods when starting a group or when new members join. Take the time for this and talk about it with the group so they will feel co-responsible.

- What do you hope to achieve (realistic, achievable, and a goal that suits them)?
- The therapeutic and working method.
- The task is extremely important: make clear what you expect from them and logically explain that it won't happen without commitment/cooperation.
- Group rules: these are logical extensions of what you explained earlier.
- Clearly ask for consent: 'Is this okay for you? Can you participate this way?' This establishes a contract, an agreement to participate in the group.

4. Use potential cohesion or strengthen cohesion

- Help find commonalities ('You are all struggling to participate because you are being forced to; I can imagine that you find it rather unpleasant').
- Connect members with each other ('Kelly, is it true that you think Keith's goal might also suit you?').

5. If you get stuck

- Understand their limited motivation and commitment.
- In doing so, explain that it will not work if they don't cooperate and that you need them to commit.
- Tell them that if they don't cooperate, they risk having to stop treatment and will suffer all the related consequences.

6. Attitude
It is important to adopt a suitable attitude during this extra attention to the task and group goals. A guiding attitude expresses empathy and understanding of the situation and subsequent lack of motivation but also confronts the member with the need to make a choice. According to motivational discourse, 'guiding' lies between steering and following (Miller, 2004). The group therapist guides by regularly switching between a LEADING and a HELPING attitude.

Notes

1 Tip from fellow group therapist Hans Fisher.
2 Tip from fellow group therapist Charles Pohl.
3 Tip from fellow group therapist Charles Pohl.

References

AGPA (2007) *Practice guidelines for group psychotherapy*. New York: American Group Psychotherapy Association.

Arendsen Hein M (1998) Overdrachts-, en tegenoverdrachtsverschijnselen in behandelteams. In: *Handboek groepstherapie*. Houten: Bohn Stafleu van Loghum: 1–18.

Asch S (1952) *Social psychology*. New York: Prentice Hall. In: Nijstad B A (2009) *Group performance*. Hove and New York: Psychology Press: 31–33.

Bales R F (1950) A set of categories for the analysis of small group interaction. *American Sociological Review* 15 (2): 257–263.

Bales R F (2001) *Social interaction systems*. New Brunswick and London: Transaction Publishers.

Barron R (2004) *Group process, group decision, group action*. New York: Open University Press.

Baumeister R and Leary M (1995) The need to belong: Desire for interpersonal attachments as a fundamental human motivation. *Psychological Bulletin* 117 (3): 497–529.

Bellerby M (2017) Picturing an organisation: The building blocks of organization design. In: Bellerby M (ed) *Organisation designs from start-up to global: Dynamic designs for growth*. E-book Collection: K.R. Publishing.

Benne K and Sheats P (1948) Functional roles of group members. *Journal of Social Issues* 4: 41–49.

Bennis W G and Shepard H A (1956) A theory of group development. *Human Relations* 9: 415–457.

Berk T (1992, Maart) Resonantie en spiegeling. *NVGP Bulletin*.

Berk T (2005) *Leerboek Groepspsychotherapie*. Utrecht: De Tijdsstroom.

Bettencourt B A and Sheldon K (2001) Social roles as mechanism for psychological need satisfaction within social groups. *Journal of Personality and Social Psychology* 81: 1131–1145. In: Forsyth D R (2017) *Group dynamics* (7th Ed). Boston: Cengage: 177.

Billow R M (2001) Therapist's anxiety and resistance to group therapy. *International Journal of Group Psychotherapy* 51 (2): 225–242.

Billow R M (2003) *Relational group psychotherapy*. London and New York: Kingsley Publishers.

Bion W R (1961) *Experiences in groups and other papers*. New York: Basic Books.

Bloch S and Crouch E (1985) *Therapeutic factors in group psychotherapy*. Oxford: Oxford University Press.

Bogdanoff M (1978) Role lock. *International Journal of Group Psychotherapy* 28 (2): 249–262.

Bollen K and Hoyle R (1990) Percieved cohesion. *Social Forces* 69 (2): 479–504.

Booij A (2019) Hoofdstuk 15 Het leerproces tot groepsbehandelaar. In: Koks R and Steures P (eds) *Praktijkrichtlijnen Groepsbehandeling voor de (Geestelijke) Gezondheidszorg.* Utrecht: Nederlandse vereniging voor groepsdynamica en groepspsychotherapie: 181–192. (in the text abbreviated as NVGP, 2019)

Bowlby J (1969) *Attachment.* London: Hogarth Press.

Bowlby J (1988) *A secure base: Parent-child attachment and healthy human development.* London: Routledge.

Boyd R and Silk J (2008) *How humans evolved.* New York: Norton.

Brewer M and Caporael L (2006) A evolutionary perspective on social identity: Revisiting groups. In: Schaller M et al. (eds) *Evolution and social psychology.* New York: Psychology Press: 143–161.

Brusa J A et al. (1994) A sociometric test to identify emergent leader and member roles: Phase 1. *American Journal of Group Psychotherapy* 2: 249–262.

Burlingame G and Jensen J (2017) Small group process and outcome research highlights: A 25-year perspective. *International Journal of Group Psychotherapy* 67: 194–218.

Burlingame G and Strauss B (2021) Chapter 17 efficacy of small group treatments: Foundation for evidence-based practice. In: Barkham M et al. (eds) *Bergin & Garfield's handbook of psychotherapy and behavior change.* Hoboken: Wiley: 583–624.

Burlingame G et al. (2018) Cohesion in group therapy: A meta-analysis. *Psychotherapy* 55 (4): 384–398.

Carron A (1988) Group cohesion and adherence to physical activity. *Journal of Sport and Exercise Psychology* 10: 127–138.

Carron A et al. (1985) The development of an instrument to assess cohesion in sport teams: The group environment questionnaire. *Journal of Sport Psychology* 7: 244–266.

Carson R C (1969) *Interaction concepts of personality.* Chicago: Aldine.

Cartwright D and Zander A (eds) (1968) *Group dynamics: Research and theory.* New York: Harper and Row. In: Hoijtink T A E (2001) *De kracht van groepen. Normen en rollen.* Houten: Bohn Stafleu Van Loghum: 42–44.

Cauffman L (2003) *Oplossingsgericht management & coaching.* Utrecht: Lemma.

Chapman N and Kivlighan D M (2019) Does the cohesion–outcome relationship change over time?: A dynamic model of change in group psychotherapy. *Group Dynamics: Theory, Research, and Practice* 23 (2): 91–103.

Chemers M M (2000) Leadership research and theory: A functional integration. *Group Dynamics: Theory, Research & Practice* 4: 27–43.

Cialdini R (2014) *Invloed.* Den Haag: Academic Service.

Claassen A M and Janzing C (2014) Het effect van samenhangend behandelen: introductie van een model voor multidisciplinair werken in de GGz. *Groepen* 9 (4): 25–40.

Claassen A M and Leferink op Reinink M (2019) Chapter 11 group treatment as part of a multidisciplinary treatment design. Therapy. In: Koks R and Steures P (eds) *Practice guidelines for group treatment in (mental) healthcare.* Utrecht: Nederlandse vereniging voor groepsdynamica en groepspsychotherapie: 42–57. (in the text abbreviated as NVGP, 2019)

Corsini R and Rosenberg B (1955) Mechanisms of group psychotherapy: Processes and dynamics. *Journal of Abnormal and Social Psychology* 51: 406–411.

Crano W (2000) Milestones in the psychological analysis of social influence. *Group Dynamics* 4 (1): 68–80.

Daemen M and Van Paassen F (2019) Hoofdstuk 7 Beëindiging en afscheid bij groepsbehandeling. In: Koks R and Steures P (eds) *Praktijkrichtlijnen Groepsbehandeling voor de (Geestelijke) Gezondheidszorg.* Utrecht: Nederlandse vereniging voor groepsdynamica en groepspsychotherapie: 85–95. (in the text abbreviated as NVGP, 2019)

Dawkins R (2009) *Het grootste spektakel ter wereld – Bewijs voor evolutie*. Amsterdam: Nieuw Amsterdam.

De Dreu C and Weingart L (2003) Task versus relationship conflict, team performance, and team member satisfaction: A meta-analysis. *Journal of Applied Psychology* 88 (4): 741–749.

De Haan C and Pol S (2019) Chapter 9: Destructive group processes and negative effects of group treatment. In: Koks R and Steures P (eds) *Practice guidelines for group treatment in (mental) healthcare*. Utrecht: Nederlandse vereniging voor groepsdynamica en groepspsychotherapie: 18–29. (in the text abbreviated as NVGP, 2019)

De Haas W (1987) Een poliklinische nazorggroep. *Maandblad Geestelijke Volksgezondheid* 11: 1252–1257.

De Haas W (2008) *Groepsbegeleiding en Groepsbehandeling in de Gezondheidszorg*. Soest: Nelissen.

De Haas W (2020) *Groepsbehandeling en Teambegeleiding in de Zorg*. Amsterdam: Boom.

De Haas W and Van Hest K (2019) Hoofdstuk 2 De organisatie van een succesvolle behandelgroep. In: Koks R and Steures P (eds) *Praktijkrichtlijnen Groepsbehandeling voor de (Geestelijke) Gezondheidszorg*. Utrecht: Nederlandse vereniging voor groepsdynamica en groepspsychotherapie: 30–38. (in the text abbreviated as NVGP, 2019)

De Jong C A J, Van den Brink W and Jansma A (2000) *ICL-R: Handleiding bij de vernieuwde Nederlandse versie van de Interpersonal Checklist (ICL)*. Sint Oedenrode: Novadic.

De Jong K and Spinhoven P (2008) De Nederlandse versie van de OQ 45: een crossculturele validatie. *Psychologie en gezondheid* 36 (1): 35–45.

De Waal F (2005) *De aap in ons. Waarom we zijn wie we zijn*. Amsterdam: Contact.

De Wolf M (2002) *Inleiding in de psychoanalytische psychotherapie*. Bussem: Coutinho.

Dion K L (2000) Group cohesion: From 'field of forces' to multidimensional construct. *Group Dynamics: Theory, Research and Practice* 4: 1–26

Durkin J (1981) *Living groups*. New York: Brunner/Mazel.

Elwyn G et al. (2012) Shared decision making: A model for clinical practice. *Original Research* 27: 1361–1367.

Erikson E (1968) *Identity, youth and crisis*. New York: Norton.

Evans C and Dion K (2012) Group cohesion and performance: A meta-analysis. *Small Group Research* 43 (6): 690–701.

Factsheet Groepstherapie (2019) *Nederlandse Vereniging voor Psychotherapie*. https://www.groepspsychotherapie.nl/research-groepstherapie/factsheet-groepstherapie/

Fay N et al. (2000) Group discussion as interactive dialogue or as serial monologue: The influence of group size. *Psychological Science* 6: 481–486.

Festinger L (1950) *Social pressures in informal groups*. Stanford: Stanford University Press.

Flores P and Porges S W (2018) Group psychotherapy as a neural exercise: Bridging polyvagal theory and attachment theory. In: Marmarosh (ed) *Attachment in group psychotherapy*. New York: Routledge: 47–66.

Forman M (1975) Movie: *One Flew Over the Cuckoo's Nest*.

Forsyth D R (2017) *Group dynamics* (7th Ed). Boston: Cengage.

Forsyth D R (2021) Recent advances in the study of group cohesion. *Group Dynamics: Theory, Research, and Practice* 25 (3): 213–228.

Foulkes S H (1964) *Therapeutic group analysis*. New York: International University Press.

Foulkes S H (1977) Chapter 4: Concerning leadership. In: *Therapeutic group analysis*. New York: International University Press: 57.

Galtung J (1969) Conflict als een wijze van leven. *Maandblad voor Geestelijke Volksgezondheid.* In: Van Riet N (1988) *Groepswerk in het maatschappelijk werk.* Nijmegen: Dekker & Van de Vegt: 160.

Gilhuis H et al. (2014) *Psychodrama in de praktijk: Therapie op de vloer.* Amsterdam: Hogrefe.

Goffman E (1959) *The presentation of self in everyday life.* New York: Double Day. In: Forsyth D R (2017) *Group dynamics* (7th Ed). Boston: Cengage: 177.

Goudsblom J (2000) Overleving en overlevingseenheden in de mensengeschiedenis. *Groepspsychotherapie* 3: 110–124.

Groot F (2004) *Bekrachtigen, bekrachtigen, en nog eens bekrachtigen. Back to basics: positieve bekrachtiging Gedragstherapie.* Houten: Bohn Stafleu van Loghum.

Hafkenscheid A (2014) *De Therapeutische Relatie.* Utrecht: De Tijdsstroom.

Hafkenscheid A (2019) Hoofdstuk 14: Uitkomstmeting en monitoring van groepsbehandeling. In: Koks R and Steures P (eds) *Praktijkrichtlijnen Groepsbehandeling voor de (Geestelijke) Gezondheidszorg.* Utrecht: Nederlandse vereniging voor groepsdynamica en groepspsychotherapie: 167–178. (in the text abbreviated as NVGP, 2019)

Hafkenscheid A and Timmerman M E (2023) Does a three-dimensional Impact Message Inventory-Circumplex (IMI-C) enclose an indirect measure of reactance? *Clinical Psychology & Psychotherapy*: 1–8.

Hart W (2017) *Verdraaide organisaties: terug naar de bedoeling.* Deventer: Kluwer.

Helderman D (2021) *Exploring the emotional life of the mind. A psychodynamic theory of emotions.* New York: Routledge.

Helwig P (1958) *Dramaturgie des menschlichen Lebens.* Stuttgart: Klett.

Hersey P (2007) *Situationeel leiding geven.* Amsterdam: Business Contact.

Hoijtink T A E (2001) *De kracht van groepen. Normen en rollen.* Houten: Bohn Stafleu Van Loghum.

Homans G C (1966) *Individu en gemeenschap. Menselijk gedrag in groepsverband.* Utrecht: Het Spectrum.

Horowitz L M et al. (1988) Inventory of interpersonal problems: Psychometric properties and clinical applications. *Journal of Consulting and Clinical Psychology* 56 (6): 885–892.

Horowitz L M et al. (2000) *Inventory of interpersonal problems. Manual.* www.mindgarden.com

Huffstadt C and Remijsen M (2019) Chapter 12: Co-counseling and co-therapy. In: Koks R and Steures P (eds) *Practice guidelines for group treatment in (mental) healthcare.* Utrecht: Nederlandse vereniging voor groepsdynamica en groepspsychotherapie: 58–64. (in the text abbreviated as NVGP, 2019)

Janzing C (1992) Angst voor teleurstelling. *Tijdschrift voor Psychotherapie* 18 (1): 207–216.

Jongerius P J (1993) *Praktijkboek groepspsychotherapie.* Amersfoort: Academische Uitgeverij.

Kameda T and Tindale R (2006) Groups as adaptive devices: Human docility and group aggregation mechanisms in evolutionary context. In: Schaller M et al. (eds) *Evolution and social psychology.* New York: Psychology Press: 317–341.

Karakowsky L and Siegel J (1999) The effects of proportional representation and gender orientation of the task on emergent leadership behaviour in mixed gender work groups. In: Nijstad B A (2009) *Group performance.* Hove and New York: Psychology Press: 189–190.

Kauff P (2015) Psychoanalytic group psychotherapy. In: Kleinberg J L (ed) *The Wiley Blackwell handbook of group psychotherapy.* Oxford: Wiley Blackwell: 13–32.

Kiesler D J (1983) The interpersonal circle: A tachonomy for complementarity in human transactions. *Psychological Review* 90 (3): 185–214.

Kiesler D J and Schmidt J A (1993) *The impact message inventory: Form IIA octant scoring version*. Redwood City: Mind Garden.

Knippenberg D et al. (2007) Work group diversity. *Annual Review of Psychology* 58: 515–541.

Koementas-de Vos M M W et al. (2018) Does progress feedback enhance the outcome of group psychotherapy. *Psychotherapy* 55 (2): 151–163.

Krijnen I (2004) Twee kunnen meer dan één. *Groepen* 1 (1): 11–20.

Kuypers B C (1986) *Group developmental patterns* (dissertation). Utrecht: Rijksuniversiteit Utrecht.

Lapakko D (2007) Communication is 93% nonverbal: An urban legend proliferates. *CTAMJ*: 7–19.

Lawler E et al. (2002) Emotion and group cohesion in productive exchange. *American Journal of Sociology* 106 (3): 616–657.

Lawler E et al. (2014) *Relational cohesion, social commitments, and person-to-group ties: Twenty-five years of a theoretical research program*. Esmerald group.

Leary M et al. (1995) Self-esteem as an interpersonal monitor: The sociometer hypothesis. *Journal of Personality and Social Psychology* 68 (3): 518–530.

Leary T (1957/2004) *Interpersonal diagnosis of personality: A functional theory and methodology of personality evaluation*. Eugene: Resource publications: Ronald Press Company. Previously published by John Wiley & Sons.

Leszcz M and Malat J (2015) The interpersonal model of group psychotherapy. In: Kleinberg J L (ed) *The Wiley-Blackwell handbook of group psychotherapy*. Malden: Wiley: 33–36.

Levine B (1979) *Group psychotherapy: Practice and development*. Inglewood: Prentice Hall.

Lewin K (1943) Psychology and the process of group living. *Journal of Social Psychology* 17: 113–131. S. P. S. S. I. Bulletin.

Lewin K (1951/1997) *Field theory in social science*. Washington: APA.

Linehan M M (1993) *Skills training manual for treating borderline personality disorder*. New York: Guilford Press.

Lizardo O (2007) Relational cohesion theory. In: *The Blackwell encyclopedia of sociology*. Wiley Online Library: 3845–3848.

Lott A and Lott B (1965) Group cohesiveness as interpersonal attraction. *Psychological Bulletin* 6 (4): 259–309.

Markus J (2021) Mythe: Communicatie is voor 93% non-verbaal. *Nederlands Debat Instituut Blog*. www.debatinstituut.nl/bibliotheek/beinvloeden/mythe-non-verbale-communicatie/

Marmarosh C L et al. (2024) Miles away: Alliance and cohesion in online group psychotherapy. In: Weinberg H et al. (2024) *The virtual group therapy circle: Advances in online group theory and practice*. New York: Routledge: 40–51.

Mc Cullough Vaillant L (1997) *Changing character*. New York: Basic Books.

Mehrabian A (1972) *Non verbal communication*. New Brunswick: Adline Transaction.

Michaels A (2006) Ritual and meaning. In: *Theorizing rituals, volume 1: Issues, topics, approaches, concepts*. Leiden: Brill: 247–261.

Mikulincer M (1998) Attachment working models and the sense of trust: An exploration of interaction goals and affect regulation. *Journal of Personality and Social Psychology* 74 (5): 1209–1224.

Mikulincer M (2007) Attachment, group–related processes, and psychotherapy. *International Journal of Group Psychotherapy* 57 (2): 233–245.

Mikulincer M and Shaver P R (2018) Augmenting the sense of attachment security in group contexts: The effects of a responsive leader and a cohesive group. In: Marmarosch (ed) *Attachment in group psychotherapy*. New York: Routledge: 5–19.

Mikulincer M et al. (2003) Attachment theory and affect regulation: The dynamics, development, and cognitive consequences of attachment-related strategies. *Motivation and Emotion* 27 (2): 77–102.

Milgram S (1974) *Obedience to authority.* New York: Harper and Row.

Miller W (2004) A randomized trial of methods to help clinicians learn motivational interviewing. *Journal of Consulting and Clinical Psychology* 72 (6): 1050–1062.

Moeskops O (2006) Het vermogen te verdragen. *Management en Organisatie* 4: 25–39.

Moreno J L (1941) Foundations of sociometry: An introduction. *Sociometry* 4 (1): 15–35.

Mullen B and Copper C (1994) The relation between group cohesiveness and performance: An integration. *Psychological Bulletin* 115 (2): 210–227.

Nijstad B A (2009) *Group performance.* Hove and New York: Psychology Press.

Nitsun M (1992) De 'anti-groep': destructieve krachten in de groep en het therapeutisch potentieel daarvan. *Psychotherapeutisch paspoort* 1: 4/5–4/20.

Nitsun M (2004) Destructive forces in group therapy. In: Motherwell L and Shay J (eds) *Complex dilemmas in group therapy: Pathways to resolution.* New York: Brunner-Routledge: 115–125.

NVGP (2019) *Praktijkrichtlijnen Groepsbehandeling voor de (Geestelijke) Gezondheidszorg.* Utrecht: Nederlandse vereniging voor groepsdynamica en groepspsychotherapie.

Oomkes F R (2002) De teamrollen van Belbin. In: *Werken leren, leven met groepen.* Houten: Bohn Stafleu van Loghum: 1–23.

Ormont L R (1968) Group resistance and the therapeutic contract. *International Journal of Group Psychotherapy* 18 (2): 147–154.

Ormont L R (1990) The craft of bridging. *International Journal of Group Psychotherapy* 40 (1): 3–17.

Parsons T et al. (1953) *Working papers in the theory of action.* New York: Free Press. In: Forsyth D R (2017) *Group dynamics* (7th Ed). Boston: Cengage: 167.

Pesso A (1973) *Experience in action: A psychomotor psychology.* New York: University Press.

Podsakoff P et al. (1997) Moderating effects of goal acceptance on the relationship between group cohesion and productivity. In: Nijstad B A (2009) *Group performance.* Hove and New York: Psychology Press: 6.

Postmes T and Jetten J (2006) *Individuality and the group.* Sage: London.

Redl F (1963) Psychoanalysis and group therapy: A developmental point of view. *American Journal of Orthopsychiatry* 33: 135–142.

Remmerswaal J (2003) *Handboek groepsdynamica. Een nieuwe inleiding op theorie en praktijk.* Soest: Nelissen.

Remmerswaal J (2015) *Group dynamics: An introduction.* Amsterdam: Boom Nelissen.

Robbertz K and Wolters R (2019) Hoofdstuk 6 Ontwikkelingsfasen, de dynamiek van de groepsontwikkeling. In: Koks R and Steures P (eds) *Praktijkrichtlijnen Groepsbehandeling voor de (Geestelijke) Gezondheidszorg.* Utrecht: Nederlandse vereniging voor groepsdynamica en groepspsychotherapie: 72–84. (in the text abbreviated as NVGP, 2019)

Rom E and Mikulincer M (2003) Attachment theory and group processes: The association between attachment style and group related representations, goals memories and functioning. *Journal of Personality and Social Psychology* 84 (6): 1220–1235.

Sanders T (2010) Indicatiestelling groepspsychotherapie. *Groepen* 5 (3): 43–55.

Schachter S (1951) Deviation, rejection and communication. *Journal of Abnormal and Social Psychology* 46. In: Nijstad B A (2009) *Group performance.* Hove and New York: Psychology Press: 24–25.

Scheidlinger S (1982) On scapegoating in group psychotherapy. *International Journal of Group Psychotherapy* 1: 131–143.

Scheuring P (2010) Movie: *The Experiment*.

Schroder H and Harvey O J (1963) Conceptual organization and group structure. *Motivation and Social Interaction*: 134–166. In: Levine B (1979) *Group psychotherapy, practice and development*. Englewood Cliffs: Prentice-Hall: 70.

Schruijer S and Curseu P (2014) Looking at the gap between social psychology and psychodynamic perspectives on group dynamics historically. *Journal of Organisation Change Management* 27 (2): 232–245.

Schutz W (1985) *FIRO: A three dimensional theory of interpersonal behavior*. New York: Rinehart Inc.

Scott Rutan J (2021) Reasons for suggesting group psychotherapy to patients. *American Journal of Psychotherapy* 74 (2): 67–71.

Scott Rutan J et al. (2014) *Psychodynamic group psychotherapy* (5th Ed). New York: Guilford Press: 255–260.

Sedikides C et al. (2006) When and why did the human self evolve. In: Schaller M et al. (eds) *Evolution and social psychology*. New York: Psychology Press: 55–79.

Shaffer J and Galinsky M (1976) *Groepstherapie en sensitivitytraining*. Deventer: van Loghum Slaterus.

Shanon E and Weaver W (1961) *The mathematical theory of communication*. Urbana: The university of Illinois press.

Shay J J (2021) Terrified of group therapy: Investigating obstacles to entering and leading groups. *American Journal of Psychotherapy* 74 (2): 72–75.

Sherif M (1936) *The psychology of social norms*. New York: Harper. In: Nijstad B A (2009) *Group performance*. Hove and New York: Psychology Press: 31–32.

Slavson S (1964) *A textbook in analytic group psychotherapy*. New York: International University Press: 52.

Spijker J (2010) Groepstherapie in de richtlijnen. *Groepen* 5 (1): 54–57.

Sullivan H S (1940) Conceptions of modern psychiatry: The first William Alanson White memorial lectures. *Psychiatry* 3 (1): 1–17. In: Berk T (2005) *Leerboek Groepspsychotherapie*. Utrecht: de Tijdstroom: 93.

Swogger G (1981) Human communication and group experience. In: Durkin J (ed) *Living groups*. New York: Brunner/Mazel: 63–78.

Tajfel H (1971) Social categorization and intergroup behaviour. *European Journal of Social Psychology* 1 (2): 149–178.

Thye S et al. (2014) Relational cohesion, social commitments and person-to-group ties: Twenty-five years of a theoretical research program. *Advances in Group Processes* 31: 99–138.

Trimbos Instituut (2008) *Landelijke Stuurgroep Multidisciplinaire richtlijnontwikkeling in de GGZ. Richtlijn voor de diagnostiek en behandeling van volwassen patiënten met een persoonlijkheidsstoornis*. Utrecht: Trimbos Instituut.

Tuckman B W (1965) Developmental sequence in small groups. *Psychological Bulletin* 6: 384–399.

Turner J et al. (1994) Self and collective: Cognition and social context. *Personality and Social Psychology Bulletin* 20 (5): 454–463.

Van de Loo E (1995) Destructieve processen in organisaties. *Groepspsychotherapie* 29 (3): 84–88.

Van Dijk L M et al. (2019) Psychometrische kenmerken van een Nederlandse Inventory of Interpersonal Problems-Circumplex (IIP-C). *Tijdschrift voor Psychotherapie* 45 (5): 299–311.

Van Paassen F (2023) De angsten van de groepstherapeut. *Groepen* 18 (2): 23–39.

Van Riet N (1988) *Groepswerk in het maatschappelijk werk*. Nijmegen: Dekker & Van de Vegt.

Van Vught M and Ahuja A (2010) *Selected*. London: Profile Books.

Van Vught M and Wildschut M (2012) *Gezag.* Utrecht: Bruna.

Watzlawick P (1973) *De pragmatische aspecten van de menselijke communicatie.* Deventer: Van Loghum Slaterus.

Weinberg H (2024) Online group psychotherapy training. In: Weinberg H et al. (eds) (2024) *The virtual group therapy circle: Advances in online group theory and practice.* New York: Routledge: 311–327.

Weinberg H and Rolnick A (eds) (2020) *The theory and practice of online therapy: Internet delivered interventions for individuals, groups, families and organizations.* New York: Routledge.

Wermers E (2006) Een Fries recept: organisatie van ambulante groepen in de GGz. *Groepen* 1 (3): 5–14.

Whitaker D S and Lieberman M A (1964) *Psychotherapy through the group process.* Chicago: Aldine.

Whitman R M (1963) Psychodynamic principles underlying T-group processes. In: Bradford et al. (eds) *T group theory and laboratory method: Innovation and re-education.* New York: Wiley: 310–335.

Whittington M et al. (2021) Group psychotherapy as a specialty: An Inconvenient truth. *American Journal of Psychotherapy* 74 (2): 60–66.

Williams K (2007) Ostracism. *Annual Review of Psychology* 58: 425–52.

Wilson E (1975) *Sociobiology. The new synthesis.* Cambridge: Belknap Press. In: Goldsmidt T (2022) *Wolven op het ruiterpad.* Amsterdam: Atheneum: 17–22.

Winnicott D (1986) *Home is where we start from.* Norton: New York.

Wrangham R (2019) *The goodness paradox.* New York: Penguin Random House.

Yalom I D (1975) *The theory and practice of group.* New York: Basic Books.

Yalom I D and Leszcz M (2020) *The theory and practice of group psychotherapy* (6th Ed). New York: Basic Books.

Zimbardo P G (1969) The human choice: Individuation, reason, and order versus deindividuation, impulse, and chaos. *Nebraska Symposium on Motivation* 17: 237–307.

Name Index

Subject Index

Note: Page numbers in *italics* indicate a figure and page numbers in **bold** indicate a table on the corresponding page.